H$_2$-Receptor Antagonists

The publication of these proceedings has been made possible by a grant from Smith Kline & French USA.

Further Experience with
H₂-Receptor Antagonists

in Peptic Ulcer Disease and Progress in Histamine Research

European Symposium
Capri, October 18-20, 1979

Editors:
A. Torsoli
P.E. Lucchelli
R.W. Brimblecombe

1980
Excerpta Medica, Amsterdam - Oxford - Princeton

International Congress Series No. 521
ISBN Excerpta Medica 90 219 9467 4
ISBN Elsevier North-Holland 04 449 0147 7

Library of Congress Cataloging in Publication Data
Main entry under title:

Further Experience with H_2-Receptor Antagonists in Peptic Ulcer Disease and Progress in Histamine Research.

(International congress series; no. 521)
Includes bibliographies.
Includes index.
1. Peptic ulcer--Chemotherapy--Congresses.
2. Cimetidine--Physiological effect--Congresses.
3. Histamine receptors--Congresses.   4.   Antihistamines--Congresses.
I. Torsoli, Aldo. II. Lucchelli, P. E.   III.   Brimblecombe, R.W. IV. Series.
[DNLM: 1. Peptic   ulcer--Drug   therapy--Congresses.   2.   Histamine H_2-receptor blockaders--Therapeutic use--Congresses. 3. Guanidines--Therapeutic use--Congresses. 4. Anti-ulcer agents--Therapeutic use--Congresses.   W3 EX89 no. 521 1979 / QV157 F992 1979]
RC821.F87   616.3'43061   80-15620
ISBN 0-444-90147-7 (Elsevier North-Holland)

Publisher:
Excerpta Medica
305 Keizersgracht
1000 BC Amsterdam
P.O. Box 1126

Sole Distributors for the USA and Canada:
Elsevier North-Holland Inc.
52 Vanderbilt Avenue
New York, N.Y. 10017

Printed in The Netherlands by Casparie, Heerhugowaard

Contents

Recent results with cimetidine treatment (II)

Progress in histamine research
Chairmen: R.W. Brimblecombe (Welwyn Garden City, United Kingdom)
         G. Bertaccini (Parma, Italy)

Foreword

The developments that have led to the discovery of the H_2-receptor antagonists have been a long succession of hopes and disappointments. As was recalled in a recent article*, many problems, not only of a scientific but also of a social nature, had to be tackled and solved. Now, however, we have at our disposal a drug, cimetidine, which is capable of dramatically changing the concept of treatment in one area of human pathology, and we owe it not to good luck but to the logical elaboration of ideas and to the joint efforts of chemists and biologists.

The introduction of cimetidine has changed the quality of life of many patients, and it has had important socioeconomic effects. Of even greater importance, it has prompted reconsideration of a number of chapters on physiology and clinical medicine. Many owe much to the few who from 1964 on have planned and guided a program that promises so much. At that time, none of them would have believed that it would take so long.

The European Symposium at Capri, the proceedings of which are published in the present volume, constitutes a further proof of the twofold value of cimetidine: on the one hand as a drug for the treatment of peptic ulcer and related conditions, on the other as a tool for the study of the normal and pathological physiology of histamine. In the pages that follow, the latest results are reported of controlled clinical studies in various areas of esophageal, gastric and duodenal pathology, data are presented on the side effects and the safety of the drug, and the results and prospects are described of studies of the histamine receptors in the digestive tract and other systems.

The combined contributions of scientists belonging to different disciplines and from many countries testify in their turn to the value and the efficiency of interdisciplinary and international cooperation.

Aldo Torsoli

---

*Duncan, W.A.M. and Parsons, M.E. (1980): Reminiscences of the development of cimetidine. *Gastroenterology 78,* 620-625.

Changes and perspectives in the management of peptic ulcer disease since the introduction of H$_2$-receptor antagonists

Chairmen: J.H. Baron *(London, United Kingdom)*
L. Barbara *(Bologna, Italy)*

Cimetidine in duodenal ulcer: the present position

K.D. Bardhan
District General Hospital, Rotherham, United Kingdom

Introduction

It is only 4 years since cimetidine became generally available, yet during this time it has radically transformed the treatment of duodenal ulcer and added greatly to our knowledge. The purpose of this paper is to provide a summary of the results achieved with cimetidine so far and to point to some directions for future research.

Past problems with medical treatment

In the past, the value of medical treatments for ulcer disease was uncertain, for 4 main reasons.

First, the cause of ulcer disease was unknown. Indeed, there are likely to be several different causes, the relative importance of which varies from patient to patient. Consequently, there was no firm rational basis for treatment.

Second, the disease is benign and runs a spontaneously relapsing and remitting course. Therefore, the value of a medical treatment can only be judged in double-blind clinical trials. Though such trials are now commonplace, it is often forgotten that they are a fairly new development. Some trials are still defective; in particular, the number of patients studied is frequently small. In a disease like duodenal ulcer, where about one-third of patients heal spontaneously in a short period, to show that a given treatment doubles the healing rate, approximately 80 patients are required in the study, half treated with placebo and the other half with the compound under investigation. Even then, there is a 20% chance that the benefit of the treatment may not be seen in the population of patients studied (the 'rogue' population). To reduce this chance to a more acceptable 5%, the sample size would need to be 140 patients. Very few studies, even with cimetidine, are of this size [1].

Third, there is often a lack of correlation between ulceration and symptoms. Ulcers are often asymptomatic when they recur; by the time symptoms develop, the ulcer has been present for weeks or even months [Bardhan, unpublished observations]. In other patients, ulcers cause troublesome symptoms but some relapses are virtually silent. Also, symptoms often disappear before healing is complete. Finally, there is no relation between the number or size of ulcers and the severity of symptoms. Therefore, relief of symptoms alone cannot be taken as a measure of ulcer healing.

Fourth, to determine whether a treatment influences duodenal ulcer healing, objective evidence is required. This is possible only by using fibreoptic endoscopy; double-contrast barium meal X-ray examinations, though accurate for making a diagnosis of duodenal ulcer, are not sensitive enough to follow its healing. Forward-viewing endoscopes allowing a proper yet easy examination of the duodenum became widely used in Britain only in the early and mid 1970's; indeed, the first study on duodenal ulcer healing using endoscopic assessment was published only in 1972 [2]. Therefore, the conclusions of earlier studies on duodenal ulcer healing, before endoscopy became available, may not be accurate. It is ironical that, had cimetidine been discovered in the 1960's, before the wider use of endoscopy, it would have been difficult to confirm its ulcer healing effect.

The significance of acid

Though the cause(s) of ulcer remain unknown, it has been recognised for many years that the presence of acid is essential for the development of ulcer. It is presumed that mucosal integrity is maintained by a balance between 'attacking factors' consisting of acid and possibly pepsin and bile, and 'defence factors' which presumably lie in the innate nature of the mucosa itself, and mucus. When the balance is tilted in favour of the attacking factors, ulceration results; when the balance re-establishes itself, healing follows. Little is known of the nature or mechanism of mucosal defence; rather more is known about acid. Therefore, not surprisingly, the main direction of anti-ulcer treatment has been to try and reduce acid.

Medical treatment before cimetidine

Medical treatment before the introduction of cimetidine consisted of antacids, anticholinergics, rest, diet and sedation, given singly or in combination.

Antacids do reduce acid, but only when given in large amounts. However, it has been wrongly assumed that antacids have little effect on ulcer healing [3, 4] and, therefore, they have traditionally been used in small amounts, and only to relieve symptoms. Anticholinergics reduce acid secretion, but their use is limited by side-effects [5]; there is no firm evidence that these compounds increase ulcer healing, though they may reduce recurrence when treatment is continued [6]. Bed rest has long been known to relieve symptoms, and recent evidence from cimetidine trials, albeit indirect, suggests that it increases ulcer healing as well [7]; though effective, taking time off work can be expensive for the patient. Restricted diets and milk-based diets have commonly been used in the mistaken belief that they buffer acid more effectively than ordinary food; in fact, the effect is similar [8]. Such diets may help in relieving symptoms, but there is no evidence that they increase ulcer healing. They also have the disadvantage of placing a burden on the domestic arrangements of patients. Sedation has been frequently recommended, but its value has not been proven.

A different approach was to use carbenoxolone, to increase mucosal defence; the first time this agent was studied, however, it was not found to be effective [2]. Colloidal bismuth in the form of tricitrato-dipotassium-bismuthate supposedly acts by providing a protective coating for the ulcer; in studies using endoscopic assessment, it was shown to increase ulcer healing [9].

The effect of cimetidine on acid secretion

It was against this background of largely ineffective ulcer treatment and the failure to reduce acid secretion effectively by medical means that the development of the histamine H_2-receptor antagonist cimetidine took place; the story of this development has been recounted elsewhere [10-12].

The most striking effect of cimetidine is reduction in gastric acid secretion. Basal and nocturnal secretion are profoundly reduced and maximal secretion, evoked either by food or by pharmacological stimuli, is greatly lessened. Over 24 hours, acid secretion is reduced by about two-thirds [13, 14]. Thus, for the first time, it became possible to achieve acid inhibition by a drug, of an order produced by vagotomy. The dose of cimetidine required for this was 1 g/day, administered in 3 daily doses of 200 mg and 400 mg at bedtime.

The effect of cimetidine on ulcer healing

Having determined that cimetidine reduced acid secretion, the next step was to investigate if it healed duodenal ulcer. This was done in numerous short-term studies conducted in many parts of the world; the trials were organised by Smith Kline & French and had a similar design (for a review of these trials, see [7]).

Patients with duodenal ulcer proven by endoscopy were randomly assigned to treatment with either cimetidine or placebo. The dose of cimetidine varied from 800 mg to 2 g daily, but the doses most commonly used were 1 g and 1.2 g daily. The duration of treatment varied from 2 to 12 weeks, but was generally 4-6 weeks. At the end of this period, endoscopy was repeated. The results were judged by 2 principal criteria: first, by comparing the proportions of patients in the 2 treatment groups whose ulcers had healed; second, by comparing the degree of symptomatic improvement.

The results of trials in Britain were similar. In 4-6 weeks, about 30% of patients on placebo healed spontaneously, compared with 60-80% of those on cimetidine. The relief of symptoms was dramatic, the majority of cimetidine-treated patients becoming pain-free or nearly so within a week. Similar results were obtained in the trials conducted in Italy, Sweden, Denmark and Australia.

Virtually all of the studies confirmed that cimetidine accelerates ulcer healing; the exceptions were the trials conducted in Norway [11], Switzerland [15] and the United States of America [16]. In these studies, though cimetidine produced a higher healing rate, the placebo healing rate was so high that the difference was not statistically significant. The study from the U.S.A. was the largest single trial; the high placebo healing rate may have been due to the large amounts of antacids taken by patients in this group, which is known to increase ulcer healing [17].

Pooling the results of the different trials, the main finding is that, in 4-6 weeks, approximately 40% of out-patients will heal spontaneously, whereas with cimetidine the figure rises to about 75% and symptomatic relief is much more rapid.

Failure to heal rapidly

The majority of patients heal rapidly; what happens to the remainder? There is much speculation as to whether such patients form a distinct subgroup of duodenal ulcer disease.

Some investigators present at the Capri symposium mentioned that their patients did not heal with continued cimetidine treatment, i.e., they had a resistant ulcer. My experience has been different: with continued treatment, the majority of patients heal, about 70% in 1 month, about 80% in 2 months, about 90% in 3 months, and 95% or more in 4 months. These differences in results are not readily explained, but may have something to do with studying different populations of patients.

Some patients are undoubtedly 'slow-healers' and take several months to heal with each course of cimetidine; however, this is only a very small group. In other patients, successive recurrences take progressively longer amounts of time to heal with cimetidine, giving the impression that the patient is becoming resistant to the drug; however, the reverse is also true. In the majority, 'slow-healing' is simply a matter of definition; those that have not healed fully in a few weeks have nevertheless either partially or almost completely healed, and are generally asymptomatic. If healing is nearly complete and cimetidine is stopped, healing generally goes on; cimetidine has helped to restore the balance between attack and defence, which is then sustained.

Non-compliance is another reason for slow healing; patients taking cimetidine soon become asymptomatic, and the urge to continue treatment then lessens. However, it is difficult to be certain how important a role this plays.

Patients with Zollinger-Ellison syndrome may present with a resistant ulcer though, in many, the standard dose of cimetidine produces healing [18]. Hypercalcaemia due to hyperparathyroidism has also been reported to cause apparent resistance to treatment [19]. Both conditions are very rare and there is little to be gained in the routine measurement of acid secretion and blood gastrin levels. In my experience, patients with slow healing have normal gastrin levels and a wide range of acid and pepsin secretion similar to those who heal more quickly.

Management after the ulcer has healed

While the value of short-term treatment of duodenal ulcer with cimetidine is no longer in doubt, further management is controversial since, when the drug is stopped, the patient is prone to relapse. There are 3 options available: first, further treatment for a fixed duration, second, long-term maintenance treatment, and third, intermittent treatment.

Further treatment for a fixed duration

The basis for this option is that, though short-term treatment does not influence the natural history of the disease, a longer period of treatment may do so.

In various studies, patients whose ulcers had healed following treatment with cimetidine were kept on the drug for periods of up to a year, with doses of up to 1 g/day. While on treatment, the relapse rate was low, but after the drug was withdrawn there was a high rate of relapse, similar to that in patients who had received only a short course of treatment [20-24].

In a large study which is still continuing, patients with duodenal ulcer who had healed within 1 month of beginning cimetidine treatment were randomly allocated to further treatment either with placebo, or with cimetidine for either 2 or 5 months, followed by placebo [25]. Endoscopy was carried out every 3 months in asymptomatic patients, and earlier if symptoms developed. Preliminary results show that the proportion of patients who relapsed on placebo was similar in all 3 groups: during the first 22 months of follow-up, 55-60% had a symptomatic relapse, and 70-77% had a silent recurrence; the rate of relapse in the different groups was also similar.

Thus, there is generally no advantage to extending treatment for a fixed duration, as this does not influence the subsequent relapse rate. The exceptions are: first, to keep a patient in remission until definitive ulcer surgery, and second, and this is much less certain, to tide a patient over a stressful period (for example, when undergoing surgery on some other part of the body, or if ill for another reason, since an ulcer relapse at this time could be particularly troublesome).

Long-term maintenance treatment

This has been investigated in several studies, and all confirm that maintenance treatment markedly reduces the relapse rate (for review, see [7]). In these trials, patients whose duodenal ulcer had just healed in short-term studies were randomly allocated to further treatment with either placebo or cimetidine. The dose of cimetidine varied from 400 mg nightly to 400 mg both at night and in the morning; the duration of treatment was generally 6-12 months. Patients were seen frequently; if symptoms recurred, endoscopy was carried out, but if not, only a final check gastroscopy was done at the end of the study. The 2 criteria used to judge the results were: comparing the proportion of patients in the 2 groups whose ulcers recurred with symptoms, and comparing the proportion of patients with an asymptomatic ('silent') relapse.

The trials were organised by Smith Kline & French and were of similar design. The results of the various studies when taken together show that, amongst those on placebo, 47% had a symptomatic relapse within 1 year, compared with only 13.4% of those on cimetidine 400 mg nightly and 13% of those on cimetidine 400 mg twice daily. The corresponding figures for silent ulceration were 30%, 5.3% and 9.3% [26].

These differences are remarkable and clearly indicate the value of maintenance treatment as a prophylaxis against ulcer recurrence. Nevertheless, there are several problems which need investigation.

First, will maintenance treatment remain effective? Approximately 1 out of 7 patients on cimetidine relapse in the first year. Will similar proportions relapse in subsequent years? In 1 study where patients were maintained on cimetidine 1 g/day for up to a year, the relapse rate steadily increased with the passage of time [20]. If this is confirmed, then maintenance treatment is merely delaying the relapse rather than abolishing it. Alternatively, will the majority of those who relapse on maintenance treatment do so in the early period? If so, such patients could then be selected for surgery. Unfortunately, no data exists on the results of treatment for longer than a year.

Second, for how long should treatment be continued? The tendency to relapse can last a life-time; therefore, maintenance treatment may need to be permanent. However, the majority of patients run a more limited course: symptoms steadily increase, reaching a peak 5 to 10 years after the onset; thereafter, there is a strong tendency for remission [26, 27]. Therefore, treatment is required for a shorter period, only for as long as relapse is likely. The problem is that there is no method by which the natural history of the disease can be predicted in individual patients.

Third, does maintenance treatment cure duodenal ulcer disease or merely suppress it? On the evidence so far, it merely suppresses. However, with prolonged treatment, the natural history of the disease may be altered.

Fourth, what is the optimal dose? Maintenance with 400 mg nightly fails to prevent all relapses. Surprisingly, the 800 mg dose is no more effective. Will a higher dose produce better results? And also, will combination with other drugs improve results?

Fifth, do all patients need maintenance treatment? Clinical experience shows that many patients have only occasional attacks; such patients probably do not require prolonged treatment. How should candidates for maintenance treatment be selected at the outset?

Sixth, cimetidine has so far been very safe. But will it remain so with very long-term treatment?

These questions will take many years to answer.

Intermittent treatment

Intermittent treatment, given as and when symptoms recur, is commonly used in practice, but its value has not been formerly investigated. I studied this method in 125 patients who were treated with cimetidine until healing was complete, which generally took 1-2 months. Thereafter, their progress was followed for up to 22 months. During this time, 83 patients relapsed and, of these, 21 defaulted. The remaining 62 patients were re-treated until healed, but 36 later relapsed again.

The pattern of relapse and remission for the group as a whole was similar on both occasions, confirming that a short course of treatment does not alter the natural history of the disease. The likelihood of relapsing was 9% at 1 month or less, 23% at 3 months or less, and 40% at 6 months or less. Conversely, 60% were likely to be in remission at 6 months, 48% at 9 months, and 38% at 12 months. But in individual patients, there was little correlation between remission periods. Some who relapsed within 1-2 months after 1 course of cimetidine relapsed after 12 months or more following the second course; the reverse was equally true.

Amongst patients I see, the majority have 1, 2 or sometimes 3 significant attacks a year. In most, symptoms develop only gradually and there is therefore enough time to intervene with a short course of cimetidine, which terminates the attack, provides rapid relief and produces quick healing. However, not everyone is suited for such treatment. Those who in the past have bled or perforated without warning, or who usually develop severe symptoms abruptly, should not be treated in this manner as there is not sufficient time to intervene. Intermittent treatment is also best avoided in the elderly or those with severe associated disease, such as cardio-respiratory problems, for there is a small but unavoidable risk of bleeding or perforation with each ulcer recurrence, which in this group could have serious consequences. Overall, about one-fifth of patients are not suited for such treatment.

Despite these limitations, intermittent treatment is simple, is cheaper than maintenance treatment as less drug is used, and allows detection of 'rapid relapsers' who can then with confidence be selected either for maintenance treatment or for surgery [29].

The severity of ulcer disease and the method of and criteria for referral to specialist units varies from place to place. Therefore, the results of intermittent treatment may also vary from centre to centre. Thus, in one study, continuous treatment was preferred to intermittent treatment [30]; in my practice, on the other hand, intermittent treatment provides an adequate alternative to maintenance treatment for the majority of patients.

Other drugs

Cimetidine has not only transformed the treatment of duodenal ulcer, but cimetidine trials have established methods for investigating other potential anti-ulcer drugs. There has recently been renewed interest in ulcer disease after many years of stagnation, and several drugs have been investigated, including some which in the past had been rejected. The important ones are antacids, carbenoxolone, and colloidal bismuth.

Antacids in large doses (1000 mmol, or about 200-250 ml daily in divided doses) have now been shown to markedly reduce gastric secretion and to accelerate ulcer healing, the results being similar to those achieved with cimetidine [31-34]. Despite initial negative results, it has been confirmed that carbenoxolone also increases ulcer healing, the results also matching those of cimetidine [35-37]. The value of colloidal bismuth has been confirmed, and this agent has been found to be as effective as cimetidine as well [9, 38-41].

However, these compounds have limitations. Large-dose antacid treatment is inconvenient and frequently causes diarrhoea; carbenoxolone can cause sodium and fluid retention, hypertension and hypokalaemia; colloidal bismuth has an unpleasant odour.

Other drugs have also been investigated, such as prostaglandin analogues, proglumide, pirenzepine and tri-imipramine; though they increase ulcer healing, the results are not as impressive as those reported with cimetidine (for a review, see [6]). Inevitably, new histamine H_2-receptor antagonists have been developed. Ranitidine markedly reduces acid secretion, its action lasts longer than that of cimetidine and, on a molar basis, it seems more potent [42-44]; however, the results of clinical trials have not yet been published. In animal studies, ICI-125211 has proven to be very powerful [45].

A personal practice

Having confirmed the diagnosis, I treat patients with cimetidine 1 g/day until healed. The majority of the patients are then treated intermittently, as and when significant symptoms develop; in between, if they have minor symptoms, they are advised to use antacids only. If attacks are infrequent, then the individual episodes are treated with a short course of cimetidine. If on the other hand the attacks are frequent, or if intermittent treatment is contra-indicated, the patient is started on low-dose maintenance treatment.

The long-term management of those on maintenance treatment is problematical. In the elderly or those who also have other serious disease, I have no hesitation in continuing them on cimetidine; the alternative treatment, namely surgery, carries substantial mortality and morbidity. But the decision is not so easy with those patients who are fit for elective surgery since, while the risk and the value of surgery is known, the consequences of long-term cimetidine treatment are not.

Until recently, I used to refer such patients for surgery. Once this decision was made, the patients would be kept on cimetidine until surgery; as they stayed asymptomatic, the urgency to operate was removed. However, as more is known about cimetidine, and partly because of the enormous demand for such treatment in preference to surgery, increasing numbers of patients are being put on maintenance treatment. Consequently, elective gastric surgery in my hospital has been reduced by about one-third.

For the small group whose ulcer does not heal within 3 months on cimetidine 1 g/day, either on the first exposure or in subsequent courses, I try the effect of a 2 g dose. This generally produces healing but, should it fail, and if symptoms are troublesome, I then use the combination of rest in hospital, cimetidine 2 g/day, carbenoxolone (in position-release capsules) 200-300 mg/day and large frequent doses of antacids (a combination of aluminium and magnesium compounds; 25 ml both 1 hour and 3 hours after meals, 50 ml at bed time, and 50 ml at any time pain arises). Should this fail and symptoms continue, there is no alternative to surgery.

So far I have used endoscopic assessment to guide intermittent treatment, but this is not strictly necessary. Providing the diagnosis of duodenal ulcer is proven beyond doubt by initial endoscopy, the recurrence of typical symptoms generally indicates re-ulceration. Cimetidine can then be started; a 1-2 month course usually produces healing, and there is generally no need for endoscopic confirmation [7]. By reducing the need for endoscopy intermittent treatment can be used much more widely, particularly in general practice where most of the ulcer patients are seen. Endoscopy can be reserved for the few patients with atypical symptoms where there is doubt about ulcer recurrence, and for those with symptoms which persist despite treatment. In those patients on maintenance treatment, even if they are asymptomatic, I do a check endoscopy every 6 months to ensure healing is maintained; several are found to have a silent ulcer. Again, such frequent endoscopy may turn out to be unnecessary, but given the fairly limited amount of information on maintenance treatment available at present, this method, though laborious, is probably the safest.

References

1. Clark, C.J. and Downie, C.C. (1966): A method for the rapid determination of the number of patients to include in a controlled clinical trial. *Lancet 2*, 1357-1358.
2. Brown, P., Salmon, P.R., Thien-Htut and Read, A.E. (1972): Double-blind trial of carbenoxolone sodium capsules in duodenal ulcer therapy, based on endoscopic diagnosis and follow-up. *Br. Med. J. 3*, 661-664.
3. Doll, R., Price, A.V., Pygott, F. and Sanderson, P.H. (1956): Continuous intragastric milk drip in the treatment of uncomplicated gastric ulcer. *Lancet 1*, 70-73.
4. Gudjonsson, B. and Spiro, H. (1978): Response to placebos in ulcer disease. *Am. J. Med. 65*, 399-402.
5. Ivey, K.J. (1975): Anticholinergics: do they work in peptic ulcer? *Gastroenterology 68*, 154-166.
6. Walan, A. (1979): Anticholinergics in the treatment of peptic ulcer. *Scand. J. Gastroenterol. 14, Suppl. 55*, 84-95.
7. Bardhan, K.D. (1978): Cimetidine in duodenal ulceration. In: *Cimetidine: the Westminster Hospital Symposium*, pp. 31-56. Editors: C. Wastell and P. Lance. Churchill Livingstone, Edinburgh.
8. Lennard-Jones, J.E. and Barbouris, N. (1965): Effect of different foods on the acidity of the gastric contents in patients with duodenal ulcer: a comparison between two 'therapeutic' diets and freely chosen meals. *Gut 6*, 113-117.
9. (1975): Tri-potassium di-citrato bismuthate. *Postgrad. Med. J. 51*, Suppl. 55.
10. Wood, G.J. and Simkins, M.A. (Editors) (1973): *International Symposium on histamine H_2-receptor antagonists*. Deltakos (U.K.) Ltd., London.
11. Burland, W.L. and Simkins, M.A. (Editors) (1977): *Cimetidine: proceedings of the*

second International Symposium on histamine H₂-receptor antagonists. Excerpta Medica, Amsterdam-Oxford-Princeton.

12. Duncan, W.A.M. and Parsons, M.E. (1980): Reminiscences of the development of cimetidine. *Gastroenterology 78,* 620-625.
13. Keenan, R.A., Hunt, R.H., Vincent, D., Wright, B. and Milton-Thompson, G.J. (1978): Case for high dose antacid therapy in duodenal ulcer. *Gut 19,* A974. ·
14. Deering, T.B. and Malagelada, J.-R. (1979): Fate of oral neutralising antacid and its effect on post-prandial gastric secretion and emptying. *Gastroenterology 77,* 986-990.
15. Peter, P., Gonvers, J.J., Pelloni, S. et al. (1978): Cimetidine in the treatment of duodenal ulcer. In: *Cimetidine: proceedings of an International Symposium on histamine H₂-receptor antagonists,* pp. 190-198. Editor: W. Creutzfeldt. Excerpta Medica, Amsterdam-Oxford-Princeton.
16. Binder, H.J., Cocco, A., Crossley, R.J. et al. (1978): Cimetidine in the treatment of duodenal ulcer. A multicentre double-blind study. *Gastroenterology 74,* 380-388.
17. Fordtran, J.S. and Grossman, M.I. (Editors) (1978): Third Symposium on histamine H₂-receptor antagonists: clinical results with cimetidine. *Gastroenterology 74, 2,* 338-488.
18. McCarthy, D.M. (1978): Report on the United States experience with cimetidine in Zollinger-Ellison syndrome and other hypersecretory states. *Gastroenterology 74,* 453-455.
19. McCarthy, D.M., Peikin, S.R., Lopatin, R.N. et al. (1979): Hyperparathyroidism — a reversible cause of cimetidine resistant gastric hypersecretion. *Br. Med. J. 2,* 1765-1766.
20. Cargill, J.M., Peden, N., Saunders, J.H.B. and Wormsley, K.G. (1978): Very long-term treatment of peptic ulcer with cimetidine. *Lancet 2,* 1113-1115.
21. Hansky, J., Korman, M.G., Hetzel, D.J. and Shearman, D.J.C. (1979): Relapse rate after cessation of 12 months' cimetidine in duodenal ulcer. *Gastroenterology 76,* 1151.
22. Dronfield, M.W., Batchelor, A.J., Larkworthy, W. and Langman, M.J.S. (1979): Controlled trial of maintenance cimetidine in healed duodenal ulcer: short- and long-term effects. *Gut 20,* 526-530.
23. Fitzpatrick, W.J.F., Blackwood, W.S. and Northfield, T.C. (1979): Does cimetidine alter subsequent natural history of duodenal ulcer? *Gut 20,* A905.
24. Don, G., Hetzel, D.J., Korman, M.G., Hansky, J. and Shearman, D.J.C. (1979): Does twelve months' cimetidine treatment influence the natural history of duodenal ulcer? (Presented at the Annual Science Meeting of the Gastroenterology Society of Australia, Brisbane.) (Abstract A21).
25. Bardhan, K.D., Cole, D.S., Hawkins, B.W. and Sharpe, P.C. (1980): Extended treatment with cimetidine at full dose does not influence duodenal ulcer recurrence. [To be presented at the 11th International Congress of Gastroenterology, Hamburg, June 1980.] *Acta Hepato-gastroenterol. Belg.,* A197. (In preparation.)
26. Burland, W.L., Hawkins, B.W., Horton, R.J. and Beresford, J. (1978): The longer-term treatment of duodenal ulcer with cimetidine. In: *Cimetidine: the Westminster Hospital Symposium,* pp. 66-78. Editors: C. Wastell and P. Lance. Churchill Livingstone, Edinburgh.
27. Fry, J. (1964): Peptic ulcer: a profile. *Br. Med. J. 2,* 809-812.
28. Griebe, J., Bugge, P., Gjorup, T., Lauritzen, T., Bonnevie, O. and Wulff, H.R. (1977): Long-term prognosis of duodenal ulcer: a follow-up study and survey of doctors' estimates. *Br. Med. J. 2,* 1572-1574.
29. Bardhan, K.D. (1979): Intermittent treatment of duodenal ulcer with cimetidine. *Gut 20,* A905.
30. Hetzel, D.J., Hecker, R. and Shearman, D.J.C. (1979): The long-term treatment of duodenal ulcer with cimetidine: intermittent or continuous therapy? (Presented at a meeting of the Gastroenterology Society of Australia, Adelaide.) (Abstract.)
31. Petersen, W.L., Sturdevant, R.A.L., Frankl, H.D. et al. (1977): Healing of duodenal ulcer with an antacid regime. *N. Engl. J. Med. 297,* 341-345.
32. Ippoliti, A.F., Sturdevant, R.A.L., Isenberg, J.I. et al. (1978): Cimetidine versus intensive antacid therapy for duodenal ulcer. A multicentre trial. *Gastroenterology 74,* 393-395.

33. Shaw, G., Korman, M.G., Hansky, J., Schmidt, G.T. and Stern, A.I. (1979): Comparison of short-term Mylanta II and cimetidine in healing of duodenal ulcers. (Presented at a meeting of the Gastroenterology Society of Australia, Adelaide.) (Abstract.)
34. Malagelada, J.-R. and Carlson, G.L. (1979): Antacid therapy. *Scand. J. Gastroenterol. 14, Suppl. 55,* 67-83.
35. Davies, W.A. and Reed, P.I. (1977): Controlled trial of Duogastrone in duodenal ulcer. *Gut 18,* 78-83.
36. Sahel, J., Sarles, H., Boisson, J. et al. (1977): Carbenoxolone sodium capsules in the treatment of duodenal ulcer. An endoscopic controlled trial. *Gut 18,* 717-720.
37. Brown, P., Salmon, P.R., Neumann, C.S., Whittington, J.R. and Read, A.E. (1979): Comparison of carbenoxolone sodium (Duogastrone) and cimetidine (Tagamet) in duodenal ulceration. *Gut 20,* A904.
38. Coughlin, G.P., Kupa, A. and Alp, M.H. (1977): The effect of tri-potassium di-citrato bismuthate (De-Nol) on the healing of chronic duodenal ulcers. *Med. J. Aust. 1,* 294-298.
39. Lee, S.P. and Nicholson, G.I. (1977): Increased healing of gastric and duodenal ulcer in a controlled trial using tri-potassium di-citrato bismuthate. *Med. J. Aust. 1,* 808-812.
40. Martin, D.F., Hollanders, D., Miller, J.P., May, S.J., Tweedle, D.E.F. and Ravenscroft, M.M. (1979): Comparison between cimetidine and De-Nol in duodenal ulcer healing. *Gut 20,* A904.
41. Cowen, A.E., Pollard, E.J., Kemp, R. and Ward, M. (1979): A double-blind comparison of cimetidine and De-Nol in the treatment of chronic duodenal ulceration. (Presented at a meeting of the Gastroenterology Society of Australia, Adelaide.) (Abstract.)
42. Peden, N.R., Saunders, J.H.B. and Wormsley, K.G. (1979): Inhibition of pentagastrin-stimulated and nocturnal gastric secretion by ranitidine, a new H_2-receptor antagonist. *Lancet 1,* 690-692.
43. Hagenmuller, F., Zeiter-abu-Ishira, A. and Classen, M. (1979): Inhibition of gastric acid secretion by the new histamine H_2-receptor antagonist AH 19065 (ranitidine) and cimetidine. A double-blind trial. *Gut 20,* A905.
44. Walt, R.P., Mate, P.J., Rawlings, J. et al. (1979): 24-hour intragastric acidity in duodenal ulcer patients on a new twice-daily H_2-receptor antagonist. *Gut 20,* A904-905.
45. Yellin, T.O., Buck, S.H., Gilman, D.J., Jones, D.F. and Wardleworth, J.M. (1979): ICI-125211: a potent new antisecretory drug acting on histamine H_2-receptors. *Pharmacologist 21,* 266.

Discussion

Northfield (London): I have some data on 2 of the questions raised by Dr. Bardhan. The first question is whether relapse is being prevented or simply postponed — that is, whether the subsequent natural history of the disease is altered once cimetidine administration is stopped. The second question is about optimal dose.

I have carried out 2 different studies in collaboration with Dr. Fitzpatrick and Dr. Blackwood. In the first, which has been published in the *Lancet**, patients were randomly allocated to bedtime maintenance treatment either with cimetidine 800 mg or with placebo. In the second study, which has not been published, patients were first treated for 6 months with cimetidine 800 mg and were then randomly allocated either to placebo or to a lower dose of cimetidine (400 mg).

The placebo relapse rates, assessed endoscopically rather than symptomatically, were identical in the 2 studies. This means that cimetidine 800 mg administered for 6 months had not altered the subsequent natural history once the cimetidine was stopped. Cimetidine had postponed the relapse, but had not permanently prevented it.

In our first study, there was a marked reduction in endoscopic relapse rate with cimetidine 800 mg as compared with placebo. In the second study, the same relapse rate on cimetidine 800 mg was observed but there was a sharp rise in relapse rate when the patients subsequently received the lower dose of cimetidine (400 mg). There was much less difference between the cimetidine and placebo relapse rates in the second study. Although these were 2 different studies, their identical placebo relapse rates provide some justification for comparing their cimetidine results, which imply that cimetidine 400 mg is probably not as effective a maintenence dose as cimetidine 800 mg.

We are now planning to carry out a study in which the same patients are randomly allocated to either cimetidine 400 mg or 800 mg, to confirm this difference.

Giacosa (Genoa): In our experience, we have never seen such a high healing rate as 95% after 4 months' treatment. After the second or third month, a rate of healing has been reached which is a maximum and is never improved upon.

Bardhan: I take the point. However, I must emphasise that we are dealing with different populations. It may well be that the patients seen by Dr. Giacosa and others are highly selected patients — it is generally the less-severely affected patients who are referred to the gastroenterologist, while those for whom there is no hope are referred to the surgeon. I tend to see patients with milder disease, and it is quite possible that the good results I have shown simply reflect this fact. It is very difficult to truly randomise a trial taking these variables into account. For example, what exactly is meant by 'mild' and 'severe'?

---

*Blackwood, W.S., Maudgal, D.P. and Northfield, T.C. (1978): Prevention of bedtime cimetidine of duodenal ulcer relapse. *Lancet I*, 626-627.

Indications for surgery in duodenal ulcer nonresponders to cimetidine

C.W. Venables

Newcastle University Hospitals, Newcastle-upon-Tyne, United Kingdom

Introduction

The management of duodenal ulceration has clearly been affected by the introduction of histamine H_2-receptor antagonists, such as cimetidine. These have, for the first time, made it possible to control acid secretion by the stomach for a prolonged period, without the need for frequent medication or surgical intervention. Their efficacy in healing duodenal ulceration has been consistently demonstrated in controlled trials [1-4]; in addition, several trials have demonstrated that ulcer remission can be maintained by the use of small doses given regularly for several months [5-7].

The major impact of the introduction of these agents has been felt by gastric surgeons who, prior to their introduction, were the only doctors who could offer long-term control of the symptoms of duodenal ulceration. Initially, treatment with histamine H_2-receptor antagonists led to a rapid fall in the number of patients being referred for operation, but, more recently, it has been recognized that not all patients will benefit from treatment with these drugs, and that surgery is still needed in some cases.

At this time, 3 years after the release of cimetidine onto the market, it is an opportune moment to examine and assess the relative roles of surgery and cime-

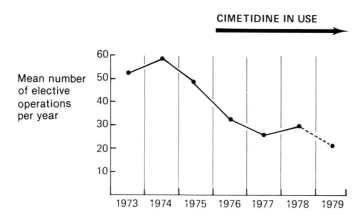

Fig. 1. Mean yearly numbers of elective operations for duodenal ulcer in our unit, from January 1973 to September 1979. (Broken line indicates a partial year.) Cimetidine was first used regularly in March 1976.

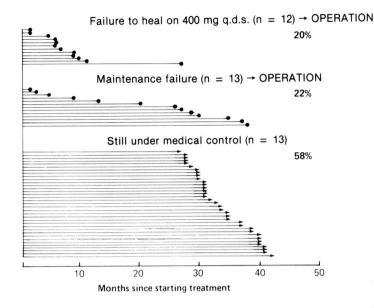

Failure to heal on 400 mg q.d.s. (n = 12) → OPERATION
20%

Maintenance failure (n = 13) → OPERATION
22%

Still under medical control (n = 13)
58%

Months since starting treatment

Fig. 2. Follow-up information on 60 patients from our long-term trial, as of September 1979. Patient entry began in March 1976 and ended in June 1977. Thirteen patients were lost to follow-up.

tidine in the long-term management of duodenal ulceration.

Our department has been in a unique position to assess these relative roles, being a surgical department with a long-standing interest in histamine H_2-receptor blockade and its role in duodenal ulcer management. Our interest in medical treatment has been spurred by the disappointing results seen in some patients in our long-term prospective studies of the results of gastric surgery in Newcastle since 1966.

To examine the overall impact of the use of cimetidine on surgical management, we have looked at the number of patients undergoing elective surgical treatment for duodenal ulcer on our unit since 1973 (Fig. 1). From 1973 to 1976, when cimetidine therapy was first introduced, the mean number of operations was 54 per year. Since then, this has fallen to a mean of 29 per year, an overall reduction of 47%. Additional support for this figure comes from the follow-up of patients in our long-term trial [8] (Fig. 2): of the 73 originally entered in the long-term study, we have follow-up data on 60; 58% of these are still being controlled on continuous treatment with low doses of cimetidine, while 42% have come to operation for the reasons shown in the Figure.

Indications for operation

Before considering the impact of cimetidine therapy on surgical management, it is clearly necessary to review how its use has affected the indications for operation. Prior to the introduction of this drug, the usual indications for surgery were those outlined in Table I. The most common indication was the failure of medical treatment: in our unit, this accounted for 408 of the 566 patients undergoing vagotomy for duodenal ulcers between 1966 and 1977. Complications of the ulcer accounted

Table I.   Indications for operation before the advent of cimetidine.

1. Failed medical treatment (72%)
   a. severe symptoms
   b. frequent attacks
   c. loss of work
2. Complications of the ulcer (24%)
   a. stenosis
   b. perforation
   c. bleeding (acute and recurrent)
   d. possible malignancy
3. Social reasons (4%)
   a. access to medical care difficult
   b. hazard to occupation

for most of the remaining 158 cases; in approximately two-thirds of these, pyloric stenosis was the prime indication.

Cimetidine would be expected to have its greatest impact on the group of patients not helped by medical treatment; it is unlikely, in the short run, to have a significant effect on complications of the ulcer, many of which arise in patients with no previous history.

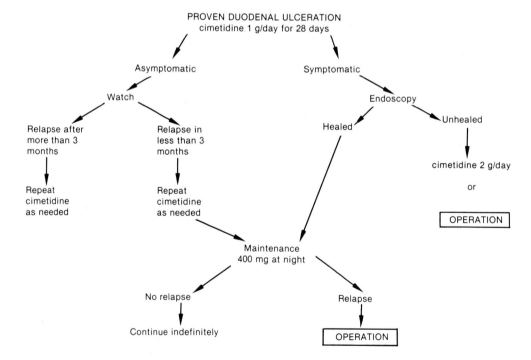

Fig. 3.   Suggested flow chart for the use of cimetidine in duodenal ulceration. Reprinted with permission from [8].

Since completion of our long-term cimetidine controlled trial, we have followed a policy based on the flow chart outlined in Figure 3. Under this regime, there are 2 major indications for operation: failure to heal even after prolonged therapy with an increased dose of cimetidine, and relapse after control on maintenance therapy. In this latter group, we have tried increasing the maintenance dose to 800 mg at night in some cases, but with only slight success to date. There is clearly a need to subject such studies to a controlled trial, as it may well be that there are some individuals who require a larger nightly dosage for maintenance.

In addition to these 2 major indications, there is also a third: intolerance of the drug. Included in this group are patients who, through poor compliance, do not take their medication regularly or effectively; patients in whom vague symptoms such as nausea and depression are noted during treatment; and patients in whom genuine side-effects (skin rashes, hepatic dysfunction, occasional central nervous system effects) occur. Under such circumstances one can hardly justify continuing treatment with the drug; if other medical measures also fail, surgery is the only available alternative.

Since January 1977, a total of 68 patients have come to surgery in our unit after treatment with cimetidine, including the 25 from our long-term controlled study who have required surgical treatment up to now (see Fig. 2). In these patients, the most common indication for surgery was failure of cimetidine to heal the ulcer (62%); maintenance failure accounted for the majority of the other patients undergoing elective surgery (30%).

Reasons for failure of cimetidine to heal the ulcer

There are a number of fairly obvious ways to explain the failure of ulcers to heal on cimetidine. The simplest is to claim that the patient is not taking the drug correctly or effectively: while we have always attempted to ensure that the patient is following treatment instructions, there is no reliable way of proving this without regular blood monitoring of cimetidine levels, and that has not been practical. However, we do not believe that many of our patients fall into this category.

In our unit, one of the demonstrable reasons for failure of cimetidine to heal an ulcer was the coexisting presence of stenosis, usually in the mid-bulb region or sometimes at the pylorus. This accounted for 11 of the 42 patients whose ulcers failed to heal on initial treatment.

Another possibility is that there may be an underlying Zollinger-Ellison syndrome. In such cases, a larger dose of cimetidine may control the ulcer disease; if this syndrome is known to be present, then adequate control may be instituted and surgery avoided. We have not, however, seen such a cause in any of our patients, although a few have had fasting serum gastrin levels at the upper limit of normal, which may be significant.

In the majority of cases, though, none of these possible causes were present, so we need to look for some other explanation for the failure of cimetidine to heal the ulcer. In our first follow-up study [8], we examined 10 patients whose ulcers failed to heal on cimetidine 1.6 g/day, administered for 4 weeks. Of these 10 patients, 5 were then randomized to cimetidine and an anticholinergic (poldine methylsulphate 4 mg q.d.s.), and 5 to cimetidine alone. The 5 given the combined drugs appeared to fare better, as all of their ulcers healed after 4 weeks of this further treatment, while only 3 healed on cimetidine alone. This suggested to us that in those patients who fail to

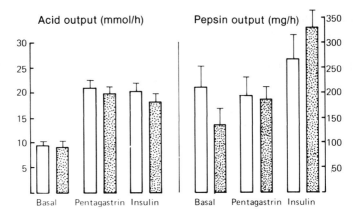

Fig. 4.   Secretory data (mean ± SE) comparing 45 patients whose ulcers healed after treatment with 400 mg cimetidine q.d.s. for 28 days (white bars) with 28 patients whose ulcers did not heal following the same treatment (dotted bars).

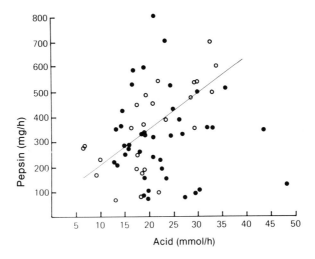

Fig. 5.   Plot of pepsin output against acid output following insulin stimulation in 45 patients whose ulcers healed (•) and 28 whose ulcers did not (○). Healed: r = 0.139 (not significant). Unhealed: r = 0.704 (p = 0.01).

heal with regular cimetidine treatment, the addition of an anticholinergic might be of some benefit. Clearly, further examination of this possibility is indicated.

Another aspect we have been investigating is whether the gastric secretory potential of those who heal on initial cimetidine therapy may be different from that of those who do not. It has previously been suggested that acid hypersecretion occurs more commonly in those who fail to heal [9]; in our own studies, however, we have not been able to confirm this suggestion. We have found no difference in the acid secretion, either in the basal or the pentagastrin- or insulin-stimulated output, between those who heal and those who do not (Fig. 4). In addition, we have been unable in this study, with more patients, to confirm our earlier suggestion that the pentagastrin/insulin ratio is lower in those who fail to heal [8]. The only secretory abnormality that we now find is one which puzzles us and for which we do not, as yet, have an explanation: after insulin stimulation, the usual relationship between acid and pepsin secretion is lost in those who heal, but is significant in those who do not (Fig. 5). Could this finding suggest that those patients who fail to heal are more responsive to vagal stimulation than those who do heal, or is it a reflection of the loss of an inhibitory mechanism, which is restored by the use of H_2-receptor blockade? Again, further study is clearly indicated.

Reasons for the failure of maintenance therapy

Twenty of our patients have come to surgery because a nightly dose of cimetidine (400 mg) failed to maintain their duodenal ulcer in remission and persistent symptoms occurred. There are a number of possible explanations for this failure of regular cimetidine maintenance therapy, including the following: noncompliance, especially in asymptomatic patients; an altered response to cimetidine due to interaction with another drug [8]; the ulcer may not have healed completely on the therapeutic dose and 400 mg at night was not sufficient to promote continued healing; or the dose was too low to control overnight acid secretion in some patients. (While we have not examined this last possibility ourselves, other workers have demonstrated that the response to a single nightly dose of cimetidine does vary from one individual to another. Further research into this point is indicated.)

In our studies, another question that has interested us is whether or not there is a secretory abnormality present in patients whose ulcers fail to be controlled on maintenance therapy. Figure 6 illustrates the mean acid and pepsin outputs in 16 patients whose ulcers are still controlled with regular cimetidine treatment, compared with 17 whose ulcers have relapsed. There were no significant differences between the 2 groups, but there was a general trend towards a lower acid and higher pepsin output following insulin stimulation in those who relapsed during maintenance therapy.

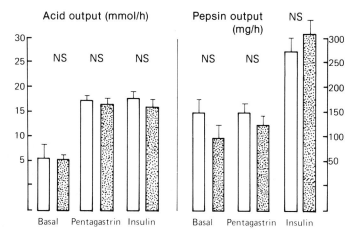

Fig. 6. Secretory data (mean ± SE) comparing 16 patients whose duodenal ulcer was controlled for 1 year on 400 mg cimetidine at night (white bars) with 17 who relapsed on maintenance therapy (dotted bars). NS = not significant.

Table II.   Results after at least 6 months' follow-up in patients who have required surgical therapy after treatment with cimetidine.

Reason for operation	Type of surgery (number)	Pain	Recurrent ulcer
Unhealed ulcers (n = 36)	Proximal gastric vagotomy (11)	1	2
	Vagotomy and pyloroplasty (23)	1	4
	Vagotomy and antrectomy (2)	0	0
Maintenance failure (n = 15)	Proximal gastric vagotomy (15)	1	1 (possible)

Follow-up results of surgical management

Should the type of surgical management of patients who 'fail' on cimetidine therapy be modified in any way? Clearly, this is an important question, and one that has yet to be answered. While it is rather early to draw any firm conclusions, we are becoming concerned by the trend we see developing in our own surgical results. Table II reports on 51 patients who underwent surgery between January 1977 and March 1979, following failure of cimetidine therapy. All have been followed up for more than 6 months. Of 36 patients treated by vagotomy after a failure to heal on initial cimetidine therapy, there have already been 6 confirmed recurrent ulcers and 2 other patients reporting pain without ulcer at endoscopy; of 15 patients surgically treated after maintenance failure, 2 have redeveloped pain, and in 1 of these a possible small ulcer was seen at endoscopy.

A recurrence rate of 16.6% in the 'failed to heal' group following vagotomy is of considerable concern, and contrasts with a 5% recurrence rate following vagotomy and pyloroplasty at 8 years and a 2% recurrence rate (1 in 41) following proximal gastric vagotomy at 2 years in our long-term follow-up studies after gastric surgery locally.

If this trend continues, we are clearly going to require a more aggressive surgical approach to these patients in the future.

Conclusions

Our studies suggest that, with the correct use of cimetidine, we can expect to reduce the need for surgical therapy in cases of severe duodenal ulcer disease by nearly 50%. The major indications for still considering an operation are: failure of the ulcer to heal on 'full therapeutic dosage', particularly if associated with duodenal narrowing; and failure of 'maintenance therapy' to prevent ulcer recurrence. In addition, there is a less significant third indication: problems with therapy.

At present, there can be no firm advice as to what specific operation should be advised for these patients, but our initial follow-up results suggest that more aggressive surgery than vagotomy may be needed.

Acknowledgements

I should like to acknowledge the many people who have assisted in this work, including Mr J.G. Stephen, who helped in our original trial; S.N. Kenny and S.E.N. Robson, who performed many of the secretion tests reported here and assisted at the endoscopies; the graphics staff of the University Audiovisual-Aids Department, who prepared the illustrations; and Miss H. Bruce, who typed the manuscript. In addition, I should like to thank the Clinical Research Department of Smith Kline & French Laboratories, who have encouraged and supported this work throughout.

References

1. Bodemar, G. and Walan, A. (1976): Cimetidine in the treatment of active duodenal and pre-pyloric ulcers. *Lancet 2,* 161-164.
2. Binder, H.J., Cocco, A., Crossley, R.J., Finkelstein, W., Font, R., Fredman, G., Groarke, J., Hughes, W., Johnson, A.F., McGuigan, J.E., Summers, R., Vlahcevic, R., Wilson, E.C. and Winship, D.H. (1978): Cimetidine in the treatment of duodenal ulcer. *Gastroenterology 74,* 380-387.
3. Gray, G.R., Mackenzie, I., Smith, I.S., Crean, G.P. and Gillespie, G. (1977): Oral cimetidine in severe duodenal ulceration — a double-blind trial. *Lancet 1,* 4-7.
4. Multicentre Trial (1979): A comparison of two doses of cimetidine and placebo in the treatment of duodenal ulcer. *Gut 20,* 68-74.
5. Bardhan, K.D., Saul, D.M., Edwards, J.L., Smith, P.M., Haggie, S.J., Wyllie, J.H., Duthie, H.L. and Fussey, I.V. (1979): Double-blind comparison of cimetidine and placebo in the maintenance of healing of chronic duodenal ulceration. *Gut 20,* 158-162.
6. Bodemar, G. and Walan, A. (1978): Maintenance treatment of recurrent peptic ulcer by cimetidine. *Lancet 1,* 403-407.
7. Burland, W.L., Hawkins, B.W., Horton, R.J. and Beresford, J. (1978): The longer term treatment of duodenal ulcer with cimetidine. In: *Cimetidine: the Westminster Hospital Symposium,* pp. 66-77. Editors: C. Wastell and P. Lance. Churchill Livingstone, Edinburgh.
8. Venables, C.W., Stephen, J.G., Blair, E.L., Reed, J.D. and Saunders, J.D. (1978): Cimetidine in the treatment of duodenal ulceration and the relationship of this therapy to surgical management. In: *Cimetidine: the Westminster Hospital Symposium,* pp. 13-28. Editors: C. Wastell and P. Lance. Churchill Livingstone, Edinburgh.
9. Hetzel, D.J., Hansky, J., Shearman, D.J.C., Korman, M.G., Hecker, R., Taggart, G.J., Jackson, R. and Gabb, B.W. (1978): Cimetidine treatment of duodenal ulceration: short-term clinical trial and maintenance study. *Gastroenterology 74,* 389-392.

Discussion

Bader (Paris): I would like to thank Mr. Venables for his very interesting data. I was especially interested in his finding of a relatively low rate of pepsin secretion in the non-healed and relapsed groups. Many years ago, together with Professor Bonfils, I studied the pepsin secretion rate and found that, when pepsin concentration in gastric juice is low, the main component of the secretory drive is gastrinergic; the extreme form of this situation is, of course, the Zollinger-Ellison syndrome.

I think Mr. Venables' data may be interpreted as showing that it is possible that groups of patients with poor healing results and/or a high frequency of relapse may have principally gastrinergic secretion and, perhaps, an increase in antral G cells. I also have a question: has Mr. Venables measured the blood level of gastrin in the groups of healed and non-healed patients and in the groups of relapsed and non-relapsed patients?

Venables: We have looked at fasting serum gastrin in all these patients, but have seen no difference in the fasting state. I would caution against accepting that as showing that gastrin has no role because, like Dr. Bader, I think that it may have some role. Even now, we do not know enough about serum gastrin. I am not sure that total serum gastrin is particularly meaningful. There are biological species of gastrin, and their biological activities are not necessarily related to their total immunoreactivity.

Speranza (Rome): As a surgeon, I believe that the use of cimetidine has fundamentally altered our assessment of the indications for surgery: in patients who are said not to have responded to conventional medical treatment, cimetidine is of significance; however, it is probably a mistake to automatically regard patients who have not responded to cimetidine as being candidates for surgery. I would say that patients who do not respond to cimetidine clearly require surgery, but not only proximal vagotomy, as is shown by the 6 patients with recurrences within 6 months of proximal vagotomy or vagotomy and pyloroplasty. It can be assumed that these patients had suffered a recurrence because cimetidine, which in practice has the same effect as vagotomy, had not proved capable of healing their ulcers.

I believe that the indication for surgery must be based upon whether or not there has been a response to treatment with cimetidine. However, 'surgery' here includes 2 specific types of operation: selective proximal vagotomy should be performed in patients who respond to cimetidine, while those who do not respond should have a vagotomy and antrectomy. Selective proximal vagotomy has no mortality, and it achieves permanently what cimetidine achieves during its administration.

Venables: I agree with Dr. Speranza up to a point, and the data I have presented confirm what he has said. He indicated that if ulcers will heal on cimetidine they will heal with proximal gastric vagotomy, and I tend to agree with this. The question then becomes one of deciding which treatment we believe should be given to these patients.

However, to assume, just because vagotomy and cimetidine both reduce acid, that they do so in exactly the same way is naive in my opinion. The effects of vagotomy on the stomach are not the same as those of cimetidine. Vagotomy does not work through H_2-receptors, but through anticholinergic mechanisms. Therefore, it comes as a slight surprise to me — although Dr. Speranza believes it has been proven — that vagotomy patients have done so much worse. I agree with what he says, which I would not have done 2 years ago.

Giacosa (Genoa): In our experience, Professor Speranza's conclusions regarding the indications for medical and surgical treatment are borne out by results from Dr. Cheli's group.

We disagree, however, on the subject of drug combinations, as we have seen cases where the combination of cimetidine with anticholinergic drugs has been effective, and some cases where anticholinergics alone have produced results. This observation must be quantified, and may indicate the existence of a group of patients with different pathophysiological characteristics.

Venables: We do not disagree, with regard to the healing of ulcer disease. Giving anticholinergics regularly with cimetidine does increase the healing rate.

Festen (Nijmegen): It is known that blood cimetidine levels vary greatly in individual patients, although the reason for this is not known. On the other hand, it is also known that the effect of cimetidine on gastric acid secretion is directly related to the blood cimetidine level. Do either Mr. Venables or Dr. Bardhan have any data on blood cimetidine levels in non-responding patients? I ask this question because, in our rather small study, we have found that out of a total of about 36 patients there were 5 relapsed patients whose blood cimetidine levels were about half those of the responders.

Venables: I would love to be able to answer that question in a positive sense. Dr. Burland knows that I have wanted to measure blood levels in all these patients for many years. Unfortunately this has, for practical reasons, not been possible.

Dodero (Genoa): We are collecting epidemiological data on non-responders. I can confirm that, after treatment for 60-90 days, there is a low incidence of non-responders. We ourselves have had about 5-6% of non-responders, with positive response defined as endoscopically-confirmed total healing of the duodenal ulcer.

Our data have not yet been analysed statistically, but I want to mention 2 observations which confirm Mr. Venables' findings. First, we noted that non-responders very often have a family history of duodenal ulceration, with one or both parents and/or brothers or sisters having been affected. Second, these are subjects with a duodenal ulcer history of at least 5 years.

Venables: We have also looked at this question of family history; it is particularly of interest in Newcastle, where our paediatricians have done a lot of work on this subject. It is impossible to find any evidence that it is only patients with a marked family history who relapse. In our own trial, the local failure-to-heal rate was only 16% at one month. This means that our results do not markedly disagree with Dr. Dodero's.

Gastric ulcer

G.F. Delle Fave, A. Kohn, C. Sparvoli and A. Torsoli
Department of Gastroenterology, University of Rome, Rome, Italy

The treatment of gastric ulcer has been and continues to be influenced by a number of factors: the uncertainty of drug efficacy, the frequent recurrence of lesions [1, 2], the possibility of diagnostic error in cases of cancer, and the possibility of neoplastic 'degeneration'.

Gastric ulcer is a non-homogeneous condition, for which reason it is difficult to arrive at a definitive clinical opinion regarding the various therapeutic measures. Variables include the age of the patient, the nature of the lesion (primary or recurrent), its etiology (ulcers associated or not associated with other morbid states or with the use of ulcerogenic drugs), its localization (prepyloric ulcer, ulcer of the corpus), the presence or absence of inflammatory or atrophic changes in the stomach, and the possibility of an influence by certain factors (smoking, alcohol, coffee, hospitalization, etc.).

The possibility of mistaken diagnosis in the case of cancer should always be considered. The presence of cancer in ulcers regarded as benign is of the order of 3-4% [3]. The occurrence of neoplastic changes in initially benign ulcers has been estimated at about 1-2%, but precise data are unfortunately not available. Based on their own experience, many surgeons would probably be disposed to suggest rather higher estimates; however, this experience is mostly derived from conventional radiology and endoscopy, and is often not supported by adequate bioptic controls. Conventional radiology may furnish false negative results in up to 40% of cases [4]. This explains why large gastric operations, even resections, are still performed for a lesion which can generally be cured by conservative means.

The advent of H_2-receptor antagonists has produced a renewed interest in the study of gastric ulceration. This renewed interest has coincided with, and has been partly determined by, a considerable development of endoscopic, histobioptic and radiological double contrast investigations. As a result, 2 important pieces of information have been reported: a) in the absence of factors which might interfere with the natural history of the disease, gastric ulcers tend to heal rapidly, with cicatrization occurring within 12-16 weeks or less [5], and b) the crater decreases exponentially over time.

This type of regression has previously been reported, based on endoscopic examination [6-8]. The results of a co-operative prospective radiologic study in which 27 gastric ulcer patients, including 15 hospital in-patients, were studied at 4 institutions, are reported here (Figs. 1 and 2). Measurements of crater width were carried out in a random order by different observers; the initial diagnosis and complete healing were controlled by endoscopy. Patients were prescribed rest and abstention from alcohol, smoking, coffee, irritating foods and drugs which alter the gastric mucous barrier. Those in whom it was not possible to obtain reliable and comparable radiologic measurements were excluded.

The exponential mode of crater reduction is a finding of notable practical and pathophysiologic interest. It permits the evaluation of disease progression according to times which may be predetermined by the course of the reduction curves. Results are independent of the initial size of the crater. It also permits both the calculation of the half-life of the lesion and the forecasting of the date of complete healing with considerable accuracy. Finally, it is probably an indicator of the simple nature of the morbid process. Curves significantly deviating from this type of regression have been observed in cases of malignant ulceration and in cases associated with duodenal ulcer or bezoar. If this is confirmed, then the ascertainment of the exponential mode of crater reduction could, together with negative endoscopic and bioptic data, constitute a useful criterion for the continuation of medical treatment.

In gastric ulceration, the H_2-receptor antagonists have primarily been used in short-term treatment, compared against a placebo or other drugs. Results of short-term experience against placebo have been ambiguous [9-13]: some trials have produced results statistically in favor of the use of the antagonists, other trials have had negative results. Nevertheless, arithmetical values, the effect on the pain syndrome and the consumption of antacids all indicate a benefit in favor of cimetidine-treated patients. It is possible that, in some series, the efficacy of cimetidine has been obscured by the relatively small number of cases, by the simultaneous use of potent antacids, or by enhanced response to the placebo.

Fifteen hospitalized patients in the present study were randomized, double-blind, either to cimetidine 1 g/day (7 patients) or a placebo (8 patients); complete healing was obtained in both groups within 70 days (Fig. 3), but the half-life of the ulcer was shorter in the cimetidine group (Fig. 4).

The role of cimetidine in the short-term treatment of gastric ulcer is, therefore,

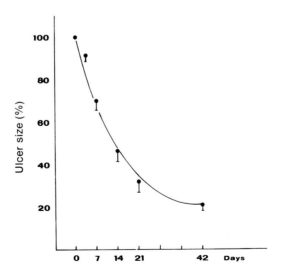

Fig. 1. *Reduction of ulcer size. 100% = ulcer size at beginning of study. Each point represents the mean (± SEM) in 27 patients with benign gastric ulcer.*

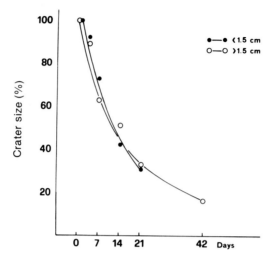

Fig. 2.   Reduction of ulcer crater, as against initial size of the ulcer. 100% = crater size at beginning of study. Twenty-seven patients were studied.

still undefined, and further studies are required. The problem of long-term treatment is also of great importance for the future, and there are already some encouraging results [14, 15]. However, surgery will remain a fundamental option for the treatment of gastric ulceration, at least until it has been unequivocally demonstrated that we are capable of preventing recurrences with medical management.

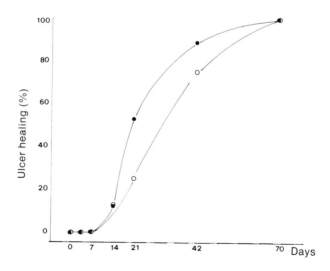

Fig. 3.   Percentage of ulcer healing in 7 patients receiving cimetidine 1 g/day (•——•) and 8 patients receiving placebo (o——o).

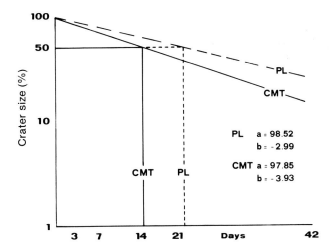

Fig. 4. Logarithm of the percentage of reduction of the ulcer crater in 7 patients receiving cimetidine 1 g/day (CMT) and 8 patients receiving placebo (PL).

References

1. Piper, D.W., Shinners, J., Greig, M., Thomas, J. and Waller, S. (1978): Effect of ulcer healing on the prognosis of chronic gastric ulcer. *Gut 19,* 419-424.
2. Halse, S.A., Kristensen, E., Jense, O.M. and Morkbak, N.K. (1977): Prognosis of medically-treated gastric ulcer: a prospective endoscopic study. *Scand. J. Gastroenterol. 12,* 489-495.
3. Fordtran, J.S. et al. (1978): Round table discussion on gastric ulcer. *Gastroenterology 74,* 431-434.
4. Mountford, R.A., Brown, P., Salmon, P.R., Neumann, C.S. and Read, A.F. (1978): Gastric cancer detection in gastric ulcer disease. *Gut 19,* 10 (A981).
5. Richardson, C.T. (1973): Chronic gastric ulcer. In: *Gastrointestinal disease.* Editors: M.H. Sleisinger and J.S. Fordtran. W.B. Saunders, Philadelphia.
6. Domschke, W., Domschke, S., Lux, G. and Demling, L. (1976): Kinetics of duodenal ulcer healing: effect of treatment with cimetidine. *Acta Hepato-gastroenterol. 23,* 441-443.
7. Scheurer, V., Witzel, L., Halter, F., Keller, H.M., Huber, R. and Galeazzi, R. (1977): Gastric and duodenal ulcer healing under placebo treatment. *Gastroenterology 72,* 838-841.
8. Torsoli, A. (1978): Progressi nella terapia medica dell'ulcera peptica. In: *Cimetidina,* pp. 47-56. Smith Kline & French, Milan.
9. Bader, J.-P., Morin, T., Bernier, J.J. et al. (1977): Treatment of gastric ulcer by cimetidine. A multicenter trial. In: *Cimetidine: proceedings of the second International Symposium on histamine H₂-receptor antagonists,* pp. 287-292. Editors: W.L. Burland and M.A. Simkins. Excerpta Medica, Amsterdam-Oxford-Princeton.
10. Frost, F., Rambek, I., Rune, S.J., Jensen, K.B. et al. (1977): Cimetidine in patients with gastric ulcer: a multicentre controlled trial. *Br. Med. J. 2,* 795-799.
11. Ciclitira, P.J., Machell, R.J., Farthing, M.J.G., Dick, A.P. and Hunter, J. (1977): A controlled trial of cimetidine in the treatment of gastric ulcer. In: *Cimetidine: proceedings of the second International Symposium on histamine H₂-receptor antagonists,* pp. 283-286. Editors: W.L. Burland and M.A. Simkins. Excerpta Medica, Amsterdam-Oxford-Princeton.
12. Landecker, K.D., Hunt, J.H., Gillespie, P. et al. (1978): Cimetidine and the gastric ulcer.

A double-blind controlled trial. *Gastroenterology 74,* 426-430.

13. Navert, H., Larose, L. et al. (1978): Cimetidine is effective in the treatment of gastric ulcer. *Gastroenterology 74,* 1072.
14. Jensen, K.B., Mollman, K.M. et al. (1979): Prophylactic effect of cimetidine in gastric ulcer patients. *Scand. J. Gastroenterol. 14,* 175-176.
15. Machell, R.J., Ciclitira, P.J., Farthing, M.J.G., Dick, A.P. and Hunter, J. (1979): The prevention of gastric ulcer relapse with cimetidine. *Gastroenterology 76,* 1191.

Discussion

Speranza (Rome): I want to ask Professor Torsoli if he can give me further information on the kind of gastric ulcer involved in his study. Were they Johnson type I gastric ulcers of the vertical part of the lesser curvature, or were they prepyloric or associated with duodenal ulcers?

Torsoli: As has been mentioned, the number of cases we were able to study was very
small; in this field, it is difficult to get a well-documented series. However, we certainly looked at these points and we found no differences in the incidence of ulcers
of the body and prepyloric ulcers between the cimetidine and placebo groups.

Ciammaichella (Rome): Duodenal ulcers do not become malignant, and many workers in gastroenterology believe that the presence of a duodenal ulcer is almost a
guarantee that a malignant gastric ulcer will not occur. I would like to know if Professor Torsoli agrees with this.

Torsoli: I think I can say that it is now the commonly held view that the presence of
a duodenal ulcer does not exclude malignancy in a gastric ulcer.

Missale (Parma): What have been the results of controlled trials comparing cimetidine and antacids?

Torsoli: As I have not myself made that comparison, I cannot say.

Missale: It has been said that gastric ulcers are not always associated with gastritis.
In my experience, however, I have found atrophic gastritis in all cases of gastric ulceration. What is Professor Torsoli's experience?

Torsoli: I do not have this information yet. About 16 biopsies were taken from our
patients at the 2 endoscopies, but these are still being studied.

Bianchi (Milan): Professor Torsoli's approach to this problem should produce
much valuable data. This precise method for the study of gastric ulceration seems
extremely interesting and new. I had thought that such precision would, technically,
be a very difficult thing to achieve.

   Having said this, I would like to ask Professor Torsoli for his comments on an impression which I have. Sometimes, at endoscopy, I see very large ulcers with raised
edges, probably with a large amount of underlying scar tissue. Is this type of ulcer
different from that which he has described, or should they all be included together?
Is the percentage of healing which can be obtained in this type of ulceration the
same? And finally, are such ulcers included in his trial?

Torsoli: I think that what Professor Bianchi has said is of great importance. The
technical difficulties involved in this kind of study are certainly great. We need high-

quality, usually double-contrast, radiology and an initial examination to decide precisely what orientation should be used for subsequent assessments; this decision is not easy to make.

In this trial, we included ulcers on the basis of negative histology and endoscopy. If the endoscopist felt that there was an element of doubt concerning the nature of the ulcer, ethical considerations precluded this type of study and the patient was immediately operated on, even with negative histology.

Montori (Rome): I would like to ask Professor Torsoli if he considers that, in addition to the biopsy to which he has referred, the use of another collateral technique (such as cytology) with the endoscopy is important in defining this condition. Also, he has said that, in about 95% of cases, gastric ulcer can be cured with medical treatment. Will he tell us clearly what action he takes in the other 5% of cases? When does he think that these patients must be operated on?

Torsoli: In response to the first question: ours is a quantitative study, and is therefor not concerned with cytology. It is obvious that, from the quantitative point of view, the endoscopic method is as important as the radiological method, if not more so.

As regards Dr. Montori's second point, we use the following criteria: we think it acceptable to treat a patient with a gastric ulcer medically if there are no radiological, endoscopic or biopsy features to suggest malignancy, and, in addition, if the reduction in crater volume is exponential. Provided these criteria are present, I believe that a patient can continue to be treated medically. It is clear that the definitive answer comes from biopsies with total healing, but we all know that sometimes, just when there has been full healing, a biopsy will become positive and the patient will have to have an operation.

Capurso (Ancona): I would like to ask Professor Torsoli what his experience has been with regard to malignant recurrence after complete endoscopically- and histologically-confirmed healing on cimetidine.

Torsoli: The literature shows that there are cases in which, with total healing, even before a recurrence, the histology is positive and there are signs of immediate recurrence at the same site. This obviously raises strong suspicion that the lesion is malignant in nature.

Cheli (Genoa): Professor Torsoli, there are several things which I want to know. First, going back to what Dr. Montori said about the extreme importance of cytology: this is a really fundamental criterion and I would say that, in assessing whether or not an ulcer is benign, if we add this parameter we can avoid mistakes in at least 95-96% of cases, combining cytology, endoscopy and biopsy.

Second, I would like to know from you how you measured the size of the ulcer. If I understand you correctly, you did this radiologically and not at endoscopy. At endoscopy there are methods of measurement which are now accepted, particularly the Erlangen method.

Third, you certainly have presented a variety of cases of gastric ulceration, even if not a large series. The statistical conditions necessary to decide on Johnson types I, II and III were not present. However, it is fundamentally important to know whether these patients, treated with cimetidine and antacids, were in- or out-patients. If the patients were all in hospital during treatment, then another curative element must be added to the series.

Torsoli: I repeat that I am in agreement with what you say about the importance of cytology, assuming you have a good cytologist, but this is not what we are talking about today. We are actually talking about a measurement system.

Regarding your second point: there have been studies comparing width (on X-rays) and depth of the lesion. We found that we can have confidence in assessment based on measurement of the maximum diameter of the base of the ulcer; we did this in 27 cases. We need to look further at this; the best method is probably to measure the greatest diameter of the ulcer in a double-contrast examination, but I am not prepared at present to discuss this problem.

With reference to the third question: certainly, we have always known that an ulcer can be cured by admission to hospital, but you know that recent data have accrued to contradict this. Neither hospitalization nor non-hospitalization has been shown to be superior in patients treated for gastric ulceration, either with cimetidine or with placebo. Our own schedule involves admission to hospital or else rest.

Cimetidine treatment and the Zollinger-Ellison syndrome*

P. Bianchi and M. Quatrini
Clinica Medica I, University of Milan, Milan, Italy

Introduction

Zollinger and Ellison described, in 1955, a syndrome characterized by the presence of severe peptic ulcer disease, marked gastric acid hypersecretion and pancreatic non-beta islet cell tumor, and postulated that a secretagogue humoral factor was produced by the tumor [1]. It was later established that this factor was gastrin, and that the tumor was sometimes located outside the pancreas or associated with other endocrine neoplasias as part of the multiple endocrine neoplasia syndrome.

Radical resection of the tumor is impossible in the majority of these patients, and mortality and morbidity are due to the consequences of gastric hypersecretion more than to the tumor itself; since, before the advent of treatment with H_2-receptor antagonists, there was no appropriate medical therapy available, total gastrectomy was generally accepted as the standard treatment for this disease [2]. Total gastrectomy, even if it did not interfere with the tumor's growth, produced the longest patient survival; it carried, however, a high mortality and morbidity, particularly in high-risk patients [3].

As soon as it became known that H_2-receptor antagonists could effectively inhibit gastric acid secretion, treatment of the Zollinger-Ellison syndrome with these agents was attempted. Impressive symptom improvement and ulcer healing were reported in many cases. However, some failures of H_2-receptor antagonist treatment were also described. Due to the rarity of the condition, the series reported were usually small, and overall experience has been limited.

The safety of long-term cimetidine at the high doses sometimes required for effective treatment of the Zollinger-Ellison syndrome has still not been established; as a result, exact indications for the introduction of this therapy instead of surgical intervention have not yet been defined.

In this paper we report on cimetidine treatment in 4 patients with Zollinger-Ellison syndrome, continued for 14-38 months with apparent success; the available literature is also reviewed.

Case reports

Case 1

A 48-year-old woman had pulmonary thromboembolic (PTE) episodes following a

*This work was supported by grant CT 770124404 from the Consiglio Nazionale delle Richerche, Rome, Italy.

cesarean section in 1958 and the removal of renal calculi in 1961 and 1963; beginning in 1971 she had diarrhea, epigastric pain, weight loss and vomiting.

In 1976, Zollinger-Ellison syndrome was diagnosed, based on a basal acid output (BAO) of 27 mEq/hour (mean of 3 tests), a peak acid output (PAO) of 58 mEq/hour, and basal gastrin of 200 pg/ml with a post-secretin increase of more than 500%. Enlargement of gastric folds and duodenal ileum was evident, multiple gastric and duodenal erosions were present, calcium was elevated, PTH plasma level was 5.5 μg/ml (the normal value is < 1.5), and galactorrhea was observed. The tumor could not be localized by duodenoscopy or ultrasound, but selective pancreatic arteriography revealed a small area in the pancreas body which was suspect, but not sufficiently so to insist on laparotomy. Parathyroidectomy and laparotomy were refused by the patient, because of the 3 previous PTE episodes.

Cimetidine 1 g/day was started in September 1976, and produced a rapid and marked improvement in symptoms and in the X-ray and endoscopy pictures. Three months later, BAO measured 12 hours after cimetidine was 14 mEq/hour. Because of symptoms recurrence, the cimetidine dose was increased to 1.4 g/day, and then later to 1.6 g/day (Fig. 1), when anticholinergics were also administered with advantage.

Gastrin levels remained stationary for about 13 months after starting treatment, but later increased steadily up to 1,250 pg/ml. BAO measured at the last symptoms recurrence was 28 mEq/hour; however, a 70% reduction in BAO was noted 60 minutes after ingestion of cimetidine 400 mg (Fig. 2). The prolactin level in January 1978 was 90 ng/ml. Secretin tests repeated after 3 and 13 months on cimetidine treatment showed a more prolonged gastrin increase than the initial test (Fig. 3).

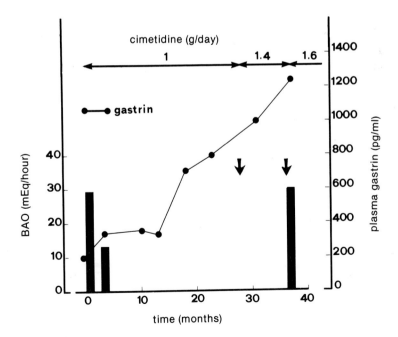

Fig. 1. *Basal acid output and plasma gastrin levels before and during cimetidine treatment in case 1. The arrows indicate symptoms recurrence.*

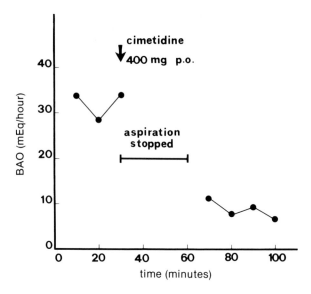

Fig. 2.   Effect of an oral dose of cimetidine 400 mg on BAO in case 1. This test was performed after 37 months of continuous cimetidine treatment; the drug was discontinued 12 hours prior to testing.

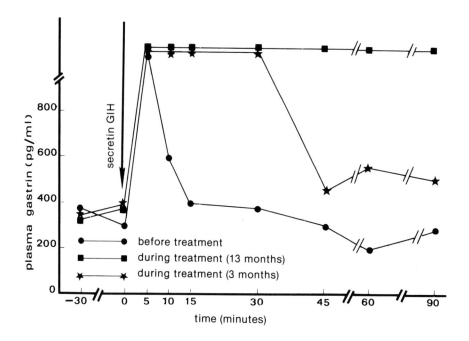

Fig. 3.   Gastrin levels at different times after an intravenous injection of a secretin bolus, before and during cimetidine treatment in case 1. The drug was discontinued 12 hours before each test.

Treatment has been given, as of this writing, for over 38 months and is still effective. The patient reports some symptoms recurrence when she is under emotional stress.

Case 2

A 51-year-old woman started to have epigastric pain, repeated bleeding episodes and vomiting in 1957. Duodenal and jejunal ulcers were present. Since 1966, bone cysts have been observed. Partial gastrectomy and truncal vagotomy were performed in 1972, followed a short time later by resection of the pancreas tail, where a nodule was found. A thyroid follicular adenoma and two adenomatous parathyroids were removed in 1976.

By 1977, when we first saw this patient, galactorrhea and multiple anastomotic and jejunal ulcers were present, PTH plasma level was 3.5 μg/ml (normal value is <1.2), and basal gastrin was over 10,000 pg/ml.

Cimetidine 1 g/day was started in 1977, and produced a marked improvement in symptoms and ulcer healing. Repeated temporary discontinuation of the treatment, due to patient noncompliance, caused immediate recurrence of symptoms, including bleeding. Two years later, the prolactin level is 48 ng/ml and the drug is still effective.

Case 3

A 58-year-old man started to have epigastric pain in November 1977. Eighteen months later he underwent gastric resection and truncal vagotomy. Pain recurred after 1 month, and a large jejunal ulcer was found. Basal gastrin was 300 pg/ml with a post-secretin increase of 400%. BAO was 3.5 mEq/hour, and it was not reduced by secretin injection. The tumor could not be localized by computed tomography (CT) or ultrasound. Arteriography was not accepted, and laparotomy not performed.

Cimetidine 1 g/day was started in September 1978, and produced marked relief of ulcer symptoms and ulcer healing. As of this writing, treatment has been given for 14 months and is still effective.

Case 4

A 63-year-old woman started to have epigastric pain and repeated hematemesis in 1967; a duodenal ulcer was found, and truncal vagotomy and repeated gastric resections were performed (7 operations). In 1977, multiple anastomotic and jejunal ulcers were present; basal gastrin was 400 pg/ml with a 500% post-secretin increase. The tumor could not be localized by arteriography, CT or ultrasound, and laparotomy was not performed.

As of this writing, cimetidine 1 g/day has been administered for over 34 months, and all symptoms have completely disappeared. Basal gastrin after 3 months' treatment was 1,500 pg/ml; secretin stimulation repeated 3 months after treatment began showed a more prolonged gastrin increase than before treatment, as in case 1.

Review of the literature

Since 1975, many reports have appeared describing the effect of treatment with metiamide and, when it became available, cimetidine, on patients with the Zollinger-Ellison syndrome. The treatment induced marked improvement and ulcer healing in many cases; in some of them, total gastrectomy was later performed, but in others where surgery was either not possible for various reasons or was refused, long-term drug treatment (up to 2-3 years at the time of this writing) was instituted, and has shown a continuous beneficial effect [4-14].

On the other hand, some authors have reported failures in up to 50% of their patients, either in emergency situations or on long-term therapy [15-18]. Bonfils et al., for example, have suggested that cimetidine is useful only in selected cases: they propose dividing Zollinger-Ellison syndrome patients into acute and chronic subgroups, and administering cimetidine to acute patients only as a preparation for surgery [16]. Of 7 chronic cases treated for 2-18 months in their study, they have reported 2 failures.

The 2 largest studies of Zollinger-Ellison syndrome treated with cimetidine that have been published to date are McCarthy's series in the United States [11] and the Stadil and Stage series in Sweden [14].

Of the 61 cases reported by McCarthy, 48 were still taking cimetidine at the time of analysis, and 31 had been treated for more than 12 months. Treatment dosage usually ranged from 1.2 to 1.6 g/day, but in some cases 2.4 g/day was given; anticholinergics were occasionally added. Problems included noncompliance (3 cases), bowel obstruction (3 cases), and bleeding (1 case, not due to acid); only 1 treatment failure was reported, and that was due to underdose. Five cases of gynecomastia and 3 of transient liver dysfunction were observed; according to McCarthy, drug tachyphylaxis did not occur. There were 4 tumor deaths.

Stadil and Stage described 15 cases seen prior to May 1978; additional cases are presently being studied. Treatment lasted from 1 week to 27 months, with doses from 1.0 to 1.6 g/day administered. No drug failure was reported. Ten patients were still taking cimetidine as of May 1978. Five patients were operated, and metastases were found in 1, in whom cimetidine was continued with the addition of streptozocin. Four patients, on the basis of the results of selective venous catheterization and gastrin assay, were submitted to Whipple's operation; 3 of these patients were apparently cured and their cimetidine treatment was discontinued, while in the fourth, serum gastrin remained elevated and cimetidine administration was continued. Gynecomastia was reported in only 1 case. Two patients died from tumor progression.

Discussion

Some failures of H_2-receptor antagonists have been reported in the treatment of severely ill patients with Zollinger-Ellison syndrome. In many of these cases, it seems probable that underdose was the cause of the inadequate acid secretion control. Cimetidine doses of 0.8-1.6 g/day were used, but, according to McCarthy, as much as 3.6 g/day may sometimes be necessary [12]. In rare cases, an entero-enteric bypass may explain oral drug inefficacy [14]. Acid output and required dosage may increase after re-establishment of the hydroelectrolytic balance [12].

Since total gastrectomy in Zollinger-Ellison patients may result in very high (over 20%) mortality [3], cimetidine treatment at the required dose ascertained by repeated secretory studies should be attempted. It should be noted, however, that patients may on very rare occasions be resistant to high cimetidine doses [18], and that arterial bleeding from an ulcer may occur despite low acidity [11].

In some cases of long-term treatment of the Zollinger-Ellison syndrome with H_2-receptor antagonists, BAO measured 12 hours after the last drug administration appeared to have decreased, as compared with pretreatment values (see case 1). Richardson and Walsh suggested that this was due to a reduction of the parietal cell mass secondary to prolonged histamine antagonism, or to a spontaneous variation of acid secretion [6]. Bonfils et al. suggested that this 'prolonged secretory inhibition' is an indication of the stability of the therapeutic success [15, 16]. Stage et al. noted that BAO increased over 82 hours after discontinuing treatment, and suggested that prolonged secretory inhibition may be due to persistent traces of the drug [13].

In many cases symptoms and ulcers may recur after a period of favorable response lasting up to several months (see case 1). This effect is probably due, not to a decreased effectiveness of the drug, as proposed by Richardson and Walsh [6], but to an increase of the acid output [10, 11]. Bonfils called this 'secondary inefficacy' or 'escape phenomenon' [15, 16]. The effect is probably due to an increase of tumor size and gastrin levels, as in case 1; in other cases, plasma gastrin is unvaried and an increased sensitivity of the parietal cell mass has been postulated [10].

Stress factors and development of hyperparathyroidism may increase resistance to treatment [12]; parathyroidectomy is known to reduce acid secretion in patients with Zollinger-Ellison syndrome and hyperparathyroidism, and must be considered as a preliminary step to treatment. In nearly all cases, however, acid secretion can be recontrolled by a cimetidine dose increase; very high doses may be necessary, however, and the safety of such doses is still unknown.

Secretin plasma levels have been used to monitor the cimetidine dose required to reduce gastric acidity in Zollinger-Ellison patients [19]. Anticholinergics, if not contra-indicated for other reasons, may be useful in some (but not all) cases in decreasing the required cimetidine dose [11]; more than 50% of all patients can be well controlled with cimetidine 1.2 g/day for many months, and probably for some years, with very few side-effects [11].

Gynecomastia and galactorrhea have been reported in Zollinger-Ellison syndrome cases as the most common side-effects of cimetidine treatment. It is of interest to note that in 2 of the cases reported above (cases 1 and 2), galactorrhea pre-existed the treatment, as part of a multiple endocrine neoplasia syndrome.

Elective total gastrectomy carries a mortality risk of 5-11%, greatly reduces the patients' quality of life, and seems presently unacceptable in view of the low morbidity of cimetidine treatment in the majority of patients. However, when cimetidine requirements are greater than 2.4 g/day [14], or in cases of noncompliance, partial gastrectomy should probably be considered. Some authors have observed that total gastrectomy can cause a halt in tumor growth and even a regression, in accordance with the theory that the stomach can produce a tumor-stimulating factor [3]. However, this observation was not confirmed by subsequent studies [12]. Data on the survival of patients treated with cimetidine compared with those undergoing total gastrectomy are not yet available.

About 26% of pancreatic gastrinomas are single, but less than half of these are located in the tail of the pancreas and are easily resected [2]. About 13% of Zollinger-Ellison syndrome cases are due to a duodenal wall tumor, only half of which are single and resectable [20]. Despite the fact that gastrinomas are only rarely single and resectable, all possible attempts should be made to identify such cases. Hypotonic duodenography, duodenoscopy, ultrasound, selective pancreatic arteriography and CT are often unsuccessful in localizing tumors, and even when they are successful do not exclude the existence of metastasis or other tumors. Transhepatic selective catheterization of the portal vein tributaries and gastrin assay have been successful in localizing gastrinomas in more than 80% of patients [21, 22]. Exploratory laparotomy with the special techniques used to search for small multiple tumors (duodenotomy, exploration of the lesser sac, exposure of the pancreas, spleen hilum, omentum) probably does not have a greater yield in patients whose tumors have not been localized pre-operatively, but it may reveal metastasis and is advocated by some authors [15], but not by others [14, 23]. Antral G-cell hyperplasia and retained antrum should always be differentiated by antral biopsy and other appropriate tests (meal and secretin challenge) since they can be cured by simple resection [24-26].

If a tumor in the duodenal wall or in the pancreas tail is detected, it should be removed, as the mortality risk in this procedure is low and the chance of curing the patient has been reported to be 20% (duodenal wall) and 40% (pancreas tail) [23]. A decision regarding major pancreatic resection is more difficult, as the higher surgical mortality and the possibility of failure must be balanced against the low risk of long-term cimetidine treatment. The validity of the cure should only be judged after a period of 1 or more years' observation; in this respect secretin challenge is probably more reliable than the simple basal gastrin values. If pre-operative techniques are unable to detect the tumor, laparotomy is not performed and long-term cimetidine treatment is instituted, attempts to localize the tumor should be repeated every year [23].

Cimetidine treatment has opened up new possibilities for cancer-directed surgery in patients with Zollinger-Ellison syndrome, since in cases of failure total gastrectomy, which is incompatible with major pancreatic resection, is generally no longer necessary. However, for the patients with multiple or metastatic tumors, cimetidine treatment remains the treatment of choice. Cytotoxic chemotherapy, usually streptozocin with or without fluorouracil, is effective in about 30% of cases, but due to its considerable toxicity it should probably be reserved for use in association with cimetidine in patients with symptoms produced by the tumor mass itself.

References

1. Zollinger, R.M. and Ellison, E.H. (1955): Primary peptic ulcerations of the jejunum associated with islet cell tumors of the pancreas. *Ann. Surg. 142,* 709.
2. Wilson, S.D. (1973): Ulcerogenic tumors of the pancreas: the Zollinger-Ellison syndrome. In: *The pancreas,* p. 295. Editor: L.C. Carey. The C.V. Mosby Company, St. Louis.
3. Fox, P.S., Hofmann, J.W., Decosse, J.J. and Wilson, S.D. (1974): The influence of total gastrectomy on survival in malignant Zollinger-Ellison tumors. *Ann. Surg. 180,* 558.
4. Halloran, L.G., Swank, M. and Haynes, B.W. (1975): Metiamide in Zollinger-Ellison syndrome. *Lancet 1,* 281.
5. Thompson, M.H., Venables, C.W., Miller, I.T., Reed, J.D., Sanders, D.J., Grund, E.R. and Blair, E.L. (1975): Metiamide in Zollinger-Ellison syndrome. *Lancet 1,* 35.
6. Richardson, C.T. and Walsh, J.H. (1976): The value of a histamine H_2-receptor antagonist in the management of patients with the Zollinger-Ellison syndrome. *N. Engl. J. Med. 294,* 133.
7. Shumaker, J.B. (1976): H_2-receptor antagonists for Z-E syndrome. *N. Engl. J. Med. 294,* 1010.

8. Fleischer, D. and Samloff, I.M. (1977): Cimetidine therapy in a patient with metiamide-induced agranulocytosis. *N. Engl. J. Med. 296,* 342.
9. Orchard, J.L. and Peternel, W.W. (1977): Cimetidine therapy in Zollinger-Ellison syndrome. *J. Am. Med. Assoc. 237,* 2221.
10. Lamers, C.B.H., Festen, H.P.M. and Van Tongeren, J.H.M. (1978): Long-term treatment with histamine H$_2$-receptor antagonists in Zollinger-Ellison syndrome. *Am. J. Gastroenterol. 70,* 286.
11. McCarthy, D.M. (1978): Report on the United States experience with cimetidine in Zollinger-Ellison syndrome and other hypersecretory states. *Gastroenterology 74,* 453.
12. McCarthy, D.M., Peikin, S.R., Lopatin, R.N., Crossley, R.J. and Harpel, H.S. (1978): H$_2$-receptor antagonists in gastric hypersecretory states. In: *Cimetidine: proceedings of an International Symposium on histamine H$_2$-receptor antagonists,* p. 153. Editor: W. Creutzfeld. Excerpta Medica, Amsterdam-Oxford-Princeton.
13. Stage, J.G., Stadil, F. and Fischerman, K. (1978): New aspects in the treatment of the Zollinger-Ellison syndrome. In: *Histamine H$_2$-receptor antagonists,* p. 137. Editor: W. Creutzfeld. Excerpta Medica, Amsterdam-Oxford-Princeton.
14. Stadil, F. and Stage, J.G. (1978): Cimetidine and the Zollinger-Ellison (Z-E) syndrome. In: *Cimetidine: the Westminster Hospital Symposium,* p. 91. Editors: C. Wastell and P. Lance. Churchill Livingstone, Edinburgh.
15. Bonfils, S., Mignon, M., Jian, R. and Kloeti, G. (1977): Biological studies during long-term cimetidine treatment. In: *Cimetidine: Proceedings of an International Symposium on histamine H$_2$-receptor antagonists,* p. 311. Editors: W.L. Burland and M.A. Simkins. Excerpta Medica, Amsterdam-Oxford-Princeton.
16. Bonfils, S., Mignon, M., Rigaud, D. and Gratton, J. (1979): Prolonged treatment of Zollinger-Ellison by cimetidine. *Nouv. Presse Med. 8,* 1403.
17. Carratú, R., Miglioli, M., Delle Fave, G.F., Salera, M., Corinaldesi, R. and Kohn, A. (1978): Trattamento con cimetidina della sindrome di Zollinger-Ellison. In: *Cimetidina: farmacologia e clinica,* p. 81. Editor: P.E. Lucchelli. Smith Kline & French S.p.A., Taormina.
18. Groarke, J., Haggstrom, G.D., Halpern, N.B. and Hirschowitz, B.I. (1979): Zollinger-Ellison syndrome unresponsive to cimetidine. *Am. J. Gastroenterol. 72,* 168.
19. Strauss, E., Greenstein, R. and Yalow, R.S. (1978): Plasma-secretin in management of cimetidine therapy for Zollinger-Ellison syndrome. *Lancet 2,* 73.
20. Hofmann, J.W., Fox, P.S. and Wilson, S.D. (1973): Duodenal wall tumors and the Zollinger-Ellison syndrome. *Arch. Surg. 107,* 334.
21. Passariello, R., Rossi, P., Simonetti, G., Tonelli, F. and Ciolina, A. (1977): Il cateterismo portale trans-epatico nella localizzazione di tumori funzionali del pancreas. *Atti Soc. Ital. Chir. 1,* 207.
22. Burcharth, F., Stage, J.G., Stadil, F., Jensen, L. and Fischermann, K. (1979): Localization of gastrinomas by transhepatic portal catheterization and gastrin assay. *Gastroenterology 77,* 444.
23. Fang, M., Ginsberg, A.L., Glassman, L., McCarthy, D., Cohen, P., Geelhoed, G.W. and Dobbins, W.O. (1979): Zollinger-Ellison syndrome with diarrhea as the predominant clinical feature. *Gastroenterology 76,* 347.
24. Ganguli, P.C., Polak, J.M., Pearse, A.G.E., Elder, J.B. and Hegarty, M. (1974): Antral-gastrin-cell hyperplasia in peptic-ulcer disease. *Lancet 1,* 583.
25. Korman, M.G., Scott, D.F., Hansky, J. and Wilson, H. (1972): Hypergastrinaemia due to an excluded gastric antrum; a proposed method for differentiation from Zollinger-Ellison syndrome. *Aust. N.Z. J. Med. 3,* 266.
26. Gray, G.R., Gillespie, G. and Gordon, I. (1976): Extragastric gastrinoma or G-cell hyperplasia of the antrum? The preoperative diagnosis in a case of hypergastrinaemia. *Br. J. Surg. 63,* 596.

Discussion

Baron: Earlier, we discussed the common duodenal ulcer and whether cimetidine is as effective as vagotomy in acid reduction and in ulcer healing, and whether patients who fail on one treatment would fail on the other. These problems were not resolved because, of course, sufficient information is not available about variabilities in drug level, in absorption and in response of acid to cimetidine, and about all the factors necessary to heal an ulcer.

Dr. Bianchi has discussed the perhaps one in 1,000 duodenal ulcers where the cause is known as a gastrinoma. This is the situation where Zollinger made the fundamental discovery of the syndrome and stated that, if the stomach is completely removed in such a patient, the syndrome is also removed. Dr. Bianchi has put strong arguments, based on his own experience and on his review of the Danish, French and American literature, that cimetidine acts as a safe and effective medical form of total gastrectomy.

It would be interesting to hear from anyone who disagrees with this viewpoint. Is there any surgeon here who still feels that he wishes to do a total gastrectomy on patients?

Bianchi: May I apologise for not completely reviewing all the literature? There are many cases reported in the literature which I have not reviewed.

Speranza (Rome): I do not agree entirely about the similarity between cimetidine and total gastrectomy, even though my personal experience is limited. I can report 3 cases of the Zollinger-Ellison syndrome, in 2 of whom, despite a dose of 2.4 g, I had to perform an emergency operation because the ulcer had perforated.

If I may go on, I asked to speak in order to ask Professor Bianchi whether, in Zollinger or supposed Zollinger cases, he attaches importance not only to the calcium test and to the secretin test but more especially to another test which we use extensively, the bombesin test. In 100 post-operative peptic ulcers (i.e., following resection), 80% had no hypergastrinaemia and 20% did. Of those 20 cases, only 5 had the Zollinger-Ellison syndrome, with gastrinomata; in the other 15 cases there were excluded or retained antra which had, especially the former, an ulcerogenic potential which did not differ greatly from that of a gastrinoma.

This is why I was asking whether it should not be stressed that it is not sufficient to study the gastrin response after secretin and that, in all cases, we should add the calcium test and the bombesin test.

Bianchi: I agree that the calcium and bombesin tests are both useful; I mentioned only the secretin test because it is the one most widely used and it is the only one which provides a mechanism different from that of the meal test. The meal test and the secretin test differentiate pancreatic tumours from antral hyperplasia or retained antrum in 95% of cases; the remaining 5% are more complicated cases, which require more complex investigation. However, I would like to say that over the last few years there has been a change in opinion about these tests, and they are now seen as less important. McCarthy and the Nordic group, for example, no longer use them routinely. This is not our position; the tests seem to me to be very useful.

As regards that more interesting question on the discrepant results: that is the problem which interests us! There are patients so severely ill with bleeding that they must have immediate surgery. Even in the American series there was a patient who had a bleeding ulcer which had to be operated on as an emergency. However, it seems that cimetidine can resolve the situation in 90% of instances.

Naturally, the surgeon probably sees a selection of acute cases, whereas I see mild, non-acute cases.

Baron: We have heard about duodenal ulcer, and the world data on acute and maintenance treatment are quite clear. We have heard about the great variation in gastric ulcer data with cimetidine, and about the clear-cut results of cimetidine in the Zollinger-Ellison syndrome. We will now turn to a much less clear topic: the problem of the use of cimetidine in emergencies in peptic ulcer disease. Professor Barbara will clarify this problem.

Emergencies in peptic ulcer disease

L. Barbara, M. Miglioli, D. Santini, M. Salera and G. Biasco
Department of Gastroenterology, University of Bologna, Bologna, Italy

Introduction

The use of H_2-receptor antagonists has been proposed and validated for the treatment of severe diarrhea induced by massive acid hypersecretion, as in gastrinoma, systemic mastocytosis and the short bowel syndrome [1-3], and to reduce the risk of severe acid-base and electrolytic imbalances due to the loss of gastric secretions, as in gastric outlet obstruction and prolonged nasogastric drainage [2, 4]. More recently, cimetidine has been proposed for the prophylaxis of pulmonary acid aspiration in patients submitted to emergency anesthesia [5].

The primary use of the H_2-receptor antagonists, however, has been in the treatment and prevention of upper gastrointestinal (GI) bleeding; in this paper we will discuss these 2 areas, and review and analyze the results of recent published studies.

The treatment of upper GI bleeding

The mortality rate from acute GI bleeding has progressively lessened over the last 50 years, as a result of the establishment of special medical and surgical units specifically trained in the care of bleeding patients, the considerable progress in diagnostic methods, and a more rational and individualized therapeutic approach to the patient. However, there is still no specific treatment which can be considered as usually effective, and this could explain why, recently, the mortality rate from GI bleeding has stabilized.

Various treatments aimed at controlling or preventing continuing or recurrent bleeding have been investigated, such as gastric hypothermia [6, 7], vasoconstrictor agents [8] and antiprotease agents [1], but the results have not been impressive. Uncontrolled studies, however, have suggested that the powerful action of H_2-receptor antagonists in inhibiting gastric secretion could be of value in patients with upper GI bleeding [9-11].

Most deaths in patients with gastrointestinal hemorrhage are tied to the hazards of continuous bleeding or rebleeding, which coexist with major diseases that render the patient a high risk for emergency intervention [12, 13]. The pathogenesis of the rebleeding episodes is controversial but, in general, it can be either the same cause which was responsible for the primary hemorrhagic lesion or any other causes which are acting on the coagulation process, rendering it insufficient.

The first major defense against uncontrolled bleeding, aside from the transient vasoconstriction which follows vascular injury, is platelet aggregation and the formation of a platelet plug. The platelet plug can secure adequate hemostasis for several hours, except in lesions of the major vessels; thereafter the plug disintegrates, unless it has been reinforced by a fibrin clot.

In vitro, hydrochloric acid has a marked inhibitory effect on platelet aggregation and increases the disaggregation of stable platelet aggregates [14]. Pepsin has an additive effect with regard to this last phenomenon in a pH range of 5.0-5.5, where its proteolytic activity is relatively low. Moreover, both hydrochloric acid and pepsin adversely affect fibrin clot generation and thrombin formation [15].

Thus, it is possible that rebleeding is partly induced by the access of both these factors to the evolving vascular hemostatic nidus and to the incapacity of endogenous buffers to maintain pH above the levels necessary for hemostatic integrity. It is these observations which constitute the principal basis for the use of antacids and H_2-receptor antagonists in the treatment of upper GI bleeding.

Results of controlled studies

During 1978 and 1979, 6 studies in which the efficacy of cimetidine was compared with that of placebo in a random clinical trial have been published, some with only preliminary results [8, 16-20]. The principal characteristics of these studies are summarized in Tables I and II.

Table I shows the criteria for admission and exclusion of patients, patient stratification, the treatment schedules used and the distribution of causes of hemorrhage in the 6 study groups.

Some differences were present in the various criteria for admission, such as the age of the patient and the last evidence of bleeding, whereas all studies excluded patients with bleeding due to upper GI malignancies or varices, patients with hepatic or renal failure, and patients with hemorrhage secondary to another major disease.

In all of the studies, the most frequent source of hemorrhage was the presence of either duodenal or gastric ulcer, distributed evenly between the cimetidine and placebo groups except in the study by Dykes et al. [16]. The other causes of hemorrhage appeared much less frequently.

Patients were stratified into age groups of up to 60 or 65 years of age and over in 4 of the 6 studies; Colin et al. separated patients into age groups of above and below 50 years [19], and MacDougall and Williams did not stratify patients with regard to age [20].

Stratification according to the severity of the hemorrhage was considered in all studies except those of Colin et al. and MacDougall and Williams, and the criteria used to define severe bleeding were similar in these 4 cases. Severe bleeding approached 40% in the studies conducted by Hoare et al. [8], Dykes et al. [16], and Pickard et al. [17], while it was less than 20% in the patients studied by LaBrooy et al. [18]. Severely-hemorrhaged and older patients were equally distributed between the cimetidine and placebo groups.

In 3 of the studies, cimetidine was initially administered intravenously at a dosage of 200 mg 4-hourly, followed by varying oral doses [8, 16, 19]; in 1 study [17], an intravenous dose of 250 mg was given every 6 hours, after an initial 200 mg injection; in the MacDougall and Williams study, cimetidine 200 mg 6-hourly was administered either intravenously or orally; and in the LaBrooy study cimetidine was only administered orally: 400 mg initially, then 200 mg 6-hourly.

These differences rule out combining the results of the 6 trials [21]. Some differences were present in the definition of treatment response as well, and these are listed in Table II, together with the results obtained.

Table I. Controlled clinical trials on the efficacy of cimetidine in the treatment of upper gastrointestinal bleeding.

Ref.	Patients admitted	Stratifications	Treatment schedule	Source of hemorrhage						
				GU	DU	Ero-sions	Stomal and other ulcers	Esophag-itis	Mallory-Weiss	Other or not seen
[8]	Over 45 years admitted with acute upper GI bleeding, excluding those with trivial bleeds, GI malignancies, serious liver or renal disease, bleeding secondary to another major disease.	Age: up to 65 and over. Severity: severe bleeding in presence of 2 or more of these factors: pulse rate >100/minute; syst. b.p. <100 mm Hg; fresh melena; hematemesis of >1 liter of fresh blood; shock.	Cim. 200 mg IV 4-hourly for 48 hours, then 400 mg orally 6-hourly for 7 days.	14	20	0	0	0	0	0
			Placebo	19	13	0	0	0	0	0
[16]	Significant upper GI bleeding, excluding patients with blood dyscrasias, bleeding abnormalities, GI malignancies, renal failure, liver disease, bleeding secondary to a separate major clinical problem, bleeding from varices.	Age: 45-64 years and over 65. Severity: severe bleeding in presence of 2 or more of these factors: pulse rate >100/minute; syst. b.p. <100 mm Hg; shock; fresh melena; hematemesis of >2 pints.	Cim. 200 mg IV 4-hourly for 48 hours, then 1 g/day orally for 7 days.	18	9	3	5	4	0	2
			Placebo	11	16	6	3	3	1	1
[17]	Upper GI hemorrhage; last evidence of bleeding less than 72 hours before admission.	Age: up to 60 and over. Severity: severe bleeding in presence of syst. b.p. <100 mm Hg; pulse rate >110/minute; hemoglobin < 8 g/dl.	Cim. 200 mg IV immediately, then 250 mg 6-hourly for 48 hours, then orally 100 mg thrice and 800 mg at bedtime for 5 days.	13	4	1	0	7	6	1
			Placebo	15	8	3	0	5	2	3

Ref	Criteria	Treatment							
[18]	Hematemesis or melena or both in preceding 24 hours, excluding pregnant women and patients < 16 years or with GI malignancies, renal or hepatic failure, bleeding from varices. Age: above or below 60. Severity: severe bleeding in presence of hypovolemic shock; pulse rate > 100/minute; syst. b.p. < 100 mm Hg.	Cim. 400 mg orally immediately, then 200 mg 6-hourly for 7 days.	13	22	6	5	3	2	6
		Placebo	12	19	3	10	2	1	4
[19]	Hematemesis in preceding 24 hours or presence of blood in stomach at endoscopy and 1 or more GU or DU at endoscopy, excluding patients with stress, renal failure, GI malignancies, bleeding from varices, Mallory-Weiss syndrome, previous treatment with anticoagulants, and age < 18 years. Age: above or below 50.	Cim. 200 mg IV 4-hourly for 72 hours, then 1 g/day orally for 4 days.	11	24	0	12	0	0	0
		Placebo	11	24	0	10	0	0	0
[20]	Bleeding from gastric erosions at endoscopy in patients with decompensated cirrhosis, with portal hypertension and varices, acute alcoholic hepatitis or fulminant hepatic failure.	Cim. 200 mg IV 6-hourly for 24 hours, then 200 mg 6-hourly IV or orally for 1-12 days.	0	0	14	0	0	0	0
		Placebo	0	0	10	0	0	0	0

GU = gastric ulcer; DU = duodenal ulcer; syst. b.p. = systemic blood pressure; Cim. = cimetidine.

Table II.   Results of controlled clinical trials on the efficacy of cimetidine in treatment of upper GI bleeding.

Ref.	Definition of treatment failure	Treatment group	All cases	DU	GU	Severe hemorrhage (All cases / DU)	Severe hemorrhage (GU / Age >60)	Age >65/>60/>50 (DU)	Age >65/>60/>50 (GU)
[8]	Continued or further bleeding as shown by: hematemesis or fresh melena; aspiration of blood through a Ryles tube; changes in pulse rate or blood pressure; falling hemoglobin.	Cimetidine	8/34	6/20	2/14 }*	5/11	1/4	3/10 }**	1/10
		Placebo	15/32	5/13	10/19	2/4	6/9	5/8	6/9
[16]	Continued or further bleeding on the basis of good clinical evidence.	Cimetidine	8/41	6/18	1/9		6/21 (All cases)	2/12 }*	7/9 }*
		Placebo	14/41	3/11	11/16		8/15		
[17]	Continued or further bleeding as shown by: failure of CVP to reach 4.1 cm H_2O after 7 units of blood; fall in CVP to less than −4 cm H_2O over 2 hours or less; fresh hematemesis; sudden rise of pulse rate of >20 beats/minute or fall of syst. b.p. of >20 mm Hg; active bleeding detected by endoscopy.	Cimetidine	12/33	7/13	1/3		10/15 (All cases)		
		Placebo	10/36	6/15	2/6		5/13		
[18]	Rebleeding.	Cimetidine	15/51	8/22	2/13	3/9 (All cases)	1/6 (Age >60)	5/28 (Single/multiple GU, Age >50)	
		Placebo	12/50	7/19	4/12	5/10	4/8	9/28	
[19]		Cimetidine	5/46	2/12	0/24 }**	3/33 }** (All cases)		4/33 }** (Age >50)	
		Placebo	12/47	1/11	5/24 }**	10/35 }**		12/30 }**	
[20]	Continued bleeding assessed by clearance of the nasogastric aspirate maintained on continuous free drainage (no applied suction).	Cimetidine	2/14 (Acute erosions)						
		Placebo	3/10						

... = systemic blood pressure. * = p < 0.01, ** = p < 0.05

There was no significant difference in the incidence of continuous or recurrent bleeding between cimetidine- and placebo-treated patients in any of the studies, although a trend in favor of cimetidine was observed in 3 of them [8, 16, 19].

When the results were analyzed according to the cause of hemorrhage, hemorrhage severity, and the age of the patients, some differences were apparent between the cimetidine- and placebo-treated patients, suggesting that, although cimetidine may not have an overall advantage over placebo, it may be effective in patients with severe hemorrhage and in patients with bleeding gastric ulcers. In fact, a significant reduction of continued bleeding or rebleeding in patients with gastric ulcers was observed by both Hoare et al. and Colin et al. In both of these studies, and in the Dykes study as well, the percentage of treatment failures was significantly lower in patients treated with cimetidine.

The lack of success in the LaBrooy and Pickard studies can be tied to the lower doses of cimetidine which were administered: according to Barbezat and Bank, such treatment regimens will suppress basal acid secretion for about 100 minutes, thus not guaranteeing continuous suppression of hydrochloric acid secretion [22].

These studies do not furnish conclusive data on the efficacy of cimetidine in gastrointestinal hemorrhage secondary to lesions other than peptic ulcer. In particular, it is not possible to confirm the favorable results obtained in uncontrolled studies on hemorrhage due to acute gastroduodenal erosions [9, 11]. Again, the results obtained with cimetidine were superior to those with placebo, but the small number of cases treated limit the possibility of drawing a valid conclusion.

To date, the efficacy of cimetidine in hemorrhage due to acute gastroduodenal erosions has been analyzed only in patients with decompensated cirrhosis, acute alcoholic hepatitis and fulminating hepatic failure [20]. Preliminary results relative to the first 24 patients treated have been published, and the percentage of hemorrhagic arrest in patients treated with cimetidine (84%) and with placebo (70%) are not statistically different. It is therefore interesting to note that, in patients treated with cimetidine but not in those treated with placebo, the recurrence of bleeding was not due to reappearance of acute lesions. This reinforces the results obtained in an earlier study by the same author on the efficacy of the H_2-receptor antagonists in preventing hemorrhage arising from acute lesions of the gastro-duodenal mucosa [23].

The prevention of acute gastroduodenal bleeding

Acute gastroduodenal lesions have been cited as one of the more common causes of severe upper GI bleeding [6, 24]. They occur with significant frequency in several severe diseases and produce a high mortality rate [25-28].

The pathophysiology of acute erosions remains complex and is probably multifactorial. However, the presence of hydrochloric acid does appear to play a basic role in their development [27, 29], even though conflicting results have been obtained as to the amount of acid secretion in patients with stress erosions [30].

On the other hand, several pathophysiological disturbances have been noted both in experimental models and in patients, such as the presence of specific damaging agents in gastric content [29], the release of mast cell histamine [31, 32], and disturbances in gastric mucosal blood flow [13] and energy metabolism [24]. One or more of these factors have been considered important in determining damage and disruption of the gastric mucosal barrier. Thus, the principal rational basis for the

Table III.   Controlled clinical trials on the efficacy of cimetidine in the prevention of acute bleeding erosions.

Ref.	Patients admitted	Treatment schedule	Definition of treatment response	Results		
				Group	Development of GI bleeding	Survival
[23]	Fulminant hepatic failure with grade IV hepatic coma.	Metiamide or cimetidine 150 mg/dose, repeated to maintain intragastric pH above 5; or placebo.	Bleeding: fresh blood in nasogastric aspirate; endoscopy in all patients who bled.	Cimetidine Placebo	1/25 (4%) 11/21 (53%) } *	6/25 (24%) 3/21 (15%)
[32]	Controlled respiration (≥ 8 hours duration); polytrauma (≥ 3 body regions).	Cimetidine 200 mg IV 4-hourly; or placebo.	Bleeding: endoscopy in all cases of bleeding.	Cimetidine Placebo	0/10 (0%) 2/9 (23%)	7/10 (70%) 4/9 (45%)
[33]	Severe brain injury (grade III coma) excluding those with previous ulcer disease, concomitant gastric surgery, pregnancy, age < 12 years.	Cimetidine 300 mg IV 4-hourly; or placebo.	Bleeding: significant coffee ground material or bright red blood in nasogastric aspirate.	Cimetidine Placebo	3/17 (17.7%) 15/16 (94%) } *	
[34]	Respiratory insufficiency; neurosurgery; burns; head injury; postoperative complications; cerebrovascular lesions; polytrauma.	Cimetidine 200 mg IV or orally 6-hourly for 10 days; AMH 5 ml hourly; or placebo.	Bleeding: endoscopy in all patients who bled.	Cimetidine AMH Placebo	0/26 (0%) 0/25 (0%) 7/36 (19.5%) } ** } **	
					Development of acute lesions	
[35]	Coma with controlled respiration (≥ 4 days); acute respiratory insufficiency (PaO$_2$ ≤ 80 mm Hg); chronic respiratory insufficiency (PaO$_2$ ≤ 50 mm Hg on controlled respiration); acute renal	Cimetidine 20 mg/kg/24 hours IV for 3-14 days; or placebo.	Development of acute erosions (endoscopy after 7 days). Bleeding: hematemesis or melena.	Cimetidine Placebo	18/21 (86%) 14/19 (74%)	

failure; major thoracic surgery; polytrauma; septicemia; shock; excluding those with acute lesions before treatment and age < 16 years.

			Development of bleeding	Healing of erosions
[35] As above, but including patients with acute lesions before treatment.	Cimetidine 20 mg/kg/24 hours IV for 3-14 days; or placebo.	Bleeding: hematemesis or melena. Healing of acute lesions (endoscopy after 7 days).		
	Cimetidine		1/27 (0.4%) *	13/27 (48%) *
	Placebo		6/33 (18.2%)	6/33 (18.2%)
			Development of acute lesions	
[36] Head injury with grade IV coma, excluding those with history of ulcer disease, or presence of DU or GU at endoscopy before treatment.	Cimetidine 200 mg IV 4-hourly for 7 days; or placebo.	Development of acute lesions (endoscopy after 3 and 7 days).		
	Cimetidine		1/10 (10%)	
	Placebo		4/10 (40%)	

AMH = aluminum magnesium hydroxide; DU = duodenal ulcer; GU = gastric ulcer. * = $p < 0.001$; ** = $p < 0.01$.

use of cimetidine in preventing stress erosions remains its powerful inhibitory effect on gastric acid secretion. It remains to be clarified, however, whether this drug has some beneficial action on the gastric mucosal barrier or on the gastric mucosal blood flow.

Results of clinical trials

The efficacy of cimetidine in preventing stress erosions has been analyzed in 6 controlled clinical trials [23, 32-36], 2 of which have only published preliminary results [32, 34]. The principal characteristics and results of these 6 studies are summarized in Table III.

The major differences in study designs were the criteria used for identifying high-risk patients and the methods for evaluation of patient response.

Fulminating hepatic failure was the only risk factor considered in the MacDougall et al. study [23], while 2 other studies chose severe brain injury [33, 36]. A separate analysis for each of the different risk conditions was planned for the study by Fischer et al. [32], but to date results have been obtained only in patients with controlled respiration (n = 10) and in patients suffering from severe polytrauma (n = 9). In the remaining 2 studies [34, 35], diverse risk conditions were considered together and the prophylactic efficacy of cimetidine was evaluated accumulatively. Due to these different admission criteria, a large number of patients was obtained, which is important in a prophylactic trial especially if the incidence of the analyzed event is low; this advantage, however, is countered by the difficulty of defining exactly the relative importance of each predisposing condition.

With regard to treatment response, gastric erosions were considered to be evidence of treatment failure in 2 of the studies [35, 36], and in the other 4 studies treatment was regarded as having failed in patients who developed a hemorrhage; however, the parameters used to define the hemorrhage were not clearly stated or varied from study to study.

A fixed intravenous dosage of cimetidine was administered 4- to 6-hourly or continuously in all except the MacDougall study, in which a single dose of cimetidine or metiamide 150 mg was repeated to maintain gastric pH above 5.

As with the controlled trials discussed earlier, differences in study design rule out the possibility of combining the results of these clinical trials; considered individually, the results obtained indicate that cimetidine markedly reduced the appearance of digestive hemorrhage in the different conditions considered.

Some patients treated with cimetidine developed bleeding lesions, but this percentage was extremely low if compared with the development of bleeding lesions in the control groups.

The efficacy of cimetidine in preventing the development of erosions was less impressive; in the study conducted by Bouletreau et al. [35], the incidence of erosions in patients treated with cimetidine was similar to that in patients on placebo.

It is more difficult to evaluate the efficacy of cimetidine in the single-risk-factor groups. A clear benefit seems to have been established only in patients with fulminating hepatic failure and in patients with severe brain injury.

With regard to the other risk conditions, no definite conclusions can be drawn, due to the small number of patients treated and to the fact that different conditions of risk were considered together.

Table IV. Incidence of acute gastroduodenal bleeding erosions in various predisposing conditions. Data compiled from [14, 23, 26, 28, 37, 39-42].

Condition	Erosions (%)	Bleeding (%)	Severe bleeding (%)
Burns	90	—	1.5 -25
Head injury	—	—	2.7
Polytrauma	90	—	1.5 - 5
Unselected surgical intervention	—	—	0.06
Major surgery	—	24	1 - 5
Postoperative acute renal failure	—	—	15
Renal transplantation	—	4-22	15
Critically-ill patients	—	24	5
Fulminant hepatic failure	—	—	54
Chronic respiratory insufficiency	—	—	9
Acute respiratory insufficiency (acute respiratory distress syndrome)	—	—	22 -84

An aspect which has not been clearly defined is the clinical utility of prophylactic cimetidine treatment. Gastric erosions can develop extremely rapidly in several conditions and particularly in shock patients, but severe hemorrhage from this is rare [28]. Most gastric erosions heal spontaneously with minimal or no bleeding [37, 38], except in patients with fulminating hepatic failure, in which the development of erosions is almost invariably associated with severe hemorrhage, probably as a result of the underlying coagulation abnormalities [20].

In the group of patients with fulminating hepatic failure studied by MacDougall et al., there was a striking difference in the survival figures between those who bled and those who did not, and direct comparisons of survival rates in patients treated with H_2-receptor antagonists and untreated patients show a trend in favor of the former; a similar trend of survival in favor of cimetidine-treated patients can be seen in the results of the Fischer et al. study.

The same observation cannot be applied to the other risk conditions analyzed, as neither the severity of the hemorrhagic episodes nor their influence on the outcome of the patients has been determined. Indirect data suggest that only a few of the hemorrhagic episodes which occurred were severe.

Finally, some uncertainty still remains in defining those situations in which it can be useful to begin prophylactic treatment with cimetidine. Some guidelines can be derived from taking into consideration the observed incidence of bleeding lesions in the various risk conditions (Table IV).

Conclusions and perspectives

Some controversial aspects need to be pursued further. In the treatment of upper GI bleeding, the efficacy of cimetidine in patients with gastric ulcer, in the elderly and in patients with hemorrhage caused by acute gastroduodenal erosions needs to be confirmed. It remains particularly necessary to determine whether the successful results obtained by some studies [8, 16, 19] were due to the use of higher doses of cimetidine and, consequently, to the greater and more constant reduction of gastric acid secretion. The usefulness of cimetidine combined with antacids has also to be verified.

In the prophylaxis of acute erosions, where positive results have been obtained, the most important task remaining is the definition of conditions of risk in which it is useful to start cimetidine treatment. The usefulness of combining cimetidine with antacids for prophylaxis must also be considered.

The prophylactic use of H_2-receptor antagonists in other conditions, such as esophageal varices and renal transplantation, is still being evaluated.

There is still controversy as to the cause of variceal rupture and bleeding [43], with little data indicating whether explosion or erosion is most frequently responsible. Normal lower esophageal sphincter pressure has been reported in patients with cirrhosis before and after variceal hemorrhage [44] and inflammation and erosions of the esophageal mucosa have been rarely observed in patients with bleeding varices [45]. Nevertheless, the hypothesis of acid regurgitation as a causing factor in variceal rupture has not been satisfactorily eliminated and trials on the efficacy of cimetidine have begun [20].

Hemorrhage from esophageal, gastric or duodenal erosions is common in the first week after renal transplantation, and later on in patients who suffer from sepsis, rejection or surgical complications. Peptic ulcer develops later, is frequently complicated by bleeding and perforation, and can account for 7.5% of all deaths in these patients [41]. The efficacy of cimetidine in preventing bleeding erosions and peptic ulcer in transplant recipients was studied by Jones et al. [41]; no episodes of upper GI hemorrhage were observed in 30 recipients who received prophylactic cimetidine for 6 weeks after transplantation, while bleeding was observed in 6 out of a well-matched group of 33 untreated patients. No adverse effects have been observed, and the evaluation of the long-term efficacy of cimetidine in these patients is still continuing.

The powerful antisecretory effect of cimetidine has to be considered in other conditions of severe peptic disease — for example as a part of medical treatment of gastric outlet obstruction and perforated peptic ulcer (in patients with major complications or in those with the formae fruste perforation). Long-term cimetidine can be of benefit in patients treated with simple suture for acute perforation (the risk of a second surgical intervention in these patients is about 50%) [46]. Finally, the prophylactic efficacy of cimetidine in preventing ulcer relapse encourages an evaluation of its efficacy in preventing a second episode of severe bleeding in those patients who have not been operated after their first bleeding episode; it has been shown that 40% of conservatively-treated patients show recurrent severe bleeding, with a related mortality of 10%, after their first episode of severe bleeding [47]. On the other hand, the value of prophylactic surgery in aged patients after a single major bleeding episode, and in all cases after the second hemorrhage, has still not been proved.

References

1. Amdrup, E. and Olesen, S. (1972): Inhibition of gastric and duodenal proteases in the

treatment of haemorrhage from peptic ulcer. *Scand. J. Gastroenterol. 7,* 273-277.

2. McCarthy, D.M. (1978): Report on the United States experience with cimetidine in Zollinger-Ellison syndrome and other hypersecretory states. *Gastroenterology 74,* 453-458.

3. Stadil, F. and Stage, J.G. (1978): Cimetidine and the Zollinger-Ellison (Z.E.) syndrome. In: *Cimetidine: the Westminster Hospital Symposium,* pp. 91-104. Editors: C. Wastell and P. Lance. Churchill Livingstone, Edinburgh.

4. Barton, C.H., Vaziri, N.D., Ness, R.L. et al. (1979): Cimetidine in the management of metabolic alkalosis induced by nasogastric drainage. *Arch. Surg. 194 (1),* 70-74.

5. Dobb, G. (1978): Pulmonary acid aspiration syndrome: prophylaxis with cimetidine. In: *Cimetidine: the Westminster Hospital Symposium,* pp. 235-245. Editors: C. Wastell and P. Lance. Churchill Livingstone, Edinburgh.

6. Palmer, E.D. (1969): The vigorous diagnostic approach to upper gastrointestinal tract hemorrhage. *J. Am. Med. Assoc. 207,* 1477-1480.

7. Simonian, S.J. and Curtis, L.E. (1976): Treatment of hemorrhagic gastritis by antacid. *Ann. Surg. 184,* 429-433.

8. Hoare, A.M., Bradby, G.V. and Hawkins, C.F. (1979): Cimetidine in bleeding peptic ulcer. *Lancet 2,* 671-673.

9. Burland, W.L. and Parr, S.N. (1977): Experiences with cimetidine in seriously-ill patients. In: *Proceedings of the second International Symposium on histamine H_2-receptor antagonists,* p. 345-357. Editors: W.L. Burland and M.A. Simkins. Excerpta Medica, Amsterdam-Oxford-Princeton.

10. Dykes, P.W., Kang, J.Y., Hoare, A., Hawkins, C.F. and Mills, J.G. (1977): Treatment of upper gastrointestinal hemorrhage with cimetidine. In: *Proceedings of the second International Symposium on histamine H_2-receptor antagonists,* pp. 337-345. Editors: W.L. Burland and M.A. Simkins. Excerpta Medica, Amsterdam-Oxford-Princeton.

11. MacDonald, A.S., Steele, B.J. and Bottomley, M.G. (1976): Treatment of stress-induced upper gastrointestinal haemorrhage with metiamide. *Lancet 2,* 68-70.

12. Allan, R. and Dykes, P. (1976): A study of factors influencing mortality rates from gastrointestinal haemorrhage. *Q. J. Med. 180,* 533-550.

13. Cheung, L.Y. and Chang, N. (1977): The role of gastric mucosal blood flow and H^+ back diffusion in the pathogenesis of acute gastric erosions. *J. Surg. Res. 22,* 357-361.

14. Fogelman, M.J. and Garvey, J.M. (1966): Acute gastrointestinal ulceration incident to surgery and disease: analysis and review of 88 cases. *Am. J. Surg. 112,* 651-656.

15. Green, F.W., Kalan, M.M., Curtis, L.E. and Levine, P.M. (1978): Effect of acid and pepsin on blood coagulation and platelet aggregation. *Gastroenterology 74,* 38-43.

16. Dykes, P.W., Hoare, A.M., Hawkins, C.F. and Kang, J.Y. (1978): The treatment of upper gastrointestinal hemorrhage with cimetidine. In: *Cimetidine: the Westminster Hospital Symposium,* pp. 173-179. Editors: C. Wastell and P. Lance. Churchill Livingstone, Edinburgh.

17. Pickard, R.G., Sanderson, C., South, M., Kirkham, J.S. and Northfield, T.C. (1979): Controlled trial of cimetidine in acute upper gastrointestinal bleeding. *Br. Med. J. 1,* 661-662.

18. LaBrooy, S.J., Misiewicz, J.J., Edwards, J. et al. (1979): Controlled trial of cimetidine in upper gastrointestinal haemorrhage. *Gut 20,* 892-895.

19. Colin, R., Galmiche, J.P., Hecketsweiler, P., Ouvry, D. and Geffroy, Y. (1979): Traitement par la cimétidine des hémorragies ulcéreuses gastroduodénales. *Proceedings of an International Congress on Tagamet, Lour Marin, 14-16 September 1979.* (In press.)

20. MacDougall, B.R.D. and Williams, R. (1978): The role of cimetidine in the management of bleeding in liver disease. In: *Cimetidine: the Westminster Hospital Symposium,* pp. 180-190. Editors: C. Wastell and P. Lance. Churchill Livingstone, Edinburgh.

21. Elashoff, J.D. (1979): Combining results of clinical trials. *Gastroenterology 75,* 1170-1172.

22. Barbezat, G.D. and Bank, S. (1977): Basal acid output response to cimetidine in man. In:

Proceedings of the second International Symposium on histamine H_2-receptor anta-gonists, pp. 110-121. Editors: W.L. Burland and M.A. Simkins. Excerpta Medica, Amster-dam-Oxford-Princeton.

23. MacDougall, B.R.D., Bailey, R.J. and Williams, R. (1977): H_2-receptor antagonists and antacids in the prevention of acute gastrointestinal haemorrhage in fulminant hepatic fail-ure. Two controlled trials. *Lancet 1,* 617-619.

24. Classen, M., Hagenmüller, L., Hoffman, L., Willards, D. and Raschke, E. (1975): Severe upper gastrointestinal bleeding. Diagnosis: endoscopy. In: *Gastrointestinal emergencies,* pp. 121-127. Editors: F. Barany and A. Torsoli. Pergamon Press, Oxford.

25. Silen, W. and Skillman, J.J. (1972): Stress ulcer, acute erosive gastritis and the gastric mucosal barrier. *Adv. Int. Med. 19,* 195-212.

26. Skillman, J.J., Bushnell, L.S., Goldman, H. et al. (1969): Respiratory failure, hypoten-sion, sepsis and jaundice. A clinical syndrome associated with lethal hemorrhage from acute stress ulceration of the stomach. *Am. J. Surg. 117,* 523-530.

27. Moody, F.G., Cheung, L.Y., Simons, M.A. et al. (1976): Stress and acute gastric mucosal lesion. *Am. J. Dig. Dis. 21,* 148-154.

28. Lucas, C.E., Sugawa, C., Riddle, J. et al. (1971): Natural history and surgical dilemma of stress gastric bleeding. *Arch. Surg. 102,* 266-273.

29. Ritchie, W.P. (1975): Acute gastric mucosal damage induced by bile salts, acid and ische-mia. *Gastroenterology 68,* 699-707.

30. Robbins, R., Idjadi, F., Stahl, W.M. et al. (1972): Studies of gastric secretion in stressed patients. *Ann. Surg. 175,* 555-562.

31. Davenport, H.W. (1970): Back diffusion of acid through the gastric mucosa and its phy-siological consequences. In: *Progress in gastroenterology,* Volume 2, p. 42. Editor: G.B.J. Glass. Grune and Stratton, New York.

32. Fischer, M., Lorenz, W., Reiman, T.H. et al. (1978): Cimetidine prophylaxis of acute gas-troduodenal lesion in patients at risk. In: *Proceedings of an International Symposium on histamine H_2-receptor antagonists,* pp. 280-291. Editor: W. Creutzfeldt. Excerpta Medi-ca, Amsterdam-Oxford-Princeton.

33. Halloran, L.G. and Silen, W. (1978): Cimetidine prevention of gastrointestinal bleeding in severe head injury. A controlled trial. *Surg. Forum 79,* 428-430.

34. Basso, N., Bagarani, M., Materia, A. et al. (1979): Cimetidine and antacid prophylaxis of acute gastroduodenal mucosal lesions in high-risk patients. *Gastroenterology 76,* 1095.

35. Bouletreau, P., Auboyer, J., Latarjet, V. et al. (1979): Ulcérations digestives hautes de stress. Traitement par la cimétidine. In: *Proceedings of an International Congress on Tagamet, Lour Marin, 14-16 September 1979.* (In press.)

36. Curzio, A., Silvestri, N. and Sala, G. (1979): Cimetidina e ulcera da stress. *Ital. J. Gastroenterol. 11,* Supplement 1, 53.

37. Czaja, A.J., McAlhany, J.C. and Pruitt, B.A. (1974): Acute gastroduodenal disease after thermal injury. *N. Engl. J. Med. 291,* 925-929.

38. Katz, D., Douvres, P., Weisberg, H. et al. (1964): Early endoscopic diagnosis of acute upper gastrointestinal hemorrhage. Demonstration of the relatively high incidence of ero-sions as a source of bleeding. *J. Am. Med. Assoc. 188,* 405-411.

39. Bouletreau, P., Petit, P. and Motin, J. (1975): Ulcère de stress et insuffisance rénale aiguë postopératoire. *Ann. Anesthésiol. Fr. XVII,* 5.

40. Hastings, P.R., Skillman, J.J., Bushnell, L.S. and Silen, W. (1978): Antacid titration in the prevention of acute gastrointestinal bleeding. *N. Engl. J. Med. 298,* 1041-1045.

41. Jones, F.H., Rudge, C.J., Bewick, M. et al. (1978): Cimetidine prophylaxis against upper gastrointestinal haemorrhage after renal transplantation. *Br. Med. J. 1,* 398-400.

42. Kamada, T., Fusamoto, H., Kawano, S. et al. (1977): Gastrointestinal bleeding following head injury: a clinical study of 433 cases. *J. Trauma 17,* 44-47.

43. Conn, H.D. (1975): Gastroesophageal varices: causes, diagnosis, treatment and progno-sis. In: *Gastrointestinal emergencies,* pp. 255-260. Editors: F. Barany and A. Torsoli. Pergamon Press, Oxford.

44. Eckardt, V.G., Grace, N.D. and Kantrowitz, P.A. (1976): Does lower esophageal sphincter incompetency contribute to esophageal variceal bleeding? *Gastroenterology 71,* 185-189.
45. Orloff, M.J. and Thomas, H.S. (1963): Pathogenesis of esophageal varix rupture. *Arch. Surg. 87,* 301-307.
46. Baekgaard, N., Lawaetz, O. and Poulsen, P.E. (1979): Simple closure or definitive surgery for perforated duodenal ulcer. *Scand. J. Gastroenterol. 14,* 17-20.
47. Johannson, K. and Barany, F. (1973): A retrospective study of the outcome of massive bleeding from peptic ulceration. *Scand. J. Gastroenterol. 8,* 113-118.

Discussion

Baron: I would like to suggest that we concentrate our discussions on the main message of Dr. Barbara's talk: the extraordinary fact that, although cimetidine will increase the rate of duodenal ulcer healing in most countries of the world, it will not help patients who are bleeding from duodenal ulcers. On the other hand, although the literature on the effectiveness of cimetidine in healing uncomplicated gastric ulcers is controversial, most studies have suggested that cimetidine is useful in elderly patients bleeding from gastric ulcer. Has anyone any suitable comments to make on that aspect, to try to resolve this particular problem?

Basso (Rome): If you are talking about haemorrhage from a duodenal ulcer, it should be stressed that gastric acid should be controlled. Also, in our experience, anatomical features of the ulcer are important. A superficial duodenal ulcer, which may still cause serious bleeding but which does not have a large component of fibrous connective tissue, may respond well to medical treatment, including cimetidine tablets. However, it is not clear to what extent cimetidine is more effective than other antacid drugs. On the other hand, there are duodenal ulders which do have a large connective tissue component, and which often have a small endoscopically-visible clot in the base occluding the bleeding vessel, which may be the gastroduodenal artery or one of its principal branches. In such cases, neither cimetidine nor other non-surgical methods of control will be effective.

Forestieri (Naples): Before the advent of cimetidine, so far as the indication for surgery was concerned, it was agreed that operation should take place much earlier in the elderly than in young subjects. I would like to ask Professor Barbara whether treatment with cimetidine has the same indications in younger patients with massive haemorrhage as in the elderly? Or, when treating the elderly with cimetidine, should we proceed to operation earlier in cases of failure on cimetidine?

I would like to know also whether Professor Barbara has any data on the use of somatostatin in combination therapy.

Barbara: In the elderly, controlled clinical trials have shown significant differences between cimetidine and placebo. Individual trials may be open to criticism, but if we do accept their validity then we should use their results. This is all the more important in these patients, who have a higher risk because of their age and the presence of other diseases; it is obvious that the mortality of a gastric operation is likely to be higher in the elderly than in younger patients. So I have accepted this result with alacrity, and I propose to use cimetidine in these patients.

Baron: The last 2 papers of this session consider the problem of cimetidine in a broader sense: having pharmacologically demonstrated a beneficial effect of cimetidine both in increasing the rate of ulcer healing and in preventing relapse, what can be done globally about its use in the general population?

Socioeconomic aspects of treatment with cimetidine in peptic ulcer disease

G. Bodemar, Ricci Gotthard, M. Ström, A. Walan, B. Jönsson* and P. Bjurulf°
*Departments of Internal Medicine and °Preventive and Social Medicine, Linköping University Hospital, Linköping; and *The Swedish Institute for Health Economics, Lund, Sweden*

The socioeconomic costs of peptic ulcer disease

In the western world, 10-15% of adult men and 4-15% of adult women are afflicted at least once during their lives with an active peptic ulcer. Because of the chronicity of this disease, which affects people often during their most productive years, its cost to society can be high.

As with any disease, the total cost of ulcer disease is composed of direct and indirect costs: the direct costs include the expense of hospitalization (including surgery), of physician care (including diagnostic procedures) and of drugs. Indirect costs include those caused by loss of productivity due to absence from work during periods of illness, and loss of *potential* productivity in cases of mortality resulting from the disease.

Studies have been reported on the costs of peptic ulceration in the United States of America in 1977 [1], The Netherlands in 1975 [2], Italy in 1976 [3] and Sweden in 1975 [4], and data on the total costs and the relative percentages of direct and indirect costs are presented in Table I. In all 4 countries, the cost for peptic ulcer disease amounted to about 1% of the total cost for all diseases.

During the years studied, the direct costs were highest in the USA (46%) and lowest in The Netherlands (21%). The cost for hospital care, which was the largest of the direct costs in all 4 countries, was also highest in the USA (33%), compared with 18% in The Netherlands and 15% in Sweden. In 1975, the hospitalization costs for peptic ulcer disease were 1.2% of the total hospital costs in the USA, compared to 0.5% in Sweden. In the same year, 1.5% of all hospital beds in the USA were occupied by peptic ulcer patients, as against 0.5% in Sweden. This figure represents a decline in hospitalization for peptic ulcer disease in Sweden: in 1964 it had been 1.3%. This decline was caused by a tendency not to hospitalize peptic ulcer patients undergoing medical treatment; the number of patients in the surgical wards did not change appreciably (46% of all peptic ulcer patients staying in hospital in Sweden in 1975 underwent surgery, compared with 48% in 1978). In the USA, a similar tendency can be observed: the number of surgically-treated patients went up from 53% in 1975 to 58% in 1977, accounting for 75% of the total hospital costs for peptic ulcer disease that year. In The Netherlands, about 45% of all hospitalized peptic ulcer patients underwent surgery in 1975.

The relative costs of physician care were higher in the USA and Italy than in The Netherlands and Sweden. However, both in the USA and in Sweden, about 0.5% of

Table I.   The cost of peptic ulcer disease before the introduction of cimetidine therapy.

	USA [1] (1977)		The Netherlands [2] (1975)		Italy [3] (1976)		Sweden [4] (1975)	
Total cost	3,224 million dollars		337 million guilders		284 billion lire		480 million croner	
Direct costs (%)	46		21		42		22	
Hospital care		33		18		24		15
Physician care		9		2		7		4
Drugs		4		1		11		3
Indirect costs (%)	54		79		58		78	
Absenteeism		41		79		58		68
Mortality*		13		0		0		10
Total (%)	100	100	100	100	100	100	100	100

*Calculated with discounts of 2.5% for the USA and 6% for Sweden; the USA estimate assumes a 2% increase in productivity and 6% inflation.

all visits to physicians in 1975 were for peptic ulceration. If patients with so-called dyspeptic symptoms are included, the figure for Sweden would rise to 2%; the liberal use of cimetidine in these patients would probably be beneficial to only a minority, while drastically increasing the total cost for drugs.

Of these 4 nations, the one spending the greatest proportion of its total on drugs during the years studied was Italy, with 11%. In the USA, by far the major portion of the 1977 drug cost was accounted for about equally by antacids and anticholinergics, with a much smaller portion spent on tranquilizers and other agents; in Sweden, antacids formed a greater part of the budget than anticholinergics (this was before the introduction of cimetidine).

In the USA, The Netherlands and Sweden, peptic ulcer symptoms cause about 1.5% of all days off work due to illness. They cost the USA 1,330 million dollars in 1975 (8.6 million working days); in 1977, about 80,000 ulcer patients in the USA were *chronically* disabled. In Sweden, about 1% of all chronic disability is due to peptic ulcer; in most cases, this disability is caused by postoperative complications. Patients who receive sick pensions in Sweden account for 25% of the total absenteeism. These figures only take actual absenteeism into account, without considering the decreased capacity to work of the patients who remain at work; although this cannot be calculated, it is probably a very important factor. The very high relative cost of absenteeism in The Netherlands (79% of the total cost of peptic ulceration) is due to the inclusion in this figure of the costs both of decreased efficiency of the *colleagues* of absent ulcer patients and of the decreased use of machines and capital, together representing fully one-third of the absenteeism costs in this country. The reason for the relatively lower costs for short-term absenteeism in the USA is that an ulcer patient with active symptoms is off work for a much shorter time: the average time off is 12 days in the USA (27 days in severe cases hospitalized for worsening symptoms, according to gastroenterologists' estimates), compared with 35 days in Italy and 45 in The Netherlands. About 20% of patients with active ulcers in The Netherlands are absent for more than 3 months, and surgical patients for an average of 3 months. In Sweden, patients in the 25-44 age group are off work for an average of 4 weeks, in the 45-54 age group for 6 weeks, and older patients for about 5 weeks. In Sweden, a 50-year-old patient with an active peptic ulcer was absent for a longer period in 1973 than in 1963 [5].

Although the mortality arising from peptic ulcer disease is low (0.9% of all deaths in Sweden and 0.4% in the USA in 1975, and 0.5% in The Netherlands in 1974), the *cost* of mortality was calculated to be 13% of the total cost of peptic ulcer disease in the USA in 1977 and 10% in Sweden in 1975, certainly not negligible amounts. Mortality from peptic ulcer disease rose in the 1960's, almost entirely because of the increased number of old people and the consequent increase in aged patients suffering from complicated ulcer disease. In Sweden, mortality from peptic ulcer reached a peak in 1971, amounting to 1.1% of all deaths recorded in that year. Since then, mortality has decreased, probably because acutely ill patients are operated on earlier. In the USA, peptic ulcer mortality declined from 8,607 in 1970 to 6,480 in 1975. The age at which patients die from the disease is increasing (in Sweden, 75% of the patients who died in 1975 were over 75 years of age), and the number of women dying from peptic ulcer disease is growing (in the USA, from 34% in 1970 to an estimated 40% in 1977).

Estimated changes in socioeconomic costs caused by cimetidine treatment

It has been suggested that treatment of peptic ulcer disease with cimetidine may decrease the costs of this disease to society [2, 6, 7]. Table II suggests potential changes in percentages for the costs described in the previous section, estimated by clinicians as being likely to result from the use of cimetidine in the USA, The Netherlands and Italy. It should be noted that the estimation for Italy has been based on the assumption that *all* peptic ulcer patients will be treated with cimetidine, and that doctors in the USA estimated that 80% of these patients will receive cimetidine. Both of these figures are perhaps too high: it is more likely that about 50% of ulcer patients will actually be treated with cimetidine, as in the Dutch calculation.

Table II. Clinicians' assumptions of cost benefit of cimetidine, expressed as percentages of the total costs.

	USA		The Netherlands	Italy
Cimetidine usage	50%	80%	50%	100%
Direct costs (%)	17	27	20	19
Hospital care	22	35	28	66
Physician care	12	18	0	0
Drugs	−25	−40	−91	−101
Indirect costs (%)	20	32	21	40
Absenteeism	22	35	21	40
Mortality	11	18	0	0
Total savings (%)	18	29	21	31

Estimation based on this 50% usage level has, therefore, also been given for the USA in the Table.

The assumption that the introduction of cimetidine therapy will decrease the costs of peptic ulcer disease despite increasing the cost for drugs is based on a presumed lesser need for hospitalization and, as a result of decreased absenteeism, a smaller loss of productivity. But absenteeism is not affected only by the use of medication: the attitudes of physicians and medical tradition also play a role. We have already pointed out the great difference in average time off work due to peptic ulcer disease in the USA and The Netherlands. We are not aware of any trial that has studied, under double-blind conditions, whether cimetidine shortens the period off work, but the often dramatic improvement in ulcer symptoms in patients undergoing treatment with cimetidine is well established. This in itself is invaluable to the individual patient, aside from any beneficial effect on the cost of the disease to society.

Absenteeism before and during maintenance treatment with cimetidine

Can maintenance treatment with cimetidine reduce absenteeism in peptic ulcer patients?

We previously reported the results of a double-blind long-term maintenance trial in 68 patients with established chronic ulcer disease [8]. Many of these patients were suffering from a severe form of ulcer disease, and many had taken time off from work due to their illness during each of the 3 years preceding the start of our study (Table III). Both the number of patients spending time away from work and the number of days per period of absence increased from year to year, probably reflecting an increase in the severity of the disease. Absenteeism during the 6 months immediately preceding the study period, however, is not included in the figures in Table III; almost all of the patients had some time off work during this half-year, due to dyspeptic symptoms of active ulceration.

To heal their ulcers, most patients received a short course of treatment with cimetidine 1 g/day; only a few of them had any remaining symptoms after 2 weeks of this treatment.

For the next year, 32 of these patients were maintained on cimetidine 400 mg twice daily and 36 received a placebo, also administered twice daily. Further

Table III.   Absenteeism from work in the 3 years preceding the 1-year maintenance study (1973-75) and during the study year itself (1976-77).

	1973		1974		1975		1976-77	
	Patients absent	Days missed per absent patient	Patients absent	Days missed per absent patient	Patients absent	Days missed per absent patient	Patients absent	Days missed per absent patient
Placebo (n = 36)	14	mean: 24.1 median: 11	19	mean: 43.7 median: 24	24	mean: 48.1 median: 41	23	mean: 52.0* median: 44*
Cimetidine (n = 32)	10	mean: 24.4 median: 15.5	14	mean: 36.2 median: 27	15	mean: 39.9 median: 42	1	79 days

*Days off work during double-blind placebo treatment and during open cimetidine treatment for healing of recurrent ulcer. Days off work awaiting surgery are not included (see text and Table V).

Table IV. The 2 treatment groups of the 1-year maintenance trial: clinical details.

	Age (years)	Sex		Prior complications (n)	Duration of disease (years)	Considered for surgery pretrial (n)	Pretrial acid secretion (mM/hour)
		M	F				
Placebo (n = 36)	50.7	30	6	11	13.6	13	BAO: 4.4 PAO: 36.3
Cimetidine (n = 32)	50.1	28	4	17	10.7	11	BAO: 4.5 PAO: 38.1

BAO = basal acid output; PAO = pentagastrin-stimulated acid output.

information on these 2 treatment groups is presented in Table IV; there were no significant differences between groups with regard to age, sex, number of patients with earlier complications, duration of disease, number of patients considered for surgery before the trial, basal acid output (BAO) or pentagastrin-stimulated acid output (PAO). In both groups, 80% of the patients were smokers.

As previously reported [8], the results of 1 year's maintenance were as follows: in the cimetidine group there were 5 patients with 1 recurrence each, 1 with 2 recurrences, none with complications and 1 who was operated; in the placebo group there were 18 patients with 1 recurrence, 12 with 2 recurrences, 4 with complications and 15 who were operated. All recurrences were documented by endoscopy; when recurrence occurred, an open course of cimetidine 1 g/day was given for 6 weeks and, at the end of that time, patients were either re-admitted to the double-blind maintenance trial or underwent surgery. All patients were allowed to take antacid tablets for relief of ulcer symptoms during the trial.

Tables III and V both show figures for days off work during this 1-year period, for both the cimetidine and placebo groups. Included in Table V are days off taken by patients with peptic ulcer symptoms during placebo treatment who had not yet developed an endoscopically-proven recurrence, by patients waiting to undergo surgery because of a lack of hospital space (these patients were treated with nightly doses of cimetidine and were asymptomatic while they were waiting, but they did not return to work until some time after operation; work loss after operation has

Table V. Absenteeism from work during the 1-year maintenance trial.

	Patients absent	Days off without recurrence during double blind treatment	Days off awaiting surgery	Days off with recurrence during open cimetidine treatment	Total days off
Placebo (n = 36)	23	428	208	769	1,405
Cimetidine (n = 32)	1	59	0	20	79

not been calculated), and by patients undergoing cimetidine treatment after endoscopy had proven a recurrence in ulceration. All 23 of the patients in the placebo group who took time off work during the year had endoscopically-proven re-ulceration.

The 769 days off work taken by patients in the placebo group who were receiving cimetidine to heal a recurrent ulcer represent a mean of 24.0 days per recurrent ulcer and a median of 20.5 days. The median value is probably more accurate than the mean, because some patients were absent from work for long periods despite the fact that their recurrent ulcers became asymptomatic. This median value during cimetidine treatment to heal re-ulceration is shorter than the figures for traditional ulcer treatment in Sweden, Italy and The Netherlands presented above.

The important finding is the number of patients maintained on cimetidine who were absent from work during the 1-year trial period: only 1 patient in this group needed to be absent from work during the course of the trial, compared with 15 in the preceding year. Treatment with placebo, however, did not change the number of patients who needed time off: of the 36 patients maintained on placebo, 24 had been absent from work during the year preceding the trial and 23 were absent for varying lengths of time during the maintenance period.

Recurrence of peptic ulceration after cimetidine

Cimetidine promotes the healing and prevents the recurrence of ulcers. But the positive effects of this agent, including its potential economic benefits, would be greatly reduced if ulcer disease was found to be aggravated after either short- or long-term cimetidine treatment is discontinued. Comparisons have been made between patients whose ulcers healed on treatment with either cimetidine or placebo, and the results have been contradictory: one study showed that there is no increased risk of recurrence after cimetidine is stopped [9], another that relapses generally occur quite rapidly when treatment is discontinued [10].

We have previously reported the results of a double-blind trial involving 71 patients with endoscopically-proven duodenal ulcers [11]. The patients were randomly allocated to 1 of 3 possible treatment regimens: 23 patients received cimetidine 200 mg 3 times daily and 400 mg at bedtime, 24 patients received a combination of 0.6 mg of a long-acting anticholinergic (l-hyoscyamine) twice daily and 10 ml of a new antacid suspension gel with a very high buffering capacity (85 mmol/10 ml) 7 times daily, and 23 patients received a placebo. Since this was a double-blind study, each patient received a total of 11 active and/or placebo tablets and 7 doses of either the antacid suspension gel or placebo 10 ml daily. Ulcer healing was controlled endoscopically.

After treatment with cimetidine for 6 weeks, 19 patients had healed ulcers; by 12 weeks this number had increased to 22. Treatment with the antacid-anticholinergic combination caused ulcer healing in 23 patients after 6 weeks; by 12 weeks the remaining patient had also healed. The healing rate on placebo was 35% after 6 weeks; by 12 weeks it was still only 50%.

In order to investigate whether peptic ulcers relapse earlier and more frequently after active treatment, patients with healed ulcers were followed up for 1 year after the discontinuation of therapy. (It may be assumed that ulcers which heal on placebo are not as severe as those which require active treatment for healing, and therefore a comparison between the clinical outcomes of placebo and active therapy would not give any information on whether the therapy itself influences the recurrence rate of peptic ulcers.) Since the number of patients whose ulcers healed on each of the 2 active treatments used in this study did not differ statistically, a difference in relapse rates after discontinuation of treatment would indicate whether either regimen itself influences relapse after discontinuation.

Twenty patients from each group have been followed either until their first symptomatic recurrence of ulceration or until the end of 1 year with no symptoms and no ulcer demonstrated at endoscopy. Twelve of the cimetidine-treated patients had a relapse after a median time of 2.5 months, and 9 of the patients treated with the combination had recurring ulcers after a median time of 4 months. The difference is not statistically significant; therefore, there does not seem to be a clinically significant rebound effect on the clinical outcome once ulcer healing with cimetidine has been completed.

In this trial, as compared to placebo, cimetidine was more effective than the antacid-anticholinergic combination in relieving pain. It is probably possible for patients on cimetidine therapy to increase their smoking and alcohol intake, take salicylic acid-containing preparations and work both day and night without increasing their ulcer symptoms. Once the treatment has been stopped, however, these etiological factors must be dealt with, to prevent aggravation of the ulcers on withdrawal of the stomach-protecting agent.

Recurrence in peptic ulceration during 2 years after cimetidine maintenance treatment

What happens after long-term treatment with cimetidine is stopped?

We followed the patients from our 1-year maintenance study, described earlier in this paper, for 2 years after the conclusion of that trial [12]. Table VI shows their clinical history during this time. When moderate or severe symptoms developed after the trial, they were well controlled by short courses of treatment with cimetidine or, in 3 patients, with almost continuous treatment.

During the 1-year trial we regularly performed control endoscopies on all patients. After the trial period was completed we did endoscopies only on patients with symptoms, so we have no reliable information on the relapse rate after treatment was stopped. However, the results presented in Table VI suggest that the severity of chronic peptic ulcer disease is favorably influenced by 1 year's treatment with cimetidine, and that this influence continues even after treatment is stopped. Many of the patients had had more than 2 episodes of bleeding ulceration before treatment, but during the trial none of the patients in the cimetidine group had a bleeding ulcer, compared with 4 in the placebo group. Fifteen placebo patients were referred to surgery because of 2 recurrences during the trial or because of the severity of symptoms at their first recurrence, whereas only 1 patient from the cimetidine group was so referred.

In the 2 years after the trial, 1 patient from each group developed a bleeding ulcer, both at 1 year after discontinuing treatment; both had had bleeding ulcers before the trial as well, and the patient in the placebo group had a bleeding ulcer during the trial. When re-ulceration occurred during the 2-year post-maintenance period, both patients were referred for surgery; the patient from the cimetidine group, however, refused surgery and was given a further short course of treatment with cimetidine.

Seven patients from the placebo group underwent surgery during the 2 years after

Table VI. Clinical outcome during and 2 years after the trial.

	Placebo group (n = 35*)	Cimetidine group (n = 31**)
During trial		
Referred for surgery	15	1
Bleeding ulcers	4	0
After trial		
Months after end of trial with mild or no symptoms mean and (range)	8.8 (1-22)	10.1 (0.5-24)
Referred for surgery	7	2
Bleeding ulcers	1	1
Not operated	13	27
No symptoms[1]	4	8
Mild symptoms[1]	2	8
Moderate symptoms[2]	7	8
Severe symptoms[3]	0	3

*One patient stopped treatment during the trial because of myocardial infarction; the patient with bleeding ulcer after the trial is included in the 7 patients who were operated on. **One patient stopped treatment during the trial because of cardiac failure; the patient with bleeding ulcer after the trial, who refused surgery, is included in the 8 patients with moderate symptoms. [1]No cimetidine administered after the maintenance trial; [2]short courses of cimetidine administered after the trial; [3]cimetidine administered almost continuously after the trial. (Reprinted with permission from [12]).

the trial, compared with 2 from the cimetidine group. Three other patients from the cimetidine group fulfilled the criteria for surgery but refused operation. Thus, considering the entire 3-year period from the beginning of the maintenance trial through 2 years after it ended, 7 of the 32 patients from the cimetidine group were or should have been operated, compared with 22 of the 36 patients from the placebo group.

In patients receiving placebo, there was a mean rise of 50% in non-stimulated acid secretion (BAO) during the 1-year trial period; this increase was statistically significant ($p < 0.05$). BAO in the cimetidine-treated patients was lower than the pre-trial values both 2 days and 3.5 months after the end of the trial. In an earlier study we found that, in patients with chronic peptic ulcer disease, there was a mean rise of 68% in BAO at the end of several years' treatment with placebo, but not after treatment with an anticholinergic for the same length of time [13]. These findings suggest that BAO rises steadily during the years when patients have active peptic ulcer disease. Our results indicate that cimetidine blocks this rise in BAO, which could partly explain the observation that cimetidine favorably influences the course of peptic ulcer disease even after maintenance treatment is discontinued.

Future aspects

A cost analysis study from Switzerland suggests that the cheapest way of treating chronic peptic ulcer patients is administration of a nightly dose of cimetidine for 15 years, only operating on patients who have a recurrence more than twice during that very long time [14]. The operation they used as a reference was selective proximal vagotomy. They based their conclusion on the fact that, in spite of the known low complication rate after this type of operation, the cost of post-surgical syndromes, including chronic disability, was 3 times higher than the initial cost for surgery. A Danish study has shown that the majority of patients probably do not need 15 years of treatment before ulceration ceases to be active [15].

Cimetidine reduces the need for surgery during treatment. If this reduction can also be achieved after discontinuation of treatment, it would substantially add to the already great economic benefits this agent offers to society. The results of very long-term toxicity studies will be decisive as to whether or not very long-term treatment with cimetidine can be undertaken.

References

1. Stanford Research Institute (1977): *Cost of ulcer disease in the United States.* On file at Smith Kline & French Corporation, Philadelphia.
2. Netherlands Economics Institute (1977): *Present cost of peptic ulceration to the Dutch economy and possible impact of cimetidine on this cost.* On file at Smith Kline & French Corporation, Holland.
3. Institute of Political Economic Studies, University of Pavia (1978): *The determination of the social costs of peptic ulcer in Italy.* On file at Smith Kline & French Corporation, Italy.
4. Hertzman, P. and Jönsson, B. (1977): *Magsårssjukdomens samhällsekonomiska kostnader.* The Swedish Institute for Health Economics, Lund.
5. Tibblin, G. and Eriksson, C.G. (1977): Ulcussjukdomens epidemiologi. In: *Ulcer and ulcer treatment,* p. 29. Editor: A. Walan. Hässle Corporation, Göteborg.
6. Robinson Associates, Inc. (1978): *The impact of cimetidine on the national cost of duodenal ulcers.* On file at Smith Kline & French Corporation, Philadephia.
7. Institute of Political Economic Studies, University of Pavia (1978): *Assessment of the social benefits deriving from the introduction of cimetidine in Italy.* On file at Smith Kline & French Corporation, Italy.
8. Bodemar, G. and Walan, A. (1978): Maintenance treatment of recurrent peptic ulcer by cimetidine. *Lancet 2,* 403.
9. Bardhan, K.D., Blum, A., Gillespie, G. et al. (1977): Long-term treatment with cimetidine in duodenal ulceration. *Lancet 1,* 900.
10. Cargill, J.M., Peden, N., Saunders, J.H.B. and Wormsley, K.G. (1978): Very long-term treatment of peptic ulcer with cimetidine. *Lancet 2,* 1113-1115.
11. Ström, M., Gotthard, R., Bodemar, G. and Walan, A. (1980): Treatment of peptic ulcer disease. A comparative study between cimetidine and combined anticholinergic and antacid therapy. *Scand. J. Gastroenterol.* (In press.)
12. Bodemar, G. and Walan, A. (1980): Two-year follow-up after one year's treatment with cimetidine or placebo. *Lancet 1,* 38.
13. Walan, A. (1970): Studies on peptic ulcer disease with special reference to the effect of l-hyoscyamine. *Acta Med. Scand. Suppl.,* 516.
14. Sonnerberg, A. and Hefti, M. (1979): The cost of postsurgical syndromes (based on the example of duodenal ulcer treatment). *Clin. Gastroenterol. 2,* 235-248.
15. Griebe, J., Buggo, P., Gjørup, P., Lauritzen, T., Bonnevie, O. and Wulff, H.R. (1977): Long-term prognosis of duodenal ulcer: follow-up study and survey of doctors' estimates. *Br. Med. J. 2,* 1572-1574.

Discussion

Baron: Thank you, Dr. Bodemar, for updating us on your previous maintenance trial of cimetidine, and also for telling us about this new and exciting trial of cimetidine with the combination of an anticholinergic and antacids.

From the socioeconomic point of view, the situation now is quite different from 25 years ago when I became a doctor, at which time patients with gastric and duodenal ulcer were all admitted to hospital for 6 weeks' bed rest. This was an enormous expense. The situation in Britain changed rapidly when carbenoxolone increased the rate of healing of both gastric and duodenal ulcer, and the medical gastroenterologist no longer admitted patients to hospital. This was not true in other countries, however.

The situation today is that there are at least 4 treatments which can increase the rate of healing of duodenal ulcer: high-dose antacids, cimetidine, antacids plus anticholinergics (as we have heard from Dr. Bodemar), and various drugs which increase mucosal resistance, such as bismuth and carbenoxolone.

It is quite clear how to heal a duodenal ulcer. The socioeconomic point of view, beautifully demonstrated to us by Dr. Bodemar's figures, is the prevention of recurrence and of operations. This was certainly achieved in the earlier trial by Walan with anticholinergics, and now by the many maintenance trials with cimetidine.

What is not clear to me is Dr. Bodemar's precise recommendations. He has shown the benefit during one year of maintenance treatment; he has then stopped the maintenance treatment and has followed the patients for 2 years. According to my interpretation of his results, there was no carryover of benefit from cimetidine. After 2 years, when long-term maintenance had been stopped in that way, there was one complication and 7 operations in the placebo group, and one operation and 5 'nearly surgery' in the other group. My logic would be not to stop cimetidine after one year, but to continue it.

Bodemar: First, several patients went to operation during placebo treatment, so the placebo group was reduced in number. If we consider the total outcome of all patients, we definitely think that there is benefit remaining after treatment has been stopped. Half of the patients treated with long-term cimetidine are still asymptomatic 2 years after stopping treatment. This is completely different from the situation in the placebo group, in which 22 of the 36 patients have been sent to operation.

We definitely believe that long-term cimetidine treatment is beneficial, but it is very difficult to say *how* long-term that treatment should be. We believe, too, that there is the possibility of a beneficial effect even if the cimetidine is given for only one or 2 years.

Baron: Dr. Bodemar, if you had a recurrent duodenal ulcer now which had been healed with cimetidine, what would you do yourself? Would you continue maintenance cimetidine indefinitely?

Bodemar: It is still impossible to answer that question. I would try to get to know the patient, to persuade him to give up smoking, for instance — which is something I believe in strongly, and which could in itself reduce the need for surgery. As a physician, I would prefer to keep the patient and not send him to operation. This is what I would do with most patients.

Reichard (Stockholm): Does Dr. Bodemar include rest from work as part of the treatment, and would he advise patients not to work when they are without symptoms but have an endoscopically-proven duodenal ulcer?

Bodemar: If a patient had no symptoms, I do not think that I would advise him not to work. If he had symptoms, I would advise rest, for about a week at least.

Baron: This is the difficulty, because some doctors think that working is bad for duodenal ulcer whereas others regard the capacity to work or not to work as unrelated to the disease, but as a reflection of the attitude of the patient and of his doctor, quite different problems scientifically.

Bodemar: It is definitely a question of the attitude of the doctors. In the United States patients are off work for an average time of 12 days, whereas in Holland, for example, they are off work for the very long time of 6 weeks. Nevertheless, patients do have symptoms, and they may be incapable of working when they have these symptoms.

Bader (Paris): I believe that the true choice is between maintenance treatment with cimetidine and proximal gastric vagotomy. Our French experience is that there is a 25% relapse rate at one year with maintenance treatment using cimetidine 400 mg/day, whereas with proximal gastric vagotomy the relapse rate is 10% over 5 years.

Bodemar: We believe that maintenance treatment with cimetidine 400 mg twice daily is necessary in some patients to keep them symptom-free. There are no data on this available, but we have a strong feeling that it is so. We are currently carrying out a trial comparing cimetidine treatment with surgery, and the results so far support that feeling.

Baron: Of course, what is needed is a controlled trial of elective operation versus elective maintenance cimetidine.

Bodemar: This is what is being done now.

Baron: We will wait to know in 5 years' time what the costs and the benefits are.

A functional view of cost/benefit analysis in peptic ulcer disease

L. Muttarini
Institute of Statistics, University of Pavia, Pavia, Italy

Introduction

The analysis of costs and benefits has, during the past decade, found numerous applications in the sphere of public health. Several critical reviews, of which the most recent was that by Joglekar [1], have been devoted to the methods used and the results obtained.

It may be said at once that such critical reviews have never been more timely. Important and tricky aspects, such as individual well-being and the management of public health, are directly involved in this field of study, and are absorbing ever-growing resources in all countries. The decision-makers who, at various levels, are called upon to assess operational projects should therefore be provided with clear information about the various alternatives which are available, and especially about the scope and limits of the results offered to them by statistical and mathematical analysis.

The various instruments of quantitative analysis inevitably lead to some simplification of reality: the important thing is that everyone is well aware of this simplification, and that the decision-maker is able to read the results with an understanding of the range of 'variables' that the analyst has actually dealt with.

In any specific case, the main aspects that cannot be taken into consideration by statistical analysis are the 'quantity' and, obviously, the 'quality' of well-being that persons affected by a given disease may obtain from a new therapy, a new method, or new and more effective means of treatment and assistance. In short, in no case will it be possible to measure the 'before and after' differential obtained as the sum of individual health 'gains' resulting from a given innovation; it is even less possible to evaluate this differential in economic terms. Attempts made in this direction have always been open to criticism [2], but the question is: what place can or could such a calculation have in an analysis of costs and benefits? The exclusion of the health-gain variable does not in fact appear to limit the analysis in itself, but rather the presupposed logic by which the analysis develops. This premise is better explained by saying that health is a primary human blessing, perhaps the greatest blessing of all, and, as such, it is not capable of measurement; the objective of modern political and social organization should be to improve the entire state of community health, so that the number of citizens who are able to develop themselves by making full use of their physical, intellectual, moral and other resources in any activity that may or may not also produce a benefit to the community (according to the criteria commonly adopted by economists) is as great as possible. From the latter statement it follows, among other things, that a given undertaking cannot be evaluated exclusively by 'number of persons affected by the disease' or 'cost of the under-taking'; in many cases the result of such evaluation would justify the rejection of a possible program on the grounds of a too-high cost/patient ratio, while the citizen who has had the misfortune to contract a rare disease has the same right to have it cured as others who have been affected by more common illnesses.

The problem posed here consists, then, of finding a suitable method for statistical and economic analysis within the public health sector. Such an analysis should be systematized in an all-round frame of reference, in a scheme of 'social accounting' (of a macro-economic kind), in which the costs to be met by the community as a whole for the treatment and cure of a certain illness can be compared with the bene-fits that can, as a whole, be recorded by the community following the introduction of an innovation and/or the realization of a program. Within a framework of this kind, costs and benefits refer to specific economic variables which may be quanti-fied according to the usual standards. It is obvious that, together with the *direct* costs that must in each case be met in order to cure the disease, it may also be necessary to calculate the *indirect* costs deriving from loss of production due to absenteeism caused by the illness or because the worker who has fallen ill has had to be replaced.

The fact that attention is focused here on the economic aspects of the problem does not mean that all other aspects of an ethical or moral nature need to be sacrificed to it. On the contrary, the latter all remain unimpaired and are bound up with the analysis. In some analyses, this conceptual separation has not been made and, as a result, conclusions have been reached which are difficult to accept. Stil-well, for example, finds that a general program of prevention would be more expensive than the treatment of specific cases of the disease, and he emphasizes slight economic advantages while ignoring the suffering of those who happen to be affected by the illness [3].

However, even if analysis *is* limited to the economic aspect of a program, it still offers various advantages. First of all, those who have to cope with specific programs involving public health will be able to check, on the basis of factors impli-cit in the analysis on either the costs or the benefits side, the reliability, coherence and stability of the objectives originally assigned to the program. Not unusually, the objectives of extensive and exacting public enterprises will be shown in the light of actual fact to have been difficult to attain or to have been made more remote with the passage of time. It might have been possible, by carefully analyzing the project-ed costs and benefits, to have fixed objectives which would have been more realistic, though perhaps less ambitious. On the other hand, it may turn out that other aims might have been pursued in addition to the primary aims, without specifying a parti-cular destination for resources and still keeping them within the range of the prin-cipal project.

It may also be useful to analyze costs and benefits in assessing resources intended for the achievement of the objectives. In particular, waste or maldistribution may be brought to light, resulting from lack of information on the part of the planners or from deficient organization of resources. In such cases, these problems must be remedied before the innovation can be introduced or the program got under way.

It follows from all this that cost/benefit analysis may be a formidable cognitive instrument, whose need will increasingly be felt as the resources available for public health increase. Such analysis should be considered within the actual context of the operation being planned, and should not be assigned objectives that it will in any case not be possible to achieve. (From this point of view, the analysis might perhaps be better defined as 'cost-efficiency' analysis.)

Another bow might be drawn at a venture in favor of such an analysis as a means of reaching a decision in public health programs, remembering what is happening at the present time in the public lives of all countries (with varying amounts of emphasis, of course, from one to the other). When public administrators, at any level, turn down or pigeon-hole a request for a program in the health field, using as their excuse the lack of sufficient available finances, they are carrying out, to a greater or lesser degree, an economic analysis, even if they restrict themselves to a calculation of the project's cost to the public without calculating the economic benefits that may accrue in the future. If the benefits were also calculated, it might be found that in the long run the community would save more than it had initially spent, and would thus acquire not only the primary benefit of a better state of health, but also a benefit in terms of purely economic resources.

Critical survey of a recent analysis of costs and benefits

In the review by Joglekar previously referred to, a study by the Netherlands Economic Institute on the costs borne by the Dutch community due to peptic ulcer and the possible benefits to be derived from the introduction of cimetidine was discussed.

In this study [4], the incidence of peptic ulcer, hospital admittances, surgical intervention and the loss of production resulting from absenteeism in the Netherlands up to 1975 were reconstructed from the historical point of view. On the basis of these data, the costs to be borne by the community on account of the disease were calculated and also, on the other hand, the reductions in costs (in terms of hospital admittance, surgical operations, reduced loss of production, etc.) that were found as a result of the introduction of cimetidine.

The degree of utilization of the drug was defined, in this study, by way of hypothesis and on the basis of the experimental results. In the first place, it was assumed that this new drug was being administered in 50% of the episodes being recorded (doctors' estimates ranged, in fact, from 50-75%); it was also assumed that 75% of the patients taking cimetidine considerably reduced their periods of absence from work, as compared to the period before cimetidine was introduced.

Joglekar contests these values, particularly the percentage by which the disease is claimed to have been reduced. From a general point of view, however, it seems that this aspect is of little relevance. Indeed, it is sufficient to interpret the estimate utilized in the Dutch study as a 'working hypothesis' in order to understand it in its true context. In dealing with a new drug, which various tests had indicated would have a truly resolutive effect (now confirmed by more extensive administration to larger numbers of patients), it would be enough to 'shift' the results a year or 2 ahead in order to accept them with fewer reservations. This is much the same as saying that, in cases such as this in which only laboratory results are available, from which only a tendency can be guessed at, it would be appropriate to proceed by true simulation, fixing 2 or 3 levels (corresponding respectively to a low hypothesis and a high hypothesis, or to a low, average and high hypothesis) and calculating the results on the basis of the means. This would have the advantage of not behaving in a way open to criticism of the 'exact' value of the estimate, and would give the decision-maker a broader view of the situation.

However, it is important here to discuss the nature of the information that can be supplied to a decision-making center where, for example, the inclusion of a drug among those guaranteed by a certain insurance scheme or the assessment of its sale price is being discussed.

It is apparent from the conclusions of the Dutch study that, during the first year in which cimetidine was administered, the 'savings' made by the community amounted altogether to 60 million guilders (US $24 million, at the 1975 rate of exchange). Does this mean that in any future year the system will save the same sum (provided values remain constant, of course), or a little less, or a little more, depending on the effective penetration of the drug into the market as compared with the original estimate of 50% penetration? Or is this a figure which should be applied to the first year only (or at most to the first and second years), and will the savings thereafter be considerably greater since the drug will have practically overcome the disease?

We have already referred to the requirement that studies of this kind should offer clear-cut guidance to the decision-maker; we need therefore to examine questions such as these. This we shall do by explicitly introducing a variable so far neglected: *time*.

'Time' in the analysis of costs and benefits

Consider a system in which, at time t, 100 persons affected by peptic ulcer are present. To simplify the situation, assume each of them suffers 1 attack each year; thus, 100 patients = 100 attacks. At the same time t, a new drug is introduced and the following hypotheses are adopted: 50% of the patients are treated with the drug, and 75% of those treated are cured.

The following simple cases can then be developed:

A. In the first instance, let us suppose that there is no further input of patients as a whole, that is, that none of them falls ill from ulcer at subsequent stages. The situation would consequently develop, at times $t + i(i = 1, 2, 3...)$, as shown in Table I, in which, for obvious reasons, the values are rounded up or down to the nearest whole number. Adopting a further, though not unrealistic, hypothesis for reasons of simplicity, that patients who are not cured (fourth row) will no longer be treated with the drug, simple calculation reveals that the patients who are available for treatment (first row) will disappear in the seventh year after the initiation of treatment with the new drug ($t + 7$). More important than this, however, is the fact that the number of patients undergoing treatment will vary from year to year, and this will lead to a modification of the factors upon which the analysis of costs is based. For example, in order to calculate the cost of treatment, account should be taken of the fact that at time t we shall have costs relating to 50 patients, while in the

Table I. *Progress of patients as a whole, on the hypothesis: new intake = 0.*

	(t)	($t + 1$)	($t + 2$)	($t + 3$)
Total patients	100	50	25	12
Treated (50%)	50	25	13	6
Cured (75%)	38	19	10	5
Not cured	12	6	3	1
Not treated	50	25	12	6

Table II.   Progress of patients as a whole, on the hypothesis: new intake = 25.

	(t)	$(t + 1)$	$(t + 2)$	$(t + 3)$
Total patients	100	75	62	56
Treated (50%)	50	38	31	28
Cured (75%)	38	28	23	21
Not cured	12	10	8	7
Not treated	50	37	31	28

following year the costs relating to 25 patients will be under consideration, and within a relatively short time a zero figure will have been reached. Obviously, other specific costs will then need to be defined, for those patients who have been treated but not cured.

B. In this case, let us more realistically assume that at each stage there will be an input of new patients, say 25 units. The situation will then develop as in Table II. Starting at time $(t + 7)$ and discounting the inevitable imprecision due to the rounding up or down, the total number of patients who are available for treatment will be 50 units; this level will be maintained at successive stages, as will the number of those treated with the new drug (25 units). At the intermediate times — that is, from (t) to $(t + 7)$ — modifications of the basic structure will follow: for example, at time $(t + 1)$ there will be a reduction from 100 treatable patients in the first year to 75, and from 50 treated and 38 cured to 38 treated and 28 cured. The number of patients treated but not cured will fall from 12 to 10, while those not treated, who will all be included in the group of treatable patients at the next stage, will fall from 50 to 37. (It should be noted, as a further complication, that the patients treated but not cured will accumulate as time passes.) In conclusion, all these modifications to the general structure will involve continuous recalculation of the costs connected with the new therapy.

We might say that the analysis has so far been conducted in a static manner, limited to a comparison between the situation at time $(t - 1)$, which summarizes the situation before the innovation, and at time (t), which expresses the post-innovation structure. We have seen, however, that analyzing the innovation is not limited to the determination of a stable change; in fact, the innovation gives rise to entirely new laws of development, the characteristics of which require investigation. These laws may of course be expressed in mathematical form, but in the present context such formalization is not necessary. We must proceed in a *functional* direction, in an attempt to supply a more detailed approach to cost/benefit analysis and thus lead to the phase of decision-making.

A functional model for studying changes due to an innovation

Essential aspects

A cost-benefit analysis of peptic ulcer was carried out in Italy on the lines of the Dutch analysis previously discussed [5-7]. In considering the results obtained and their reliability at the decision-making level, account was taken of the mistaken ideas implicit in the usual view of the problem and of the need to single out the modifications in structure consequent upon the introduction of cimetidine. The chief aspects of this research into a functional model may be summed up as follows:

1. The first problem was that of defining the probable progress of patients with duodenal ulcer in the post-cimetidine period, *had the introduction of cimetidine not taken place.* In other words, the pre-cimetidine situation had to be shifted forward in time, so as to have a coherent 'before' period for comparison with what would later be the real situation.

2. This shift, however, could not be achieved simply by extrapolating from the available historical trends (in particular, that relating to the number of attacks in each year). The patients themselves were considered as a basic aggregate or 'stock', to which new additions were periodically made and from which various deductions were made due to cure, surgical intervention, or death. The loss of stock through death included both those dying from ulcer and those who died from other causes but were suffering from an ulcer. Loss through surgical intervention is obviously a simplifying hypothesis, arising from the fact that operation did not always result in cure.

3. A further novelty as compared with the Dutch investigation was introduced with regard to the definition of the disease. Based on the methodology of an investigation which was conducted in the USA [8], patients with peptic ulcer were classified into 4 possible stages of severity, which will be specified later.

4. In order to check on the patients' progress in terms of time, a matrix was set up to indicate the intersecting of the 4 stages of severity of the illness. Using this matrix, it was possible to determine transition between the different categories (i.e., to establish whether the patients' condition improved, deteriorated or remained stationary over a given period of time), and reductions in the stock due to cure, operation or death.

Methods of collecting data

The major difficulty in a research plan of this kind is the accumulation of the necessary basic data. In order to analyze the clinical picture of ulcer with sufficient depth, it was necessary to have recourse to doctors and to their direct experience.

Having discussed various alternatives which could have been adopted, it was decided to collect data directly at a meeting convened for this purpose, to be attended by doctors with considerable experience in the treatment of ulcer and representing the various clinical trends existing in Italy.

In working this out, a sketch of the data-collection model had to be prepared, and this necessitated a limited number of meetings with clinicians in Milan. Then a questionnaire was drawn up, designed to collect information on the various aspects previously stressed, in particular on the transition of patients from one category of severity to another and on the flow of patient entry and exit. The questionnaire ultimately used, including modifications suggested by the clinicians, is presented in an Appendix to the present paper. With the organizational help of Smith Kline & French of Milan, the meeting of doctors was held in Milan on May 25-26, 1979. The participants, representatives of various 'schools' of Italian gastroenterology, had been informed only in a very general way of the investigation and its aims.

The meeting began with an explanation of the way in which the functional model worked and the procedures used to obtain the information. Subsequently, a copy of the questionnaire was given to each participant, and participants were asked to give estimated answers to each question. The extreme values thus obtained were then discussed, an effort being made to discover the basic reasons for the differences encountered and to 'weight' them in an attempt to evaluate the phenomenon as a whole. The discussion led more or less brilliantly to a more or less laborious final synthesis; in the end, a compromise was always reached on a 'mean' estimate which could be used in the model.

A few words may now be said to elucidate the significance of the term 'mean', which has just been introduced. On the basis of varying experience in this field, we are convinced that the method we followed is more valid than others adopted else-where, such as submitting the questionnaire individually to different experts and then calculating, once the data have been collected, some measurement of a central tendency. When variability between responses is very high (as happens in most cases), the mean tends inevitably to lose some of its concrete value. In our case, the same experts who supplied the original estimates also assessed the reasons for the differences that emerged. This assessment resulted from a debate, in which everyone had made notes of their own 'points of view' and their own experience, which gave a more realistic meaning to the conclusions than could have been attained by any mechanically-operated synthesis, performed a posteriori on individual estimates.

The clinical picture of ulcer in Italy in the pre-cimetidine era

We shall next discuss the estimates agreed on during the meeting in Milan and subsequently used in the proposed functional model.

Attacks of duodenal ulcer. The historical series relative to the number of attacks (cases) of peptic ulcer had already been estimated, during previous research on ulcer in Italy [5]. For the purposes of the present study, however, the number of patients was considered, rather than the number of attacks. In response to the first question of the questionnaire reproduced in the Appendix, the group of doctors in Milan agreed that 35% of patients had 1 attack per year, 45% had 2 attacks, 15% had 3 attacks, and 5% had 4 or more attacks per year.

Degrees of severity of duodenal ulcer. Reference has already been made to the classification system adopted in an investigation into the impact of cimetidine upon

Table III.   Distribution of patients according to categories of severity of the disease.

Category of ulcer	Estimate of the Italian doctors (%)	Estimate of the American doctors (%)
1	20.0	38.6
2	55.0	28.0
3	15.0	15.4
4	10.0	18.0*
Total	100.0	100.0

*Sum of American categories 4 and 5.

the social costs of ulcer in the USA [8]. Five classes of duodenal ulcer severity were singled out in that investigation; the group of Italian doctors who collaborated with us, however, only found it necessary to make use of 4 categories, consolidating the fourth and fifth classes of the American study into a single category. Other modifications were made to the American definition of each category, resulting in the second question on our questionnaire. The pre-cimetidine distribution of patients by severity of ulceration, as determined by doctors' estimates, is shown in Table III. For the purpose of comparison, the distribution found in the USA study is also presented.

Transition of patients between categories of severity of ulcer. The transition matrix constituted an important aspect of the investigation, in that it introduced the time factor. Table IV shows the estimates which emerged in Milan and were subsequently used in the model. The data refer to the status of patients after an interval of 2 years, based on results obtained with traditional forms of treatment. The choice of a 2-year interval came from a definition of 'cure' which was agreed on in Milan: a patient was considered to have been cured if he had no symptoms for 2 years. This definition of 'cure' is crucial to the model as it is presented here: a different definition of the term would, in fact, produce different results, as was found when a comparison matrix was prepared using an interval of 5 years without symptoms to define cure.

The clinical picture of ulcer in Italy in the cimetidine era

A second meeting was held in Milan on October 1, 1979, witrh the object of gathering estimates relating to the use of cimetidine. A group of doctors who had been involved in the May 25-26 meeting took part.

Table IV. Transition matrix for patients after 2 years of traditional therapy.

Initial category	Category after 2 years				Operated	Cured	Died	Total
	1	2	3	4				
1	0	0.527	0.090	0.045	0.032	0.300	0.006	1.000
2	0	0.499	0.181	0.088	0.080	0.140	0.012	1.000
3	0	0.257	0.203	0.164	0.256	0.100	0.020	1.000
4	0	0.205	0.159	0.076	0.450	0.070	0.040	1.000

Table V. Transition matrix for patients after 2 years of treatment with cimetidine.

Initial category	Category after 2 years				Operated	Cured	Died	Total
	1	2	3	4				
1	0	0.250	0.060	0.020	0.015	0.651	0.004	1.000
2	0	0.300	0.067	0.030	0.055	0.542	0.006	1.000
3	0	0.360	0.170	0.050	0.080	0.330	0.010	1.000
4	0	0.300	0.225	0.070	0.200	0.175	0.030	1.000

From the results obtained at this second meeting, a transition matrix showing th
movement of duodenal ulcer patients between categories of severity and the loss o
stock due to cure, surgical intervention or death, after an interval of 2 years o
cimetidine therapy, was prepared; this matrix is presented in Table V.

First results and future progress of the investigation

The purposes of this study were to discuss the role and the limitations of statistica
and economic analysis within the range of health programs, bearing particularly in
mind the political and social realities in Italy, and to set out some essential aspects of
a functional view of the processes underlying this analysis in an instance such as ulcer, which cannot be divorced from economic and social factors. This Symposium,
therefore, represents the first important opportunity for verifying the philosophical
line of action taken; the observations and criticisms that may derive from it will certainly be of great help for the future development of the analysis, and for its application.

The details of our results will be expounded elsewhere. We here propose to briefly
summarize the changes that would take place within 2 years after the introduction of
cimetidine therapy to Italy.

At this point, however, a few preliminary statements must be made. The first concerns the 'degree of coverage' that could be assigned to the drug: the percentage,
that is, of patients who will be cured by cimetidine. In order to assess this parameter, we can proceed in two directions: on the basis of historical data (so long as,
of course, a minimum of 'history' is available for extrapolation, however tentative),
or on the basis of statements by doctors concerning the percentage of patients they
intend to treat, or are treating, with cimetidine.

With regard to the latter method, the team pursuing this research found itself
facing various trends, in particular with reference to the treatment of patients in category I of severity of the disease (see definition in Question 2 of the appended questionnaire). Some clinicians were in favor of treating all the patients with cimetidine,
others considered that only about half of them should be so treated. This is an
important point which we hope to take up at a future date with a wider and more
representative sample of doctors; ultimately, it could supply results for 2 different
levels of employment of cimetidine in category I. It is thought that useful indications for this purpose could be obtained from an investigation into the effective
penetration of the drug in its various markets, in search of a sufficiently stable and
reliable trend.

Another quite important premise concerns the treatment to be given to patients
already treated with cimetidine but not cured. This number, as explained earlier,
will tend to 'accumulate' with time and will become increasingly more important in
the structure; obviously, it will vary in direct relation to the degree of employment
of cimetidine. From the first clinical results collected, it seems that the majority of
such patients are destined for surgical operation, as the drug to a certain degree acts
as a 'filter', leading to an immediate decision of this kind. If this is so, we should
expect a considerable increase in 'exit' due to surgical operation; however, our initial results have shown that this exit actually decreased in the short term, before
increasing later on.

We shall now proceed to deal with the results, but shall merely introduce them.

In order to facilitate understanding of the effects of cimetidine, differences between pre- and post-cimetidine transition matrices (Tables IV and V, respectively) are shown in Table VI. The numbers of patients who would be found in the various categories of severity 2 years after the introduction of cimetidine therapy and of those who would, by that time, have left the stock, are presented in the bottom section of Table VII; these numbers can be compared with those for patients undergoing traditional therapy, which are shown in the top section of Table VII.

Work proceeded on the hypothesis that 100% of the treatable patients were treated with cimetidine, over a time period of only 2 years. For a longer-term view, it would have been necessary to introduce parameters relative to patients treated with cimetidine but not cured. This is what will be done in the future, when it should also be possible to utilize more reliable estimates of the percentages of patients treated with the drug.

Table VI. Effect of cimetidine treatment.

Initial category	Category after 2 years				Operated	Cured	Died
	1	2	3	4			
1	0	−0.277	−0.030	−0.025	−0.017	+0.351	−0.002
2	0	−0.199	−0.114	−0.058	−0.025	+0.402	−0.006
3	0	+0.103	−0.033	−0.114	−0.156	+0.230	−0.010
4	0	+0.095	+0.006	−0.006	−0.250	+0.105	−0.010

Table VII. Distribution of patients after 2 years on traditional therapy (top) and cimetidine (bottom).

Initial category	Category after 2 years on traditional therapy				Operated	Cured	Died	Total
	1	2	3	4				
1	86,310	91,586	12,513	7,462	4,824	22,614	829	226,138
2	0	103,441	37,521	18,242	16,584	29,021	2,488	207,297
3	0	14,529	11,477	9,272	14,473	5,654	1,131	56,536
4	0	7,726	5,993	2,864	16,961	2,638	1,508	37,690
Total	86,310	217,282	67,504	37,840	52,842	59,927	5,956	527,661

Initial category	Category after 2 years on cimetidine				Operated	Cured	Died	Total
	1	2	3	4				
1	122,338	41,685	7,538	3,016	2,036	49,072	453	226,138
2	0	62,189	13,889	6,219	11,401	112,355	1,244	207,297
3	0	20,353	9,611	2,827	4,523	18,657	565	56,536
4	0	11,307	8,480	2,638	7,538	6,596	1,131	37,690
Total	122,338	135,534	39,518	14,700	25,498	186,680	3,393	527,661

References

1. Joglekar, P. (1979): Cost benefits of health care programs: a review of methodologies. (Paper presented at the Joint National Meeting of TIMS/ORSA, New Orleans, Louisiana, USA, May 2.)
2. Hoos, I.R. (1972): *Systems analysis in public policy: a critique*. University of California Press.
3. Stilwell, J.A. (1976): Benefits and costs of School's BCG vaccination programme. *Br. Med. J. 1*, 1002.
4. Netherlands Economic Institute (1977): *Present cost of peptic ulceration to Dutch economy and possible impact of cimetidine in this cost*. NEI, Rotterdam.
5. Istituto di Studi Politico-Economici, Università di Pavia (1978): *La determinazione dei costi sociali dell'ulcera peptica in Italia*.
6. Muttarini, L. (1978): Metodi e primi risultati di un'indagine sulla determinazione dei costi sociali dell'ulcera in Italia. In: *Cimetidina: farmacologia e clinica,* p. 21. Smith Kline & French, Milan.
7. Angelini, E. (1978): Analisi critica delle fonti statistiche sanitarie in Italia ai fini della determinazione dei costi sociali di una malattia di large diffusione. In: *Cimetidina: farmacologia e clinica,* p. 33. Smith Kline & French, Milan.
8. Robinson Associates, Inc. (1978): *The impact of cimetidine on the national cost of duodenal ulcer.*

Appendix

Questionnaire for the functional model of costs and benefits associated with ulcer

1. Attacks of duodenal ulcer

   Q. In your experience, with 100 representing the total number of patients suffering from duodenal ulcer, how many manifested 1 attack per year, 2 attacks per year, etc.? (Give the data in the following table.)

1 attack per year	%
2 attacks per year	%
3 attacks per year	%
4 attacks per year	%
more than 4 attacks per year..............	%
Total:	100.0 patients

2. Categories of severity of the ulcer

   (In an American trial, types of patients were built up, based on their symptoms. Below we give the definition of each of the categories suggested.)

   Q. Still on the basis of your own experience, can you indicate how your patients (totaling 100) can be distributed among the following categories?

Category of ulcer	Description	% of total
1	*Patients diagnosed initially* Symptoms: a. Pain at night or on an empty stomach, disappearing when food is taken b. Periodical attacks every 7-10 days c. Ulcer can be demonstrated by X-ray or endoscopy d. No hemorrhage or other contra-indications e. No previous episode f. Atypical symptoms, but ulcer can be demonstrated radiologically or endoscopically	.... %
2	*Patients with recurrent attacks, not hospitalized* a. Acutely recurrent at least once a year b. The attacks do not increase in intensity	.... %
3	*Patients with recurrent attacks, not hospitalized, whose condition is deteriorating* a. The patient was never admitted on account of ulcer b. The intensity of the attacks is increasing or persistent c. No hemorrhage or perforation	.... %
4	*Patients admitted but not operated, with hemorrhage* a. Admitted due to ulcer b. Hemorrhage, but no need for immediate intervention	.... %
		Total: 100.0 %

3. Transition between categories of ulcer

Within the categories of ulcer just defined, it may reasonably be expected that there will be movement of patients from 1 category to another, due to improvement or deterioration, in each period (year or years). For example, it could be imagined that a patient initially classified in category 3 would later be classified in category 4, etc. (By definition, no 'return' to category 1 is anticipated.)

Considering for purposes of simplicity 2 periods: a) 2 years after the first year, and b) 5 years after the first year, can you indicate on the table below how 100 patients initially classified under 1 would be distributed, how 100 patients initially classified under 2 would be distributed, etc.?

Initial category	Category at 2 years				Operated	Cured	Died	Total
	1	2	3	4				
1								100.0
2	0							100.0
3	0							100.0
4	0							100.0

Initial category	Category at 5 years				Operated	Cured	Died	Total
	1	2	3	4				
1								100.0
2	0							100.0
3	0							100.0
4	0							100.0

Discussion

Baron: Thank you for those interesting data. We have a limited amount of data regarding 2-year follow-up, we have heard about some mathematical models, and we have also heard about different approaches to maintenance treatment. The conventional approach, used in most trials, is continuous maintenance therapy, as was discussed by Dr. Bodemar. Dr. Bardhan has described the approach of most British doctors: that is, to give patients repeated courses of cimetidine therapy if they have repeated attacks. Both of these methods of maintenance treatment should decrease the loss of work — provided, of course, that the doctor takes his responsibility seriously and tells the patient that, if he is symptom-free, he can return to work. There is no economic gain from any treatment if the patient has benefit from the treatment but continues sitting around at home.

The second benefit of maintenance treatment is, of course, the avoidance of operation. There are 2 separate questions here, the answers to which depend entirely on what is believed to be the natural history of duodenal ulcer disease. Some doctors believe that the patients continue to have hypersecretion and abnormal diathesis forever, in which case they may have to consider remaining on maintenance treatment forever. Others believe that the disease burns itself out after, say, 15 years, in which case we have to consider short-term policy and might hope to stop maintenance treatment. This is where the mathematical models fail, because clinical doctors cannot provide the necessary basic epidemiological figures for accurate curves to be created. Has anyone questions on this particular problem?

Orlandi (Ancona): On looking at these results and at those in the previous report, I am struck by the apparent lack of attention given to some of the components of the clinical situation — for example, smoking. Are we not running the risk, to use an analogy, of carrying out a clinical trial of oral hypoglycaemics in diabetes without looking at compliance with diet by the various groups examined? Moreover, if we consider and stress these aspects — I am talking of smoking but I could just as well be talking of alcohol — we may be able to make strategic suggestions, in social-health terms. A drug is always a tactical response to a problem, but I think that we would all agree that the strategic response is prevention, the removal of some of the risk factors present in the population being examined.

Muttarini: Not as a doctor but as a smoker I can well understand what Professor Orlandi has said. I want to stress one aspect: the model which we have tried to build is a macro-model, a model with large aggregates; it cannot look at details, no matter how important they admittedly are. Such details would raise so many alternatives that the model would become unmanageable, and the results would be incomprehensible.

In my opinion, it is more important to offer clear possibilities to the decision-makers than to cater for all situations which can be imagined. I hope that the group of clinicians who provided the data have taken smoking into account when giving their figures.

Baron: If there was ever a revolution in Britain, and if I became the first President, I would ban the sale of tobacco, of alcohol and of white bread, as a result of which the population would become much healthier. We are, however, not in the sort of political situation where it is possible to influence these factors.

Recent results with cimetidine treatment (I)

Chairmen: W. Lorenz *(Marburg, West Germany)*
            R. Cheli *(Genoa, Italy)*

Long-term treatment of duodenal ulcer in Ireland

C.F. McCarthy, J.M. Walters, P. Crean, D. Kelly, P. Cahill, D.S. Cole, M. Whelton and D. Weir
University College, Galway; St. Finbarr's Hospital, Cork; Trinity College, Dublin, Republic of Ireland; and Smith Kline & French Research Ltd., Welwyn Garden City, United Kingdom

Introduction

Although this paper describes a study in which cimetidine was used in the short-term and long-term management of patients with duodenal ulcer, I do not wish to give the impression that the treatment of these patients in Ireland is based solely on the use of cimetidine. The general pattern of treatment is based on diagnosis by either endoscopy or barium meal or both. This is followed by informing the patient that a duodenal ulcer is present and that there is no risk of malignancy. Some advice about smoking, alcohol, and general attitude towards work is given, and the hazards of various analgesics are described. An anti-ulcer drug is then prescribed for 6 weeks, and endoscopy or barium meal is not repeated if the patient is asymptomatic after this treatment. Minor relapses are treated with antacids and rest; severe relapses are re-treated with an anti-ulcer drug, and consideration is given to long-term use of cimetidine or to surgical treatment.

Subjects and methods

Our study [1] was carried out in and in the surrounding areas of 3 University centres in Ireland: Dublin, Cork and Galway. Patients were referred by their family doctors, by consultant physicians, or by surgeons. To enter the study, a duodenal ulcer had to be demonstrated at endoscopy performed no more than 7 days prior to entry. Diagnosis by barium meal was not accepted as adequate for the purposes of this study.

A total of 128 patients entered the trial (20 in Cork, 49 in Dublin and 59 in Galway). Ninety-five were male and 33 were female. The mean age was 44.3 years, the mean duration of ulcer history was 7.8 years and the mean period since the last ulcer relapse was 3.1 months.

After 1 month's therapy with cimetidine 1 g/day, 91 patients' ulcers (71.1%) had healed. A further 18 patients (14.1%) healed following a second month of therapy, and after a third month of therapy 3 additional patients (2.4%) had healed ulcers. One patient remained unhealed, and 15 patients dropped out of the study: 9 failed to return for endoscopy at 4 weeks and 6, unhealed at 4 weeks, failed to turn up at 8 weeks.

One hundred of the patients whose ulcers had healed then entered a low-dose maintenance trial: 49 were given cimetidine 400 mg at night, and 51 were given placebo. This trial was a double-blind study.

Results

The results of our low-dose maintenance trial are shown in Table I. Over 42% of the cimetidine group remained healed, compared to 21% of the placebo group. The number of drop-outs was similar in each group, and their reasons for leaving the study are indicated in Table II. The time at which relapses and drop-outs occurred is indicated in the Figure.

Table I.   Results of maintenance study.

Treatment group	Number entered	Remained healed at 11 months*	Relapsed	Dropped out
Cimetidine	49	21 (42.9%)	13 (26.6%)	15 (30.7%)
Placebo	51	11 (21.6%)	26 (51.0%)	14 (27.5%)
Total	100	32	39	29

*Maintenance of ulcer healing was significant at $p < 0.007$ for ulcers initially healed at 1 month, and at $p < 0.02$ for those healed at 2 months [7].

Table II.   Reasons for drop-out from maintenance study (other than recurrence of ulcer).

	Treatment group	
	Cimetidine	Placebo
Noncompliance	11	10
Psychiatric admission	0	2
Pregnancy	1	1
Zollinger-Ellison syndrome	1	0
Development of gastric ulcer	0	1
Operation for small bowel obstruction	1	0
Severe duodenitis at 5th month endoscopy	1	0

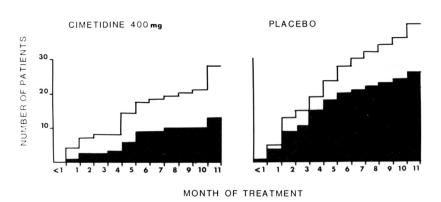

Figure   Relapses (black areas) and drop-outs (white areas) in cimetidine and control groups during study period.

Table III. Summary of abnormalities in biochemistry and haematology.

Test	Number of patients with abnormal readings	
	Cimetidine group	Placebo group
Alkaline phosphatase	15	6
Bilirubin	18	7
Creatinine	23	15
Haemoglobin	13	3
LDH	9	7
RBC	0	3
SGOT	19	8
Urea	20	10
Uric acid	13	5
WBC	11	6
Total number of abnormalities	141	70
Total patient-months of treatment	532	309
Abnormalities per patient-month	0.27	0.23

No major side-effects occurred, although minor and usually transient biochemical abnormalities occurred in both groups (see Table III).

Discussion

The frequency of healing in the first 2 months of our study is similar to that reported elsewhere [2-6]. Maintenance on cimetidine 400 mg at night reduced the incidence of relapse in patients with healed duodenal ulcer over an 11-month period. This reduction in the number of recurrences was not accompanied by serious side-effects. The relapse rate was reduced from 50% to 25%, and if this 25% recurrence rate is repeated in subsequent years of low-dose cimetidine therapy, the number remaining healed after 5 years could well fall to 23%. It is possible that recurrences may be less after the first year of maintenance, and studies are in progress to assess this and to study long-term toxicity.

The number of patients in the placebo group remaining healed at 11 months is higher than that in several other studies, and may result from a milder form of ulcer disease in the patients in our study.

Acknowledgements

We wish to thank our colleagues who referred patients to us, and those who made available haematological and biochemical estimations. We are particularly grateful to our endoscopic associates, Nurses A. Dixon, E. Shorten, E. Finnegan and S. Griffith, and to Mr David Underwood for the statistical analysis.

References

1. Walters, J., Crean, P., Kelly, K., Cahill, P., Cole, D., Whelton, M., Weir, D. and McCarthy, C. (1979): Cimetidine and duodenal ulcer: efficacy of low dosage maintenance treatment. *Gut 20*, A451.

2. Winship, D.H. (1978): Cimetidine in the treatment of duodenal ulcer. *Gastroenterology 74*, 402-406.
3. Binder, H.J., Cocco, A., Crossley, R.J., Finkelstein, W., Font, R., Friedman, G., Groarke, J., Hughes, W., Johnson, A.F., McGuigan, J.E., Summers, R., Vlahcevic, R., Wilson, E.C. and Winship, D.H. (1978): Cimetidine in the treatment of duodenal ulcer: a multicentre double-blind study. *Gastroenterology 74*, 380-388.
4. Bianchi Porro, G., Cheli, R., Dobrilla, G., Verme, G., Molinari, F., Pera, A., Petrillo, M. and Valenti, M. (1978): Treatment of active duodenal ulcer with oral cimetidine: a multicentre controlled endoscopic trial. *Digestion 17*, 383-386.
5. Hetzel, D.J., Hansky, J., Shearman, D.J.C., Korman, M.G., Hecker, R., Taggart, G.J., Jackson, R. and Gabb, B.W. (1978): Cimetidine treatment of duodenal ulcer: short-term clinical trial and maintenance study. *Gastroenterology 74*, 389-392.
6. Dronfield, M.W., Batchelor, A.J., Larkworthy, W. and Langman, M.J.S. (1979): Controlled trial of maintenance cimetidine treatment in healed duodenal ulcer: short- and long-term effects. *Gut 20*, 526-530.
7. Gehan, E.A. (1965): The generalised Wilcoxon test for comparing arbitrarily single-censored samples. *Biometrika 52*, 203.

Long-term treatment of duodenal ulcer with cimetidine: a review

G. Bianchi Porro, W.L. Burland*, B.W. Hawkins* and Maddalena Petrillo

*Gastrointestinal Unit, Ospedale L. Sacco, Milan, Italy; and *The Research Institute, Smith Kline & French Laboratories Ltd., Welwyn Garden City, United Kingdom*

Introduction

Duodenal ulcer is, by definition, a relapsing chronic disease with limited mortality, but with relatively high morbidity because of its clinical relapses and anatomical recurrences.

The traditional aims of medical treatment of duodenal ulcer, accepted by all medical authorities, are: in the short term, to relieve symptoms; in the middle term, to accelerate healing; and in the long term, if possible, to prevent recurrences.

The discovery of cimetidine brought about a complete change in the short-term treatment of duodenal ulcer and, today, cimetidine is considered first choice in this clinical situation, since it has been demonstrated in an unquestionable way that a 6-8 week course of treatment induces peptic ulcer healing in more than 80% of patients [1-5].

Until a short time ago we had no convincing evidence that medical treatment could prevent the ulcer relapsing, as demonstrated by the fact that the main indication for surgery was medical intractability. Few gastroenterologists, however, are completely satisfied with surgical treatment, which is not without mortality, albeit limited, and which presents important postoperative nutritional and metabolic complications as well as a number of recurrences. Undoubtedly, the major problem the physician has to face today is the prevention of re-ulceration once the ulcer has been healed by pharmacological means.

In this paper we will present the results of 2 long-term controlled studies which we made with the aim of preventing ulcer recurrence, analyze in detail the results of an international controlled collaborative study in which we participated, and draw definite conclusions about this very stimulating topic.

Maintenance treatment of duodenal ulcer: a personal experience

Methods

During the period 1977-79, we completed 2 long-term studies on the efficacy of cimetidine in preventing ulcer recurrence in patients whose ulcers had been healed by pharmacological means. Both studies were conducted in the Gastrointestinal Unit of Sacco Hospital, in Milan.

The first trial, a double-blind study, involved a group of 23 patients who received cimetidine 400 mg at bedtime (2 tablets of 200 mg each), and a control group of 23 patients who received matching placebo tablets. In all of these patients, endoscopic confirmation of ulcer healing had been obtained within 4 days of the beginning of the trial.

In the second trial, which was controlled but not blinded, 63 patients were admitted: 31 were treated with cimetidine 400 mg at bedtime, and 32 received cimetidine 400 gm twice daily (morning and evening).

All patients in both studies were seen every 2 months for normal routine examinations; endoscopy was carried out after 6 and 12 months of treatment and also at any time patients complained of epigastric pain lasting for more than 2 consecutive days, suggesting ulcer relapse.

Results

In the first study, we observed 14 relapses in the placebo group at 6 months (61%), and 19 relapses at 12 months (83%). In the cimetidine group, 7 relapses were observed at 6 months (30%), and 9 relapses at 12 months (39%). The difference in number of relapses between the placebo and cimetidine groups was significant, both at 6 months ($p = 0.046$) and at 12 months ($p = 0.003$).

These data are shown graphically in Figure 1: it can be seen clearly that most relapses were observed within the first 6 months of treatment. Two so-called 'silent' or 'asymptomatic' ulcers were observed in the cimetidine group, 1 at 6 months and 1 at 12 months, while 4 silent ulcers were seen in the placebo group, 3 at 6 months and 1 at 12 months.

It is worth noting that, in this trial, 1 patient in the cimetidine group and 4 in the placebo group complained of severe pain, suggesting recurrence, although there was no endoscopic demonstration of re-ulceration. This underlines the importance of endoscopic control at short, fixed intervals, even in totally asymptomatic patients; only such control will allow us to accurately judge the effectiveness of a drug. At the

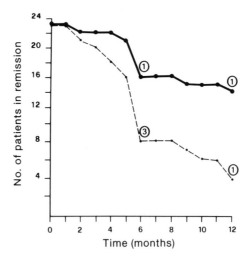

Fig. 1.   Number of duodenal ulcer patients in remission during 12 months of treatment with cimetidine 400 mg at bedtime (●—●) or placebo (●---●). The circled numbers indicate asymptomatic ulcers observed at routine endoscopy.

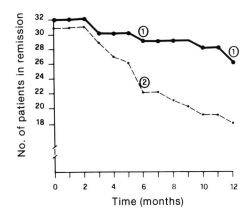

Fig. 2. Number of duodenal ulcer patients in remission during 12 months of treatment with cimetidine 400 mg at bedtime (•---•) or twice daily (•—•). The circled numbers indicate asymptomatic ulcers observed at routine endoscopy.

same time, we can be critical of those studies in which pain is considered sufficient evidence of ulcer recurrence and, thus, of treatment failure; it is possible that, in such studies, drug effectiveness will not be accurately determined.

In our second trial, there were 9 relapses in the group treated with cimetidine 400 mg at bedtime after 6 months of continuous treatment (29%), and 13 relapses at 12 months (42%). In the group treated with cimetidine twice daily we observed only 3 relapses at 6 months (9%) and 6 relapses at 12 months (19%).

These results are presented graphically in Figure 2: whilst prophylactic long-term treatment with cimetidine twice a day appeared to be superior to 400 mg nightly, the difference between the 2 groups was not statistically significant at either 6 or 12 months ($p < 0.1$). Two silent ulcers were observed in each of the study groups, 1 at 6 months and 1 at 12 months in the group of patients receiving cimetidine twice daily, and both at 6 months in the group receiving cimetidine 400 mg at bedtime.

Finally, we want to emphasize the great similarity in the percentage of relapses observed between our 2 studies in the groups treated with the same dosage (400 mg at bedtime): 30% and 29% at 6 months in the first and second study, respectively, and 39% and 42% at 12 months.

Maintenance treatment of duodenal ulcer: an international collaborative study

Methods

A total of 696 patients with healed duodenal ulcers, demonstrated by endoscopy within 7 days of the beginning of the trial, were admitted to an international collaborative study, designed with the aim of comparing cimetidine and placebo in the prevention of recurrence of ulceration [6].

Patients were randomly allocated, double-blind, to one of the following 4 treatments: cimetidine 400 mg morning and evening (184 patients), cimetidine 400 mg at bedtime (179), placebo twice daily (152) or placebo at bedtime (181).

Treatment was administered for 12 months, with the exception of one trial which included 109 patients and lasted only 6 months. The reappearance of persistent ulcer-like pain was considered an indication for re-examination by endoscopy; endoscopy was also carried out in a certain proportion of patients after 6 months and in most asymptomatic patients after 12 months.

Statistical methods.   Data were compared for symptomatic recurrence of duodenal ulcer using the generalized Wilcoxon test for comparing arbitrarily single-censored samples [7]. The χ^2 test was used to compare groups for the recurrence of asymptomatic re-ulceration.

Results

A symptomatic recurrence of duodenal ulceration during treatment occurred in 31 of the patients who received cimetidine 400 mg at bedtime (17.3%), and in 28 of those who received cimetidine twice daily (15.2%); this difference in recurrences is not significant. However, 178 of the patients receiving placebo had a symptomatic recurrence of ulceration (53.5%), and the difference between these placebo-treated patients and both cimetidine groups is very significant ($p < 0.001$).

During the course of their treatment, 277 symptom-free patients were examined by endoscopy: 8 patients receiving cimetidine 400 mg at bedtime (9.6% of those examined from that group), 17 patients receiving 400 mg twice daily (16.3%), and 24 patients on placebo (26.7%) were found to have a duodenal ulcer. The difference between placebo-treated patients and cimetidine-treated patients is significant ($p < 0.01$).

The possible influence of previous treatment is shown in Table I. Of the 290 patients who received cimetidine to heal their ulcer and were then maintained on placebo, 184 (63%) had a symptomatic recurrence of ulceration, compared with 47% of the smaller number of patients whose ulcers healed on placebo and who were then maintained on placebo; this difference is not statistically significant. The latter

Table I.   *The possible influence of previous treatment on re-ulceration in 696 patients. The short-term treatment led, in each case, to endoscopically-demonstrated ulcer healing. (Reprinted with permission from [6]).*

Short-term treatment	Long-term treatment (number of patients)	Symptomatic re-ulceration	Asymptomatic re-ulceration	
		Number (%)	Patients examined	Number (%) with re-ulceration
Cimetidine	Cimetidine 400 mg at bedtime (161)	28 (17) ⎫ 55 (18)	77	7 (9)
	Cimetidine 400 mg twice daily (149)	27 (18) ⎭	84	11 (13)
	Placebo (290)	184 (63)	77	17 (22)
Placebo	Cimetidine 400 mg at bedtime (18)	3 (17) ⎫ 4 (15)	6	2 (33)
	Cimetidine 400 mg twice daily (9)	1 (11) ⎭	5	1 (20)
	Placebo (30)	14 (47)	13	5 (38)

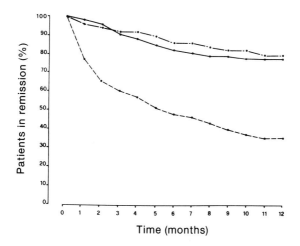

Fig. 3. Percentage of duodenal ulcer patients in clinical remission during 12 months of treatment with cimetidine 400 mg at bedtime (●——●), cimetidine 400 mg twice daily (●—-●), or placebo (●----●). (Reprinted with permission from [6]).

group, however, had a higher incidence of asymptomatic ulcer (38% against 22%); again, the difference is not significant.

The possible outcome for the whole groups of patients who began the trial is shown in Figure 3; in this projection, those patients who for different reasons did not complete the trial have also been included. Although the loss of patients did gradually reduce the population available for study, 52 of the dropouts (34%) were only lost in the last 2 months of the 12-month treatment period, and the number of patients available for review each month of treatment enables the probability of symptomatic ulcer recurrence and the time of recurrence to be estimated for the whole population.

Discussion

The relative safety of up to 12 months' treatment with cimetidine has been recently reviewed by Burland [8], who concluded that there are no effects which are likely to restrict longer-term treatment with cimetidine 400 mg, administered once or twice daily.

Of the 696 patients entering this international trial, 154 failed to complete treatment by default, 286 were withdrawn because of re-ulceration, 245 completed their allocated treatment and only 11 were withdrawn from the study owing to side-effects. Of these, 2 were receiving placebo and 9 were being treated with cimetidine 400 mg at bedtime. Both of the placebo-treated patients suffered myocardial infarctions, and 1 of them died. Of the 9 cimetidine-treated patients, 4 died (2 from myocardial infarction, 1 from a ruptured aortic aneurysm and 1 from septic shock) and 2 were withdrawn because of cardiological problems (1 developed heart failure and 1 developed tachycardia following a myocardial infarction).

Therefore, only 3 of the 363 patients treated with cimetidine in this trial (0.8% of those receiving the drug) were withdrawn for reasons which were probably drug-related: 1 developed impotence, 1 developed tremor, headache and vertigo, and 1 had elevated transaminases.

In conclusion, the results of this study indicate that cimetidine 400 mg, administered either once or twice daily, is significantly superior to placebo in the prevention of duodenal ulcer recurrence. There seems to be no reason why maintenance treatment should not be prolonged to 12 months, but more data are needed in order to evaluate treatment for periods of longer than 12 months.

Very long-term treatment of duodenal ulcer: a personal experience

We want now to take into consideration the outcome of patients in the period of time after completion of 12 months of initial prophylactic treatment. The evidence which has accumulated in the literature suggests that the relapse rate during the first 6 months after an initial period of treatment lasting 6 or 12 months is very similar to the rate which is seen in patients treated initially with only a short course of cimetidine [9-11]. Therefore, when long-term treatment is completed the patient finds himself back where he began. This observation led us to wonder whether treatment lasting an *additional* 12 months could have the same positive effect in the prevention of ulcer recurrence as the initial 12 months of treatment.

To investigate this possibility, we followed up the 18 patients whose ulcers were still healed at the end of our first long-term treatment study, which is described earlier in the present paper. After 12 months of continuous treatment, 14 patients from the cimetidine group and 4 patients from the placebo group still had healed ulcers: of the 14 patients previously treated with cimetidine 400 mg nightly, 4 were continued on this dosage for the additional 12 months and 4 had 12 months' further treatment with a reduced cimetidine dosage (200 mg nightly); the remaining 6 cimetidine patients and the 4 patients who had previously received placebo received no treatment during the 12-month follow-up period.

At the end of this second 12 months, no recurrences were observed in the 8 patients who were still receiving cimetidine 400 mg or 200 mg nightly; of the 10 patients receiving no treatment, re-ulceration was observed in 3 of the 6 who had previously received cimetidine and in 1 of the 4 who had previously received placebo.

Table II.   Very long-term treatment of duodenal ulcer in 32 patients.

Treatment during first 12 months	Treatment during second 12 months	Number of patients	Patients with re-ulceration
Cimetidine 400 mg at bedtime	Cimetidine 400 mg	7	1
	Cimetidine 200 mg	6	1
	No treatment	4	1
Cimetidine 400 mg twice daily	Cimetidine 400 mg twice daily	8	1
	Cimetidine 400 mg at bedtime	7	1

Table III.   Very long-term treatment of duodenal ulcer in 50 patients.

Treatment during first 12 months	Number	Treatment during second 12 months	Number	Symptomatic re-ulceration	
				Number	%
Cimetidine 400 mg twice daily	15	Cimetidine 400 mg twice daily	8	1	12
		Cimetidine 400 mg at bedtime	7	1	} 11
Cimetidine 400 mg at bedtime	31	Cimetidine 400 mg at bedtime	11	1	
		Cimetidine 200 mg at bedtime	10	1	10
		No treatment	10	4	} 36
Placebo	4	No treatment	4	1	

We also have some preliminary data on a similar follow-up of patients whose ulcers were still healed at the end of our second long-term trial. At the end of 12 months of continuous treatment, 18 patients who had received cimetidine 400 mg at bedtime and 26 of those who had received 400 mg twice daily still had healed ulcers; 1 of the former group and 11 of the latter were lost to follow-up. The treatment schedules and results for the 12-month follow-up of the remaining 32 patients are shown in Table II; regardless of the treatment regime followed during this second 12-month study period, 1 re-ulceration occurred in each group for a total of 5 recurrences out of 32 patients under observation.

The combined results of these 2 follow-up programs are presented in Table III. Although numbers are still too small to draw definite conclusions, the data seem very encouraging: the percentage of relapses occurring during a second year of cimetidine treatment was very similar in all cimetidine groups, regardless of the dosage administered, and was in each case considerably smaller than the percentage of relapses occurring in patients receiving no treatment during the second year.

No important side-effects were observed during follow-up.

Conclusions

From the data presented, the following conclusions emerge:
— treatment with cimetidine 400 mg at bedtime or twice daily for up to 12 months very significantly reduces recurrence of symptomatic ulceration;
— no serious untoward effects of treatment have been observed and therefore this specific treatment can be considered to be without significant hazard;
— the protective effect of cimetidine seems to last as long as the patient is on treatment;
— the natural history of duodenal ulcer remains unaltered when cimetidine treatment is stopped after 1 year.
In our opinion, aims and questions for future research could be:
— is cimetidine a sufficiently safe drug when taken for more than 1 year?

— is very long-term treatment with cimetidine simply a postponement of re-ulceration?

— or is treatment prolonged for some years able to alter the natural history of duodenal ulcer and, as a consequence, should cimetidine treatment be prolonged indefinitely?

Acknowledgments

We very gratefully acknowledge the co-operation of the clinical investigators who participated in the international collaborative study and gave us permission to publish the data. The principal investigators were P.M. Smith (Cardiff), W. Larkworthy (Lincoln), J.H. Wyllie (London), M.J.S. Langman (Nottingham), K.D. Bardhan (Rotherham), H.L. Duthie (Sheffield), B.J. Smits (Coventry), G.P. Crean and G. Gillespie (Glasgow), C.W. Venables (Newcastle), M. Whelton (Cork), D.G. Weir (Dublin), C.F. McCarthy (Galway), J. Kreuning (Leiden), M. van Blankenstein (Rotterdam), G. Bianchi Porro and M. Petrillo (Milan), J.-P. Bader (Paris), R. Lambert (Lyon), E. Aadland, A. Berstad and J. Myren (Oslo), A. Walan (Linköping), G. Strohmeyer (Dusseldorf), A.L. Blum (Zurich), S. Bank and G.O. Barbezat (Cape Town), M.G. Moshal (Durban) and R. Mekel (Pretoria).

References

1. Bodemar, G. and Walan, A. (1976): Cimetidine in the treatment of active duodenal and prepyloric ulcers. *Lancet 2,* 161.
2. Gray, G.R., Smith, I.S., MacKenzie, I. and Gillespie, G. (1978): Long-term cimetidine in the management of severe duodenal ulcer dyspepsia. *Gastroenterology 74,* 397.
3. Bianchi Porro, G., Cheli, R., Dobrilla, G., Verme, G., Molinari, F., Pera, A., Petrillo, M. and Valentini, M. (1978): Treatment of active duodenal ulcer with oral cimetidine: a multicenter controlled endoscopic trial. *Digestion 17,* 383.
4. Bardhan, K.D., Saul, D.M., Edwards, J.L., Smith, P.M., Fettes, M., Forrest, J., Heading, R.C., Logan, R.F.A., Dronfield, M.W., Langman, M.J., Larkworthy, W., Haggie, S.J., Wyllie, J.H., Corbett, C., Duthie, H.L., Fussey, I.V., Holdsworth, C.D., Balmforth, G.V. and Maruyama, T. (1979): Comparison of two doses of cimetidine and placebo in the treatment of duodenal ulcer: a multicentre trial. *Gut 20,* 68.
5. Bianchi Porro, G. and Petrillo, M. (1979): L'ulcera peptica. Prospettive di terapia a lungo termine. In: *Gastroenterologia ospedaliera,* p. 77. Editors: P.F. Baratta, G. Dobrilla and E. Belsasso. Cortina, Verona.
6. Burland, W.L., Hawkins, B.W. and Beresford, J. (1980): Cimetidine treatment for the prevention of recurrence of duodenal ulcer: an international collaborative study. *Postgrad. Med. J. 56,* 173.
7. Gehan, E.A. (1965): The generalized Wilcoxon test for comparing arbitrarily single-censored samples. *Biometrika 52,* 203.
8. Burland, W.L. (1978): Evidence for the safety of cimetidine in the treatment of peptic ulcer disease. In: *Proceedings of an International Symposium on histamine H₂-recepto antagonists,* p. 238. Editor: W. Creutzfeldt. Excerpta Medica, Amsterdam-Oxford Princeton.
9. Gudmand-Høyer, E., Jensen, K.B., Krag, E., Rask-Madsen, J. and Rahbek, I. (1978) Prophylactic effect of cimetidine in duodenal ulcer disease. *Br. Med. J. 1,* 1095.
10. Dronfield, M.W., Batchelor, A.J., Larkworthy, W. and Langman, M.J.S. (1979): Effec of maintenance cimetidine treatment in duodenal ulcer and the eventual outcome afte cessation of treatment. *Gut 20,* 526.
11. Hetzel, D.J., Shearman, D.J.C., Hansky, J., Korman, M.G., Hecker, R., Jackson, R. Gabb, B.W. and Sheers, R. (1978): Maintenance of remission of duodenal ulcer by cime tidine: a double-blind controlled trial. *Gut 19,* 442.

Discussion

Turpini (Pavia): In patients treated with cimetidine who had an asymptomatic relapse, does treatment with full doses of cimetidine clear the ulcer? Also, is the incidence of such complications as bleeding and perforation in patients with asymptomatic relapses higher than in patients on placebo?

Bianchi Porro: Obviously, the answer can be based only upon personal experience. In our study, patients who had a silent ulcer were treated again with full doses of cimetidine; they demonstrated the same sensitivity to the drug as on initial treatment, and the percentage of complications was not different overall between the group with symptomatic ulceration and the other group.

Giacosa (Genoa): I have a comment for Dr. Bianchi Porro, and a question for Professor McCarthy.

Dr. Bianchi Porro, we have been using a maintenance dose of cimetidine 200 mg in the evening and have found no significant difference from patients treated with 400 mg; this seems to be an extremely important fact, and confirmation from other groups would encourage the continuation of such a regime. A smaller dose of drug is desirable for the patient, both biologically and because of cost.

I would like some more information from Professor McCarthy on those patients removed at some stage from the maintenance group. In particular, can he clarify the characteristics of that case defined as severe duodenitis, the functional, histological, morphological, endoscopic and other features upon which the assessment was based, and also, can he specify what happened to the patient? Could he tell us, with regard to the case of gastric ulceration, how the subsequent lesion was interpreted? Finally, can he say a few words about the morphology of the 5 cases — too many, it seems to me — with a skin rash, given the known effects of cimetidine upon the skin and its lesions? What were the characteristics, have you any details of the history of the skin in these 5 patients?

McCarthy: The skin rashes in each instance were transient erythematous rashes, and they disappeared although the drug was continued. There is no proof that they were due to cimetidine. I can add nothing further to what has already been said about the rashes.

The gastric ulcer developed by one patient was a benign ulcer, which subsequently healed following treatment with carbenoxolone. The patient with duodenitis was shown at endoscopy to have the ulcer healed; however, the duodenitis was so severe that the endoscopist felt the patient should be withdrawn from the trial. He was then treated with the higher dose of cimetidine. This was not a patient treated in Galway, where I work, but in one of the other centres. I can give no further follow-up on this patient. The appearance of the duodenitis was of a red, inflamed duodenal mucosa. As far as I know, no biopsy was taken from the mucosa.

Bianchi Porro: We ourselves have treated the patients with cimetidine 200 mg only after the first year. In fact, this was a little odd: towards the end of our trial of cimetidine 400 mg versus placebo, we asked ourselves whether we should randomise the patients also with a 200 mg dose. But I should like to repeat my strong impression that, in first-year maintenance, 800 mg is better than 400 mg, although only Northfield has, to date, shown a significant difference. We still have to find out what happens between the first and second years; the group was very small, and a difference of 10-11% between 200, 400 and 800 mg is also so small that, at this point, we cannot draw any definite conclusions. We have no more than impressions.

Cheli: A fundamental point of Dr. Bianchi Porro's paper is the possibility of very low dose maintenance therapy; that has been our hope in Genoa, too, and we have in fact had some success with this regime. However, more concrete data are needed.

One small point for Professor McCarthy. When we speak of peptic disease, we often have to make distinctions between true peptic pathology and inflammatory pathology: antisecretory treatment in gastritis or in duodenitis probably does not have a pathophysiological rationale, as suppression of secretion is part of the course of gastritis, just as, in the majority of cases of duodenitis (I would say 80-90% of cases), the secretory profile is one of hyposecretion. That is a generalisation, rather than a specific comment on Professor McCarthy's paper, but it is correct at the pathophysiological level.

McCarthy: Perhaps I did not understand what Dr. Cheli said, but all the patients I reported were documented by endoscopy. It was only in one patient that the possibility of duodenitis arose. I imagine that there must be some misunderstanding either on my part or by Dr. Cheli.

Lorenz: If I understood Dr. Cheli correctly, it was a question of the morphology. I remember an Italian paper which showed that, in duodenitis, there is a great difference between the endoscopic and morphological findings. Is that right?

Cheli: Yes, thank you. Duodenitis is not an endoscopic finding, but only a histological finding on biopsy.

McCarthy: Yes, I accept that as a comment related to the one patient.

Pera (Turin): In the light of the finding that, on placebo, some 50% of the patients did not relapse within the first year, would it be appropriate to have trials of intermittent treatment with courses of the drug or, otherwise, to use long-term treatment but only after a second or third recurrence?

Bianchi Porro: I think that the answer to this is very difficult but, just as a working hypothesis, I would agree. Dr. Bardhan seems to have already done such trials. Certainly, the problem is when to give the courses: if we give the course at the next recurrence, we are back exactly to the initial position. I will stress one point again: there are certainly geographical differences but, of our 23 patients treated with placebo, only 3 did not relapse at the end of the 2 years, really a very small proportion. I do not know whether our group was particularly severe, but the 53% recurrence with placebo in this group seems to me to be very good.

Molinari (Genoa): I think that everyone now accepts the effectiveness of cimetidine. I would like to ask Dr. Bianchi Porro, who has made a particular study of the problem, whether, in patients treated with other types of antisecretory agents, there is the same or a similar percentage of recurrences as in the patients treated with cimetidine.

Bianchi Porro: I have no experience of other long-term treatments, that is the problem. We have completed one long-term treatment with pirenzepine, a German anticholinergic which has just become available in Italy, and we have carried out a long-term trial comparing placebo and pirenzepine 50 mg administered in 2 doses/day. There was no significant difference between the 2 treatments, and the percentages of recurrence with placebo in that trial were very similar to those which I have just reported — between 60 and 80%. This is an imperfect answer, but experience is very limited.

Carratù (Rome): A question about the difference, or the impression of a difference, between 400 and 800 mg: at the end of one month of acute treatment, do you pass directly (that is, overnight) from 1 g to 400 mg? Also, given that the curve of recurrences in maintenance treatment is rather sharp in the first few months and then very flat, did you find a seasonal factor, say between 3 and 6 months after the recurrence? Is this a problem in clinical practice or in controlled trials?

Bianchi Porro: The answer to the first question is yes. All our patients who were found to have a healed lesion at endoscopy started maintenance treatment at once, with the placebo or with 400 or 800 mg, without any graduation.

The answer to the second question is that I have not studied those points. I did not think of them, and I thank you for the suggestion. We will study the matter, but the problem is that our numbers are small, so I do not know if anything will come out of such a study.

Cimetidine and medicinal ulcer

A. Bitoun and J.-P. Bader*

Gastroenterology Department, Saint-Lazare Hospital, Paris; and
*Gastroenterology Department, Henri Mondor Hospital, Créteil, France

Introduction

The effectiveness of cimetidine in preventing and curing lesions in patients suffering from gastroduodenal ulcers having been proven, it was a natural next step to determine whether similar results could be obtained with gastroduodenal lesions induced by gastrotoxic substances. A number of experimental and therapeutic studies have been carried out to investigate this question, and this paper will review the results of those studies in animals and in man.

Experimental studies on animals

Mann and Sachdev have indicated that cimetidine acts as a protective agent against gastric erosion caused by various anti-inflammatory drugs in rats. The drugs involved in their studies were acetylsalicylic acid, ketoprofen, ibuprofen and naproxen, each of which produced a certain number of histologically-confirmed gastric erosions in batches of 10 animals.

These authors concluded that, when cimetidine 400 mg/kg was administered along with the gastrotoxic product, it provided full protection, reducing to zero the number of iatrogenic erosions. The only exception to this finding was seen with acetylsalicylic acid which, at a dosage of 225 mg/kg, caused a considerably higher rate of erosions than did the other anti-inflammatory drugs; when administered along with cimetidine, very slight erosion was still found.

Pharmacological studies on humans

MacKercher and colleagues studied 5 healthy volunteers to assess the protective effect of cimetidine on acetylsalicylic acid-induced gastric lesions. The 2 parameters involved in their study were: the potential difference measured in the mucosa, and the examination under microscope of a biopsic mucosa sample.

Using a base potential of 48 ± 1 mv, a suspension of 600 mg of acetylsalicylic acid in the stomach produced a drop in potential difference to 39 ± 1 mv in under 10 minutes, which returned to normal within 30-60 minutes. If an intra-gastric dose of 300 mg of cimetidine was administered 1 hour before acetylsalicylic acid, there was an initial increase in potential difference to 63 ± 2 mv, with the acetylsalicylic acid dosage then causing a drop in potential difference back to 47 ± 3 mv, i.e., the normal base value.

The authors estimated histologically, in biopsy samples from a normal stomach, that up to 2.4% of epithelial surface cells were abnormal. Ten minutes after administration of the 600 mg dose of acetylsalicylic acid, the percentage of abnormal cells rose to 19%; 1 hour later, this percentage had dropped back down to 9%. Cimetidine 300 mg administered 1 hour before acetylsalicylic acid did not alter the base situation; after the acetylsalicylic acid dosage, the percentage of abnormal cells rose only to 4.4% at 10 minutes, and to 6% at 60 minutes.

These results showed, both electrophysiologically and histologically, that cimetidine has considerable protective power against gastric lesions caused by acetylsalicylic acid in human beings.

Welch and colleagues, also studying the protective effect of cimetidine on acetylsalicylic acid-induced gastric lesions in man, concentrated on 1 parameter: decrease in fecal blood loss. Their study involved 22 patients suffering from rheumatoid, degenerative, or inflammatory complaints, each of whom was taking at least 2.6 g of acetylsalicylic acid per day. All subjects had an acid secretion, and none had hemorrhagic digestive lesions. A gaïac test showed that all had infraclinic blood loss. Each patient, in a random cross experiment, had 4 weeks on cimetidine 1-2 g/day, and 4 weeks on a placebo. Blood loss during the trial period was measured using the chromium-51 erythrocyte method.

The results were significant. During the acetylsalicylic acid and placebo phase, daily fecal blood loss was 4.1 ± 0.7 ml, whereas during the acetylsalicylic acid and cimetidine phase it was 2.2 ± 0.3 ml ($p = 0.002$).

Therapeutic studies on humans

We are only aware of 2 therapeutic studies of cimetidine treatment of peptic ulcers in patients receiving anti-inflammatory drugs: that of Davies et al., and a multi-center French trial in which we took part.

The Davies et al. study was a controlled experiment on 18 patients suffering from ulcers diagnosed by endoscopy 4 days before the beginning of the trial: 13 of these were gastric, and 5 were duodenal. Sixteen subjects had rheumatoid polyarthritis, and 2 had arthrosis. A broad range of anti-inflammatory treatments were being used, with frequent association: prednisolone, indometacin, ketoprofen, azaprop-azone, ibuprofen, benorilate, flufenamic acid and alclofenac.

In the experiment, 9 patients received a dose of cimetidine 1.6 g/day for 4 weeks, and 9 received a placebo. Anti-inflammatory treatments were continued without change, and antacid treatment was administered as requested.

After 4 weeks of treatment, a fibroscopic examination was performed to check for scarring of the ulcer. The results showed no difference between the cimetidine group and the placebo group: of the 13 gastric ulcers, 3 from the cimetidine group and 3 from the placebo group were scarred, and of the 5 duodenal ulcers, 2 from the cimetidine group and 2 from the placebo group were scarred.

More recently, a multi-center trial in France was undertaken, with the same objective: to examine the effect of cimetidine on gastroduodenal ulcers in patients taking anti-inflammatory drugs. For ethical reasons, this was an open study.

There were 37 subjects: 17 with gastric ulcers and 20 with duodenal ulcers, all diagnosed by endoscopy. Of these 37 subjects, 26 were rheumatoid, 15 had polyarthritis, 2 had chronic active hepatitis, and there were isolated cases of nephrotic syndrome, nodose periarteritis, reticulopathy, etc. The anti-inflammatory drugs being administered varied, and were often associated: prednisone, prednisolone, methylprednisolone, tetracosactide, indometacin, ketoprofen, acetylsalicylic acid and phenylbutazone.

Treatment lasted 4 weeks, extended in some subjects for an additional 4 weeks, with endoscopy checks to determine whether or not the ulcer was scarred. Anti-inflammatory treatment was continued without change, and antacid treatment was administered as requested.

At the end of the fourth week, 8 of the 17 gastric ulcer patients and 10 of the 20 duodenal ulcer patients had scarred ulcers; at the end of the eighth week, 13 of the 17 gastric ulcers and 18 of the 20 duodenal ulcers were scarred.

Discussion

This presentation of the experimental and clinical work that has been done to date on the possible effectiveness of cimetidine in the prevention or healing of gastric lesions caused by gastrotoxic drugs shows the difficulty of drawing clear, unarguable conclusions.

The experimental results for animals and humans seem to be the least debatable. They show that cimetidine protects gastric mucosa in rats from gastric erosion caused by certain anti-inflammatory drugs, and they show that, in healthy humans and in those suffering from certain rheumatic complaints, cimetidine limits the potential difference of the gastric mucosa caused by acetylsalicylic acid and protects the gastric mucosa from certain histological lesions, significantly reducing infraclinic hemorrhages also caused by acetylsalicylic acid.

The therapeutic studies, however, have been disappointing.

The Davies et al. study was negative but, because of the small sample, the short-ness of the treatment, the exceptionally high rate of scarring on the duodenal ulcers treated with placebo, the uneven distribution of smokers (3 to 1), and the wide range of anti-inflammatory drugs being used, its results are hard to interpret.

The multi-center French experiment was an open study, so that the natural history of drug-induced ulcer was unknown. Only a double-blind study will be able to clarify this point.

After 4 weeks of treatment, the scarring ratio in the cimetidine group of the multi-center trial (8 of 17 gastric ulcers and 10 of 20 duodenal ulcers) was no different from the scarring ratio in the placebo group of the Davies et al. trial (3 of 7 gastric ulcers and 2 of 3 duodenal ulcers).

With such results, we cannot say that formal proof of the curative effect of cime-tidine on gastroduodenal ulcers caused by gastrotoxic drugs has yet been demonstrated, although there are grounds for *presuming* its effectiveness by the demonstration of a certain protective quality of cimetidine in certain elementary lesions linked to these drugs.

One should, however, remember the difficulties of the situation: the relative scar-city of patients with ulcerous lesions using gastrotoxic drugs, our lack of knowledge about the spontaneous frequency of ulcers in subjects with inflammatory diseases, our lack of knowledge about the spontaneous development of these iatrogenic ulcers, and the problem of studying, in 1 experiment, lesions due to different drugs which very probably have different ulcerogenetic mechanisms.

Summary

Various pharmacological tests on animals and humans have shown that cimetidine plays a protective role with gastroduodenal lesions caused by certain anti-inflammatory drugs.

However, therapeutic studies performed to date have failed to confirm this protective effect of cimetidine, perhaps due to several difficulties encountered in the administration of such trials. We can deduce that cimetidine does have a curative effect on iatrogenic ulcers, but this has not yet been formally proven.

Bibliography

1. Bernades, P. (1979): Prévention et traitement des lésions ulcéreuses gastroduodénales chez les malades soumis à la corticothérapie. *Rev. Prat. 16,* 1343-1346.
2. Bommelaer, G. and Guth, P.H. (1978): Protection by histamine antagonists and prostaglandin against gastric mucosal barrier disruption. *Pharmacologist 20,* 208. (Abstract.)
3. Bommelaer, G. and Guth, P.H. (1979): Rupture of gastric mucosal barrier by aspirin: effect of antihistamines and prostaglandins. (French.) *Gastroenterol. Clin. Biol. 3,* 81-82. (Abstract.)
4. Davies, J., Dixon, A.J. and Beales, J.S.M. (1978): The effects of cimetidine on peptic ulceration in patients receiving anti-inflammatory therapy. In: *Cimetidine: the Westminster Hospital Symposium,* pp. 275-280. Editors: C. Wastell and P. Lance. Churchill Livingstone, Edinburgh.
5. Dodi, G., Farini, R., Pedrazzoli, S., Zannini, G., Lise, H. and Fagiolo, U. (1978): Effect of cimetidine on steroid experimental peptic ulcers. *Acta Hepato-gastroenterol. 25,* 395-397.
6. Guth, P.H., Avres, D. and Paulsen, G. (1979): Topical aspirin plus HCT gastric lesions in the rat: cytoprotective effect of prostaglandin, cimetidine and probanthine. *Gastroenterology 76,* 88-92.
7. Ivey, K.J., Brändli, H.H. and Blum, A.L. (1975): Effect of cimetidine on gastric potential difference in man. *Lancet 2,* 1072-1073.
8. Ivey, K.J., MacKercher, P.A., Baskin, W.N., Krause, W. and Jeffrey, G.E. (1977): Cimetidine protection from aspirin-induced human gastric mucosal damage. *Rend. Gastro-enterol. 9,* 79. (Abstract.)
9. Jones, R.H., Rudge, C.J., Bewick, M., Parsons, V. and Weston, M.J. (1978): Cimetidine: prophylaxis against upper gastrointestinal hemorrhage after renal transplantation. *Br. Med. J. 1,* 398-400.
10. Kenyon, G.S., Ansell, I.F. and Carter, D.C. (1977): Cimetidine and the gastric mucosal barrier. *Gut 18,* 631-635.
11. Khamis, B., Finucane, J. and Stephen-Doyle, J. (1977): The effect of oral cimetidine on pH gastric transmucosal potential difference in canine Heidenhain pouches. *Ir. J. Med. Sci. 146,* 86.
12. MacKercher, P.A., Ivey, K.J., Baskin, W.N., Krause, W. and Jeffrey, G.E. (1976): Effect of cimetidine on aspirin-induced human gastric mucosal damage. *Gastroenterology 70,* 912. (Abstract.)
13. MacKercher, P.A., Ivey, K.J., Baskin, W.N. and Krause, W.J. (1977): Protective effect of cimetidine on aspirin-induced gastric mucosal damage. *Ann. Intern. Med. 87,* 676-679.
14. Mann, N.S. (1977): Acute erosive gastritis induced by D-penicillamine: its prevention by mylanta II, metiamide and cimetidine. *Clin. Res. 25,* 314A.
15. Mann, N.S. (1977): Aspirin and colchicine-induced acute erosive gastritis: its prevention by metiamide and cimetidine. *Gastroenterology 72,* 1094. (Abstract.)
16. Mann, N.S. (1977): Capasaicin-induced acute erosive gastritis: its prevention by mylanta II, metiamide and cimetidine. *Gastroenterology 72,* 1096. (Abstract.)

17. Mann, N.S. (1977): Drug-induced acute erosive gastritis: its prevention by antacid, metiamide and cimetidine. *Am. J. Proctol. 28,* 23-28.
18. Mann, N.S. (1977): Naproxen and tolectin-induced acute erosive gastritis: its prevention by metiamide and cimetidine. *Gastroenterology 72,* 1096. (Abstract.)
19. Mann, N.S. and Sachdev, A. (1976): Prevention of aspirin, ketoprofen and ibuprofen-induced acute erosive gastritis by metiamide and cimetidine. *Gastroenterology 70,* 914. (Abstract.)
20. Mann, N.S. and Sachdev, A. (1976): Prevention of naproxen-induced acute erosive gastritis by mylanta II, metiamide and cimetidine. *Gastroenterology 70,* 914. (Abstract.)
21. Mann, N.S. and Sachdev, A. (1977): Acute erosive gastritis induced by aspirin, ketoprofen, ibuprofen and naproxen: its prevention by metiamide and cimetidine. *South. Med. J. 70,* 562-564.
22. Mann, N.S., Borkar, B., Kadian, R.S. and Narenderan, K. (1977): Effect of metiamide and cimetidine on aspirin-induced reduction of gastric electrical potential in rat. *Gastroenterology 72,* 1096. (Abstract.)
23. Rainsfort, K.D. (1978): The role of aspirin in gastric ulceration: some factors involved in the development of gastric mucosal damage by aspiring in rats exposed to various stress conditions. *Am. J. Dig. Dis. 23,* 521-530.
24. Villafane, V., Cosen, J.N., Mazure, P.A. and Apray, M.O. (1978): Lesiones gastricas por stress experimental accion del acido-acetyl-salicilico (A.A.S.) y de le cimetidina. In: *Proceedings of the VI World Congress on Gastroenterology,* p. 133. Garsi, Madrid.
25. Welch, R.W., Bentch, H.L. and Harris, S.C. (1978): Reduction of aspirin-induced gastrointestinal bleeding with cimetidine. *Gastroenterology 74,* 459-463.

Discussion

Baron (London): Could Dr. Bader tell us more about the ethical problems of his colleagues? Coming from the country of Pascal and Descartes, I would have expected them to have thought it unethical to give a treatment to a series of patients if, at the end of that treatment, it was impossible to determine whether those patients had benefited or had been harmed.

Bader: I agree that the ethical aspect is a problem. I was involved in this protocol, but I was against this type of open trial — I say that very clearly. The reason put forward by the people who decided on this type of open trial was that it was not possible to give no treatment to these very severe ulcer disease patients. Placebo treatment would probably not be justified in these patients but, in my opinion, it would be reasonable to carry out a randomised controlled trial between cimetidine and antacid treatment. That is what I shall do if I make another trial in this area.

Molinari (Genoa): In the last few years we have collected a large series of patients with drug-induced gastric lesions, especially cases of diffuse haemorrhagic gastric erosions. There were 162 cases from 1973 to 1976, rising later to 234 cases. We have treated the last 50 cases with cimetidine, because the drug was available and on the basis of the pathophysiological premise of arresting, or at least of reducing, back-diffusion of hydrogen ions.

We did not feel able to rely exclusively on cimetidine and so used other measures as well, such as antacids and supportive treatment, including of course transfusion when necessary. I emphasize that our material was different from that reported, in that the patients rarely had acute peptic ulcers, but rather diffuse drug-induced lesions. We have had experience with various types of drugs with different modes of action but, in the final analysis, the same pathological picture.

In our experience, cimetidine proved to be a good drug in this type of lesion and the cases of acute peptic ulceration were found to be similar to cases of non-iatrogenic peptic ulceration. A monograph presenting these data has been published by Piccin.

Lorenz: Why were only rats and human subjects compared? Rats differ so greatly from man. Why is it not possible to present any data, say, on guinea-pigs, which are very similar to man in this respect? For instance, rats have the enzyme histidine decarboxylase, which is strongly influenced by all the anti-inflammatory drugs mentioned by Dr. Bader, but neither man nor the guinea-pig have this enzyme. Is there any experience with other species?

Bader: I agree that there is a need for such trials.

Cimetidine treatment of duodenal ulcer in children: a controlled trial

A.S. McNeish and C.A. Ayrton*

*Department of Child Health, University of Leicester, Leicester; and *Clinical Research Department, The Research Institute, Smith Kline & French Research Ltd., Welwyn Garden City, United Kingdom*

Introduction

The incidence of peptic ulcer disease in children is not known. Estimates include 3.9 per 100,000 [1], 3.4 per 10,000 hospital admissions [2], and 1 per 4,700 hospital admissions [3]. Several workers have reported that there may have been a true increase in incidence in recent years [4, 5], but this could be explained in part by an increased awareness among paediatricians of the fact that ulcer disease can and does occur in childhood.

Most authors recognize that peptic ulceration in childhood falls into 2 broad categories: *primary* ulceration of unknown aetiology, and ulceration which is *secondary* to an underlying disease, drug, or toxic substance [6] (see Table I).

Primary ulcers are usually chronic [6], arise in the duodenum much more commonly than in the stomach, and are found most frequently in children over the age of 12 years [2, 3, 6, 7]. Secondary ulcers may be acute, and they affect infants and preschool children as well as teenagers.

Chronic duodenal ulcer (DU) is 3 [7] to 7 [8] times more common in boys than in

Table I. Conditions that cause or are associated with secondary peptic ulceration in children.

Burns
Cirrhosis
Corticosteroids
Cushing's ulcer (encephalitis, trauma, meningitis, tumour)
Cystic fibrosis
Cystinosis
Extrahepatic portal hypertension
Hypoparathyroidism
Pyloric stenosis
Salicylates
Stress (infection, dehydration, hypoglycaemia, birth)
Tetralogy of Fallot
Transection of spinal cord T_1-T_4
Truncus arteriosus with pulmonary banding
Uraemia

girls. There is a positive family history of peptic ulcer in 28-65% of first-degree relatives [2, 9]. There is a significant excess of blood group O in childhood cases of DU [7], as with adults. Studies of gastric acid output report that it is normal [4, 7]. Several studies have revealed a high incidence of psychological stress in the lives of children with DU [6, 7].

Clinically, most cases of DU present with abdominal pain, which may be atypical in younger children. Vomiting and gastrointestinal bleeding are less common, but are important presenting features.

In previous large surveys of DU in children, the ulcers have been detected radiologically [2-7]. The increasing use of endoscopy in children, as in the present study, should improve the accuracy of diagnosis.

The course of DU in children is increasingly recognized as being chronic, with frequent exacerbations [10].

Conventional medical treatment with diet and antacids has given disappointing results and, in the last decade, there has been an increasing referral rate for elective surgery. This trend has been more pronounced in the United States [5] than in Europe [10].

To date, there have been few published studies of cimetidine therapy in children with DU: Lilly and Hitch reported prompt healing of 3 children with life-threatening ulcer disease in 1977 [11]; in 1978, Dogan et al. reported that 'the majority' of 20 children with DU 'benefited' from 1 month's treatment with cimetidine 30-50 mg/kg/day [12].

The British Paediatric Gastroenterology Group is an informal group of paediatric gastroenterologists who have regular scientific meetings and discussions. The present study developed from its recently-established collaborative study of endoscopically-proven DU in children, and involved cooperation with colleagues in continental Europe. The patients in this preliminary report came from 5 centres, 4 in the United Kingdom and 1 in Belgium.

Materials and methods

A double-blind trial was designed to assess the effectiveness of 4 weeks' treatment with cimetidine in healing endoscopically-proven DU in children, as compared with 4 weeks' treatment with placebo. This paper is a preliminary report of the first 16 patients to complete the trial.

Details of the age, sex and family history of these patients are given in Table II, of their presenting symptoms in Table III, and of the duration of disease in individual patients in Figure 1. There was 1 African child in the cimetidine group, and 1 Asian Indian in the placebo group; all other children were Caucasians. The mean (and range) of weight was 34.9 (31.0-40.6) kg in the cimetidine group, and 40.6

Table II. Age, sex and family history of 16 patients completing the trial.

Treatment group	Number of patients	Age (years)		Sex		Family history of ulcer disease
		Mean	Range	M	F	
Cimetidine	8	12.0	11-14	5	3	6
Placebo	8	12.6	10-15	5	3	8

Table III.   Clinical features presenting at the beginning of the trial.

Symptom	Number of patients presenting	
	Cimetidine group	Placebo group
Abdominal pain	7	7
Acid regurgitation	1	1
Haematemesis and melaena	2*	1
Haematemesis alone	1**	0
Vomiting and diarrhoea	0	1
Vomiting alone	0	1

*Occurred 3 days before entry in 1 of these patients; **occurred 4 weeks before entry. In both of these cases, symptoms were associated with abdominal pain.

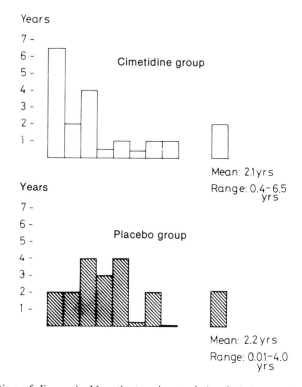

Fig. 1.   Duration of disease in 16 patients prior to their admission to the trial.

(29.4-59.0) kg in the placebo group. There were no significant differences between the 2 groups for any of these features.

Initially, the protocol for admission to the trial required that there had been no previous treatment with cimetidine, but this was later modified to allow inclusion provided that no cimetidine had been given to the child for at least 3 months prior to entry. Approval was obtained from the Ethical Committee of each participating centre, and informed consent was given by the parents of each child included in the study.

Table IV.   Scales for rating extent and severity of duodenitis, as assessed endoscopically at the beginning and end of the trial.

Rating	Severity	Extent
0	none	none
1	slight	localized, small
2	moderate	more than one area
3	severe	throughout cap

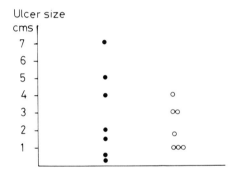

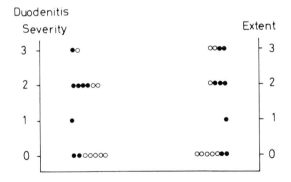

Fig. 2.   Size of duodenal ulcer, and severity and extent of duodenitis, at initial endoscopy.
• = 1 patient in cimetidine group; ○ = 1 patient in placebo group.

No more than 7 days before beginning either cimetidine or placebo treatment, an initial endoscopic assessment was performed on each subject: the number and size of duodenal ulcers was recorded, and duodenitis was rated visually according to the extent and severity scales shown in Table IV. Figure 2 shows the initial similarity of the 2 groups.

The methodology of the trial is shown in Figure 3. Patients were randomly allocated to 4 weeks' treatment with either cimetidine 20 mg/kg/day (in 3 cases modified to 25 mg/kg/day) or with a matching placebo. (At the time of the design of this study, little information was available on the use of cimetidine in children. The treatment dose that was chosen was 'extrapolated' from the standard adult dose

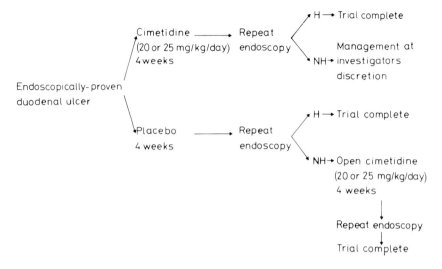

Fig. 3.   Trial methodology. (H = ulcer healed; NH = ulcer not healed.)

of 1 g/day irrespective of body weight, so that an average-sized child of 14 years would receive the full adult dosage [13].)

Only a standard antacid preparation (aluminum hydroxide) was allowed as treatment in addition to cimetidine or placebo. No dietary restrictions were imposed.

During the course of the trial, the children were seen weekly: clinical details were elicited; the consumption of drug and antacid was checked, by measuring the amounts of each of these treatment agents that were returned, and recorded; and routine haematology, serum biochemistry and urinalysis testing was performed (Table V).

All patients were re-endoscoped at the end of the 4 weeks of treatment.

Table V.   Routine investigations performed weekly on each patient throughout the course of the trial.

Haematology:	Haemoglobin
	Total WBC
	Film
Biochemistry:	SGOT/ASAT
	SGPT/ALAT
	Urea
	Creatinine
Urinalysis:	Protein
	Sugar
	Ketones
	Microscopy

Table VI.   Side-effects occurring during the trial.

Treatment group	Total number of patients experiencing side-effects	Side-effect	Number of patients experiencing side-effect
Cimetidine	3	Headache	1
		Unpleasant after-taste	1
		Nausea	1
		Vomiting	1
		Mild erythema	1
Placebo	2	Headache	1
		Vomiting	1
		Nasty taste	1

Results

There was an overall tendency for the mean number of daily episodes of abdominal pain to diminish during the trial, and the average daily consumption of antacid fell; however, no significant differences were observed between the cimetidine and placebo groups.

Side-effects were mild, and are summarized in Table VI.

Haematology, serum biochemistry and urinalysis testing was not significantly abnormal for any of the subjects during the course of the trial.

After 4 weeks of treatment, endoscopy showed complete healing of the duodenal ulcer in 5 of the 8 patients in the cimetidine group (62.5%), and in 4 of the 8 patients in the placebo group (50%).

Subsequent course of patients whose ulcers did not heal after 4 weeks' treatment with cimetidine

There were 3 patients in the cimetidine group whose ulcers did not heal after the initial 4 weeks of treatment.

Of these, 2 healed after a further 4 weeks' cimetidine treatment: 1 continued to receive a dosage of 20 mg/kg/day, and the other received 1 g/day (equivalent to 29.5 mg/kg/day).

The third child, a 12-year-old boy who had had symptoms for 4 years, also received cimetidine 1 g/day for an additional 4 weeks, but did not heal. At the beginning of the trial, a 1.5 cm DU had been found; at the end of 8 weeks of cimetidine treatment there were 2 DUs, 1 of 1.0 cm and 1 of 0.5 cm, with persisting duodenitis. Subsequently, this child had a vagotomy and pyloroplasty.

Subsequent course of patients whose ulcers did not heal after 4 weeks' treatment with placebo

There were 4 patients in the placebo group whose ulcers did not heal after the initial 4 weeks of treatment.

One of these patients had healing after 8 weeks of open cimetidine. Of the 3 who were treated with open cimetidine for 4 weeks, 1 healed, but continued to have mild duodenitis; 1 showed obvious improvement (DU reduced from 1.0 cm to 0.1 cm and duodenitis reduced in severity and extent from grade 3 to grade 1); the fourth, also given a further 4 weeks' open cimetidine (25 mg/kg/day), deteriorated. This latter patient had originally presented with haematemesis and melaena for 1 week, and had a 3.0 cm DU. After 4 weeks of treatment with placebo, the DU had reduced to 0.5 cm, but after the 4 weeks' further treatment with cimetidine it increased back to 0.7 cm; duodenitis also increased in severity and extent after cimetidine.

Discussion

Since the patients in our study were referred to us by various colleagues, with the pattern of referral being different in each centre, it is not possible to draw conclusions as to the prevalence of ulcer disease in children from our data.

The general clinical features of the children in our study resembled those of chronic primary DU described in our Introduction: all subjects were over 10 years of age, there was a preponderance of boys, abdominal pain was the predominant presenting symptom, and the majority had a family history of peptic ulcer. None had any of the conditions listed in Table I.

The diagnosis of DU in each case was made endoscopically. Although this is standard practice in adults, and the technique is being increasingly applied to children [14], there have been few systematic studies of endoscopically-proven DU in children to date. In the present study, one experienced endoscopist in each centre was responsible for the examinations.

Recently, Thompson and Lilly reported a significant reduction of gastric acid output in an infant, using cimetidine in a dose of 20 mg/kg/day [15]. Increasing the dose to 40 mg/kg/day produced a further reduction of gastric acid output, but the infant developed signs of cerebral toxicity that were reversed by stopping the drug. An older child, reported by Bale et al. [16], developed transient central nervous system dysfunction after 10 days of cimetidine 15 mg/kg/day.

In the present study, no significant adverse effect was observed in any patient, but the experiences cited above, albeit in single cases, suggest that cimetidine should be used with caution, especially in excess of 20-25 mg/kg/day.

The endoscopic findings at the onset of our trial were broadly comparable in both groups. The mean ulcer size was greater and the duodenitis scores were higher in the cimetidine group, but these differences were not significant.

The findings at the conclusion of the trial provoke 2 comments, which must be cautious because the numbers involved are small: first, a 50% healing rate with placebo is twice as high as has been reported in similar studies in adults [17, 18]; second, a high rate of spontaneous healing of DU in children in the short term has previously been reported [19], and spontaneous healing may represent a true feature of DU in this age group.

Our 62.5% healing rate after 4 weeks of cimetidine treatment (5 of 8 patients healed) is similar to the 61% healing rate that was reported in a study of adults treated with cimetidine 1 g/day [18], but is lower than the 85% healing rate achieved with the same dose in another series [19]. It is possible that cimetidine 20 mg/kg/day does not adequately inhibit gastric acid output in children; more data are needed.

Of the 7 patients who were given open cimetidine because of non-healing at the end of the initial 4-week trial period, 4 healed, 1 improved considerably, and 2 did not improve within the next 4 weeks. One of these 'failures' had a subsequent vagotomy and pyloroplasty and is now well. The other failure was given cimetidine for a further 6 weeks (total 14 weeks treatment: 4 with placebo and 10 with cimetidine); at the end of this period, the DU had healed.

The trial is continuing, and it is hoped that, with larger numbers, the results will be more clear-cut. However, the need to determine the weight-related dose of cimetidine that safely produces the most effective diminution of acid output in children will remain.

Acknowledgements

We are grateful to our colleagues for their collaboration in this trial, especially Dr R. Nelson and Dr E. Eastham of Newcastle, and Dr J. McClure of Ayr, United Kingdom; and Dr S. Cadranel of Brussels, Belgium.

References

1. Sultz, H.A., Schlesinger, E.R. and Feldman, J.G. (1970): The epidemiology of peptic ulcer in childhood. *Am. J. Publ. Health 60,* 492.
2. Deckelbaum, R.J., Roy, C.C., Lusier-Lazaroff, J. and Morin, C.L. (1974): Peptic ulcer disease: a clinical study in 73 children. *Can. Med. Assoc. J. 111,* 225.
3. Seagram, C.G.F., Stephens, C.A. and Cumming, W.A. (1973): Peptic ulceration at the Hospital for Sick Children, Toronto, during the 20 year period 1949-1969. *J. Pediatr. Surg. 8,* 407.
4. Habbick, B.F., Melrose, A.G. and Grant, J.C. (1968): Duodenal ulceration in childhood: a study of predisposing factors. *Arch. Dis. Child. 43,* 23.
5. Curci, M.R., Little, K., Sieber, W.K. and Kiesewetter, W.B. (1976): Peptic ulcer disease in childhood reexamined. *J. Pediatr. Surg. 11,* 329.
6. Nuss, D. and Lynn, H.B. (1971): Peptic ulceration in childhood. *Surg. Clin. North Am. 51,* 945.
7. Robb, J.D.A., Thomas, P.S., Orszulok, J. and Odling-Smee, G.W. (1972): Duodenal ulcer in children. *Arch. Dis. Child. 47,* 688.
8. Dogan, K., Oberiter, V., Najam, E., Dogan, S., Buneta, L., Rudar, D. and Mark, B. (1969): Some characteristics of peptic ulcer in children. *Lijec. Vjesn. 91,* 1058.
9. Prouty, M. (1970): Juvenile ulcers. *Am. Fam. Physician 100,* 814.
10. Puri, P., Boyd, E., Blake, N. and Guiney, E.J. (1978): Duodenal ulcer: a continuing disease in adult life. *J. Pediatr. Surg. 13,* 525.
11. Lilly, J.R. and Hitch, D.C. (1977): Cimetidine can control peptic ulcer disease in children. *Pediatr. Res. 11,* 445 (A444).
12. Dogan, K., Jurcic, Z., Rudar, D., Verona, E. and Lucev, Z. (1978): Experience in treatment of gastroduodenal ulcers with cimetidine (Tagamet) in children. In: *Proceedings of the VI World Congress of Gastroenterology, Madrid, 5-9 June, 1978,* p. 151.
13. Tanner, J.M., Whitehouse, R.H. and Takaishi, M. (1966): Standards from birth to maturity for height, weight, height velocity and weight velocity: British children 1965. *Arch. Dis. Child. 41,* 454.
14. Liebman, W.M. (1977): Fiberoptic endoscopy of the gastrointestinal tract in infants and children. *Am. J. Gastroenterol. 68,* 362.
15. Thompson, J. and Lilly, J. (1979): Cimetidine-induced cerebral toxicity in children. *Lancet 1,* 725.
16. Bale, J.F., Roberts, C. and Book, L.S. (1979): Ibid, 725.
17. Comparison of 2 doses of cimetidine and placebo in the treatment of duodenal ulcer. A multicentre trial. *Gut 20,* 68.

18. Gillespie, G., Gray, G.R., Smith, I.S., Mackenzie, I. and Crean, G.P. (1977): Short-term and maintenance cimetidine treatment in severe duodenal ulceration. In: *Cimetidine: Proceedings of the 2nd International Symposium on histamine H_2-receptor antagonists,* p. 240. Editors: W.L. Burland and M.A. Simkins. Excerpta Medica, Amsterdam-Oxford-Princeton.
19. Tudor, R.B. (1967): Peptic ulceration in children. *Pediatr. Clin. North Am. 14,* 109.

Discussion

Lorenz: Dr. McNeish mentioned that the optimal dose for cimetidine in children is probably not known. Has he any experience in individual children, studying those doses of cimetidine which inhibit gastric secretion?

McNeish: There are very few individual case reports in the literature. For instance, Lilly and co-workers gave a dose of 20 mg/kg/day to a baby. This dose was shown to significantly reduce maximal gastric acid output by nearly 60%. They also showed, in the same infant, that doubling the dose to 40 mg/kg/day caused a further diminution in gastric acid output. About the same time as this work was reported, however, the same group and another group each reported one child who developed signs of cerebral toxicity at a dose of 25 mg/kg/day in one case and about 40 mg/kg/day in the other.

There is need to obtain further data on optimal dose. We must proceed cautiously, however, as there is already the suggestion that if the dose is raised much above, say, 25 mg/kg/day, cerebral toxicity may be produced in children. There is the suggestion, at least from one or 2 cases, that 20 mg/kg/day or, in one case, 15 mg/kg/day will significantly reduce gastric acid output. We are therefore probably in about the right dose range.

Giacosa (Genoa): Were these patients followed up, was treatment continued or stopped?

McNeish: As I indicated, these patients were treated by various investigators in various centres. Therefore, at the completion of the trial, it again became the choice of the individual investigator as to what happened to them. I know what has happened to some patients, but overall they have been managed in a heterogeneous fashion and I have no data. For most of my colleagues I think that the principle has been that, once healing has occurred, treatment is stopped and we wait to see what happens.

Venables (Newcastle-upon-Tyne): Many of these cases came from our centre. The impression of my paediatric colleagues and of myself was that these children were not being healed as well as the adults I had seen treated with cimetidine, even those with not very large ulcers. For that reason, one or 2 of the patients — as Dr. McNeish pointed out — were treated with larger doses, with apparent healing.

This question of dosage is important. I wonder whether extrapolating from the infant situation into the young adult situation — which is where these children are — is correct. Perhaps the anxiety about using a larger dose is not really necessary. What does Dr. McNeish think about that idea?

McNeish: When we started this work we had no idea what was the right dose to use. This was why we extrapolated, but backwards. Our dose of 20-25 mg/kg/day was calculated to give the standard adult dose of 1 g/day to an average-sized 14-year-old. As paediatricians, we are very interested in that we know children come in different sizes. We have also observed that *adults* come in different sizes, but we never hear physicians relating the dose of a drug given to an adult to that adult's size. I guess that a dose of 1 g/day given to everybody in this room would have a greater variation in effect than would a dose of 20 mg/kg/day at various age ranges.

Venables: I think that this is true, except that when this point was investigated during our work in adults on cimetidine, no relationship was observed between dose and body weight.

Lorenz: From the pharmacological point of view, this is not completely true. If a dose of 1 g or 1.2 g is given, these are both within the optimum range, which means that giving a slightly higher or lower dose has less effect than a dose which is within the 50% range of the dose-response curve. We need to be careful — it is not all that easy to compare the doses.

Secondly, what about the type of operation? I think Dr. McNeish used vagotomy with pyloroplasty. It was in England that Mr. Johnston developed the nice operation of highly selective vagotomy; why was this not used?

McNeish: I cannot comment on that question because it was not my patient.

Gastric function after treatment with cimetidine

Richard H. Hunt, M.A. Melvin* and Jane G. Mills*
*Department of Gastroenterology, The Royal Naval Hospital, Haslar, Gosport; and
*The Research Institute, Smith Kline & French Research Ltd., Welwyn Garden City,
United Kingdom*

Introduction

Extensive clinical trials have confirmed the therapeutic efficacy of cimetidine, an H_2-receptor antagonist, in the short- and long-term maintenance treatment of peptic ulcer disease. It has been shown to inhibit basal and nocturnal acid output in man, as well as gastric acid stimulated by all known secretagogues [1]. The principal mechanism which prevents release of gastrin is acidification of the gastric antrum; marked inhibition of gastrin release occurs at pH values of 3 and below [2].

It has been suggested, however, that prolonged inhibition of gastric secretion by cimetidine might lead to hypergastrinaemia and a resultant increase in the parietal cell mass with rebound hypersecretion.

This paper reviews a number of studies of the effect of cimetidine treatment on gastric function in animals and, especially, in man.

Animal studies

In the rat, treatment with metiamide 800 mg·kg⁻¹ for 18 days resulted in a significant increase in the total number, total volume and volume density of parietal cells [3]. This increase correlated with an increase in stimulated gastric acid output, but no changes in fasting serum gastrin were observed after 16 days' treatment, nor was there any difference in the gastrin content of the antrum or G-cell population between treated animals and controls [4].

In another study, cimetidine given to rats in a very high daily dosage (150-950 mg·kg⁻¹) for periods of up to 2 years resulted in an increase in stomach size. A dose-dependent increase in parietal cell counts was observed, and was accounted for by the increase in surface area and thickness of the whole fundic mucosa; similar changes were also seen in the antral mucosa [5].

These animal studies used very high doses of an H_2-receptor antagonist; the data obtained from such studies are unlikely to be relevant to patients treated with conventional doses, especially since the pattern of gastric secretion in man is quite different from that seen in the rat.

Studies in man

The possibility of severe and sudden relapse of peptic ulceration within a few days of stopping long-term treatment with an H_2-receptor antagonist was raised by Saunders and Wormsley, following maintenance studies with metiamide [6]. In addition, isolated reports have been published describing perforation occurring shortly after discontinuing cimetidine treatment [7-12]. However, most of these studies were not controlled by endoscopic data, and the number of cases reported has been small, particularly when the widespread clinical use of cimetidine is considered.

Observations of 24-hour intragastric acidity in patients with duodenal ulceration have shown that treatment with cimetidine 0.8 or 1.6 g/day in divided doses leads to a marked reduction in intragastric hydrogen ion activity, throughout the study period [13]. Increasing the dose from 0.8 to 1.6 g/day made little difference in daytime intragastric acidity, but overnight a greater reduction in acid output was noted. In this study, the mean hourly intragastric hydrogen ion activity was reduced from 45.5 to 17.4 $mmol \cdot l^{-1}$ after treatment with cimetidine, which represents a rise in pH from 1.3 to 1.8, which is below the suggested threshold for release of gastrin [2]. Studies in 4 patients with complete remission of symptoms after truncal vagotomy showed a pattern of intragastric acidity similar to that observed after treatment with cimetidine [13]. A further study, in which 6 patients were studied with cimetidine both before and again 6 months after vagotomy, showed that cimetidine 400 mg reduced the mean hourly intragastric hydrogen ion activity overnight by 60% before vagotomy. Following vagotomy, mean hydrogen ion activity was reduced by 68%, from 40.7 $mmol \cdot l^{-1}$ (pH 1.39) to 13.0 $mmol \cdot l^{-1}$ (pH 1.88) [15].

These studies suggest that anacidity is not necessary to heal or prevent the recurrence of duodenal ulceration, and show that the reduction of intragastric hydrogen ion activity achieved by cimetidine is comparable to that achieved by vagotomy. Both treatments maintain the mean intragastric pH at a level below that at which gastrin is normally released, although Walsh et al. have suggested that in duodenal ulcer patients there may be a defect in the autoregulation of gastrin release. In a group of 7 healthy subjects, they found complete inhibition of meal-stimulated gastrin release when the intragastric pH was maintained at 2.5; however, in 6 patients with duodenal ulcer, gastrin release was still seen at this pH [16].

Serum gastrin after single-dose and short-term treatment with cimetidine

Studies in man have shown that cimetidine has no effect on fasting serum gastrin when given as a single oral dose. In 2 short-term studies, no change was seen 12 hours after the last dose of a 6-week course of treatment with cimetidine 1.6 g/day [17, 18]. In another study, no significant difference was seen in the mean fasting serum gastrin levels of a group of 21 duodenal ulcer patients treated with cimetidine 1.0 g/day for 4 weeks as compared with placebo, but a marked rise was seen in 4 of the cimetidine-treated patients [19].

Serum gastrin response to food is dependent on the change in intragastric pH: when the pH was maintained at a level of 5.5 by intragastric titration, cimetidine had no effect on either peak or integrated serum gastrin response [20, 21]; if, however, the pH was allowed to rise, a small but significant increase was seen during the second to third hour after the meal, with a corresponding increase in the total integrated serum gastrin response [21-23]. Following a single dose of cimetidine 300 mg, Sewing et al. reported an increase in the basal, peak and integrated serum gastrin in response to peptone meal stimulation, after 30 days' treatment with cimetidine 1.2 g/day [24]. In this study, a significant level of circulating cimetidine was observed throughout most of the study period.

Serum gastrin after long-term treatment with cimetidine

Arnold and Creutzfeldt carried out studies before and after 12 and 24 weeks' treatment with cimetidine, and reported no change in the serum gastrin response to a high-calorie liquid test meal, in the antral immunoreactive gastrin concentration, nor in the basal or stimulated gastric acid output [25].

Studies in 23 duodenal ulcer patients treated with cimetidine 1.6 g/day for 12 months have shown no effect on fasting serum gastrin. Peak serum gastrin and the integrated response to an 'Oxo' test meal were significantly increased after 12 months, in studies which were carried out only 12 hours after the last dose of cimetidine. Gastric secretory studies carried out 56 hours after the last dose of cimetidine showed a significant reduction in the basal acid output (BAO) at 3 months and no change at 1 year when compared with pre-treatment values, while peak acid output (PAO) was significantly reduced at both 3 and 12 months ($p < 0.01$) [26]. On completion of 12 months' treatment with cimetidine, patients were randomly allocated to placebo or continued cimetidine 800 mg at night, and serum gastrin responses were studied again after 24-55 weeks (mean 42.8 weeks) in 16 patients [27]. An increase in fasting serum gastrin and peak and integrated gastrin response was seen in these patients after the first year of treatment with cimetidine 1.6 g/day, but follow-up studies in 10 patients subsequently allocated to placebo showed that there were no longer any significant differences from pretreatment values.

Gastric secretory studies and their relationship to gastrin concentrations

Gastric acid secretion, fasting serum gastrin and the serum gastrin response to a meal have been measured in 17-22 duodenal ulcer patients before, during and after treatment with cimetidine 1 or 2 g/day for 4 or 8 weeks, followed by cimetidine 600 mg twice daily for 6 months [28]. No difference was seen in either the basal or maximal acid output after treatment with cimetidine. A small increase in fasting serum gastrin was observed both during (36%) and after (25%) treatment with cimetidine ($p < 0.02$). A marked increase was seen in the integrated gastrin response during treatment, but this had returned to pre-treatment levels when studied 5 days after withdrawal of the drug (Fig. 1).

Bodemar and Walan carried out gastric secretory studies before and after 1 year's maintenance treatment with cimetidine 400 mg twice daily or placebo [29]. Two days after withdrawal of treatment, a small but significant decrease in PAO was observed in 24 patients treated with cimetidine, and a decrease was still seen after 3.5 months (Fig. 2). No difference was seen in the fasting serum gastrin at the end of treatment with either cimetidine or placebo. Fasting serum gastrin measured in 22 patients during the last week of treatment with cimetidine, and again 2 days after withdrawal of treatment, showed a small but significant increase in 14 duodenal ulcer patients, but no difference was seen in the group as a whole, which also included 8 patients with prepyloric ulceration [30].

Kennedy reported increases in the serum gastrin response to a meal during treatment with cimetidine 1.0 g/day, but no significant increase was seen during maintenance therapy or on withdrawal of the drug [31].

A number of other studies have shown no alteration from pre-treatment values in maximal or peak acid output on withdrawal of cimetidine after 1-12 months' treatment with 1-1.6 g/day, nor any changes in the secretory response to a single dose of

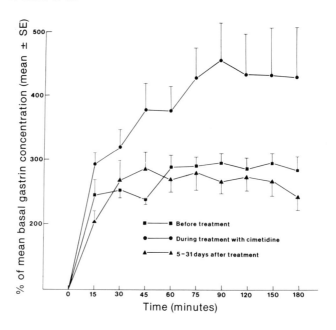

Fig. 1. *Serum gastrin concentrates, expressed as a percentage of mean basal concentration, in 17 duodenal ulcer patients after a standard meal. (Reproduced from [27] by permission of the author and the British Medical Association.)*

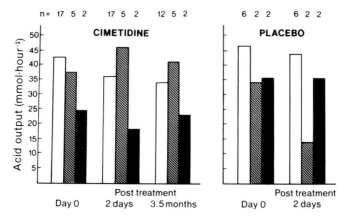

Fig. 2. *Peak acid output after 12 months' treatment with cimetidine or placebo in patients with duodenal ulcer (white bars), prepyloric ulcer (striped bars), and gastric ulcer (black bars). Adapted from [28].*

cimetidine [32-35]. Only 1 study has suggested an increase in BAO and PAO after stopping treatment: this was a comparative study with trithiozine, and the increase was not statistically significant [36].

Clinical studies

These data suggest that significant lasting hypergastrinaemia and parietal cell hypertrophy should not occur in association with cimetidine treatment in man, and that rebound hypersecretion of acid is unlikely to occur when treatment is withdrawn. These conclusions have been supported by the results of clinical studies.

Maintenance studies have demonstrated that cimetidine 400 mg twice daily or at night significantly protects against ulcer relapse [29, 37-40]. After 12 months of treatment, up to 83% of patients receiving placebo treatment had suffered a relapse, and a steady rate of relapse was seen throughout the placebo population. In none of these studies was there any evidence of a more rapid relapse rate following treatment with cimetidine.

Pooled data from 696 patients allowed comparison of the outcome in patients who, after treatment with cimetidine or placebo to heal their ulcers, were then given placebo for long-term maintenance. Throughout the follow-up, there was no evidence of a more rapid relapse in those patients whose ulcers had healed on cimetidine. Of patients who received cimetidine to heal their ulcer and were then maintained on placebo, 63% had a symptomatic recurrence of ulceration, compared with 47% of the smaller number of patients whose ulcer healed on placebo and who were maintained on placebo. This difference was not, however, statistically significant, and the latter group had a higher, though not significant, incidence of asymptomatic ulceration (38% against 22%) [41].

Treatment with cimetidine 1.0 g/day for 4 weeks produced an overall healing rate in the European trials of about 75%. In most of the unhealed ulcer cases, continuation of treatment with cimetidine results in healing of the ulcer. A number of attempts have been made to explain the relative lack of response in about 20% of the ulcers treated.

In the cat, atropine and metiamide have been shown to have an additive effect on the reduction of stimulated gastric acid secretion [42]. Studies in man, however, have failed to demonstrate any benefit from the addition of atropine or poldine to a night-time dose of cimetidine 400 mg [14, 43].

In most clinical trials, no difference in fasting serum gastrin has been seen between placebo- and cimetidine-treated groups of patients, and gastric secretory studies have proved inconclusive, probably because of the small numbers of patients whose ulcers have failed to heal after short-term treatment. Hetzel et al. showed that basal acid output was significantly higher in 5 patients whose ulcers failed to heal than in 24 whose ulcers healed [44]. Although maximal acid output was also higher, the increase was not statistically significant. They suggested that during maintenance treatment with cimetidine, some of those patients who relapsed had increased acid secretion. In another study, Cargill et al. reported that patients who remained well on cimetidine maintenance, or whose ulcers recurred late, tended to have lower acid and pepsin secretory responses than patients whose ulcers recurred rapidly after stopping treatment, but the differences were not statistically significant [45].

Our own studies of the 24-hour intragastric acidity in a group of duodenal ulcer patients treated with cimetidine 1.0 g/day has led us to suggest that 2 groups of patients can be identified by their response to cimetidine [15]. We have now studied 20 patients, 12 of whom showed a dramatic response to a 400 mg bedtime dose and were anacidic for several hours, while the other 8 showed only a small decrease in

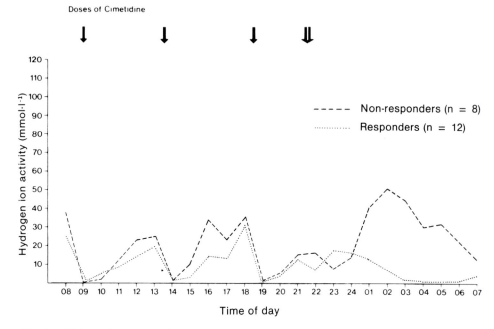

Fig. 3. *24-hour intragastric hydrogen ion activity in duodenal ulcer patients during treatment with cimetidine 1 g/day.*

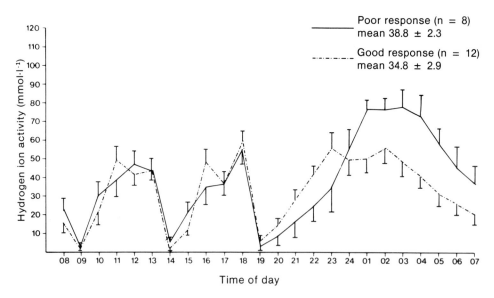

Fig. 4. 24-hour intragastric hydrogen ion activity in 2 groups of duodenal ulcer patients (good and poor responders to cimetidine) during treatment with placebo.

intragastric acidity (Fig. 3). The data for these 2 groups, when studied on placebo, show that there is a significant difference between them at night (Fig. 4). It remains to be seen whether or not these patients show any other special features with respect to their gastric secretory patterns, and if this is related to the rate of ulcer healing.

Summary and conclusions

The theoretical arguments for the development of hypergastrinaemia and a resultant increase in parietal cell mass with rebound hypersecretion are not supported by the literature. The results of studies following single-dose, short-term and longer-term treatment with cimetidine have shown no clear pattern of change in the serum gastrin response. Fasting serum gastrin may rise in some patients, but generally little change has been reported. The integrated gastrin response to food increases during treatment with cimetidine, but rapidly returns to normal on withdrawal of the drug. However, these changes in the serum gastrin response do not appear to be related to changes in gastric acid secretion. On withdrawal of treatment, either no change or a decrease in stimulated acid output has been observed.

Treatment of duodenal ulcers with cimetidine 1.0 g/day heals the ulcer in the majority of patients, but there is at the present time no way of predicting which of the patient population will fail to heal or will relapse more rapidly than others. A number of studies have suggested that differences in gastric secretory status might contribute to this variation in response. Studies of gastric acidity have shown a difference in the response to cimetidine in patients with higher acid secretion overnight. It is also possible that, in some duodenal ulcer patients, a defect in the autoregulation of gastrin release may contribute to a relative hypergastrinaemia following a small rise in intragastric pH. Further studies are required to clarify these mechanisms. In the majority of patients, however, the response to cimetidine is more predictable, and studies to date suggest no deleterious effects on the regulation of gastric function.

References

1. Burland, W.L., Hunt, R.H., Mills, J.G. and Milton-Thompson, G.J. (1979): Drugs of the decade 1970-79: cimetidine. *Br. J. Pharmacotherapy 2*, 24-40.
2. Uvnas, B. (1962): Mechanisms of gastrin release. *XXII International Congress of Physiological Science 1*, 342-347.
3. Witzel, L., Halter, F., Olah, A.H. and Hacki, W.H. (1977): Effects of prolonged metiamide medication on fundic mucosa. *Gastroenterology 73*, 797-803.
4. Witzel, L., Heitz, P.V., Halter, F., Olah, A.J., Varga, L., Werner, O. and Hacki, W.H. (1979): Effects of prolonged administration of metiamide on serum gastrin, gastrin content of the antrum and gastric corpus, and G-cell population in the rat. *Gastroenterology 76*, 945-949.
5. Crean, G.P., Daniel, D., Leslie, G.B. and Bates, C. (1978): The effects of prolonged administration of large doses of cimetidine on the gastric mucosa of rats. In: *Cimetidine: the Westminster Hospital Symposium*, pp. 191-205. Editors: C. Wastell and P. Lance. Churchill Livingstone, Edinburgh.
6. Saunders, J.H.B. and Wormsley, K.G. (1977): Long-term effects and after-effects of treatment of duodenal ulcer with metiamide. *Lancet 1*, 765-767.
7. Wallace, W.A., Orr, C.M.E. and Bearn, A.R. (1977): Perforation of chronic peptic ulcers after cimetidine. *Br. Med. J. 2*, 856-866.
8. Gill, M.J. and Saunders, J.B. (1977): Perforation of chronic peptic ulcers after cimetidine. *Br. Med. J. 2*, 1149.
9. Keighley, B.D. (1977): Perforation of peptic ulcer after withdrawal of cimetidine. *Br. Med. J. 2*, 1022.
10. Hoste, P., Ingels, J., Elewaut, A. and Barbier, F. (1978): Duodenal perforation after cimetidine. *Lancet 1*, 666.

11. Buck, J.P., Murgatroyd, R.E., Boylston, A.W. and Baron, J.H. (1979): Perforation of gastric carcinoma (at site of previous benign ulcer) after withdrawal of cimetidine. *Lancet 2*, 42.
12. Bulman, A.S. (1979): Cimetidine and duodenal ulcer. *Br. Med. J. 1*, 409-410.
13. Pounder, R.E., Williams, J.G., Hunt, R.H., Vincent, S.H., Milton-Thompson, G.J. and Misiewicz, J.J. (1977): The effects of oral cimetidine on food-stimulated gastric acid secretion and 24-hour intragastric acidity. In: *Cimetidine: Proceedings of the second International Symposium on histamine H$_2$-receptor antagonists*, pp. 189-204. Editors: W.L. Burland and M.A. Simkins. Excerpta Medica, Amsterdam-Oxford-Princeton.
14. Pounder, R.E., Hunt, R.H., Vincent, S.H., Milton-Thompson, G.J. and Misiewicz, J.J. (1977): 24-hour intragastric acidity and nocturnal acid secretion in patients with duodenal ulcer during oral administration of cimetidine and atropine. *Gut 18*, 85-90.
15. Hunt, R.H., Pounder, R.E., Williams, J.G., Vincent, S.H., Misiewicz, J.J. and Milton-Thompson, G.J. (1978): Reduction of intragastric acidity in duodenal ulcer. Cimetidine or surgery? *Acta Gastro-enterol. Belg. 41*, 458-462.
16. Walsh, J.H., Richardson, C.T. and Fordtran, J.S. (1975): pH dependence of acid secretion and gastrin release in normal and ulcer patients. *J. Clin. Invest. 55*, 462-468.
17. Siewert, R., Lepsien, G., Arnold, R. and Creutzfeldt, W. (1977): Effect of cimetidine on lower oesophageal sphincter pressure, intragastric pH and serum levels of immunoreactive gastrin in man. *Digestion 15*, 81-85.
18. Bank, S., Barbezat, G.O., Vinik, A.I. and Helman, C. (1977): Serum gastrin levels before and after 6 weeks of cimetidine therapy in patients with duodenal ulcer. *Digestion 15*, 157-161.
19. Vantini, I., Ederle, A., Bovo, P., Vaona, B., Piubello, W., Benini, L., Cavallini, G. and Scuro, L.A. (1978): Serum fasting gastrin levels after short-term treatment with cimetidine in patients with duodenal ulcer. *Acta Hepato-Gastroenterol. 25*, 376-379.
20. Pounder, R.E., Williams, J.G., Russell, R.C.G., Milton-Thompson, G.J. and Misiewicz, J.J. (1976): Inhibition of food-stimulated gastric acid secretion by cimetidine. *Gut 17*, 161-168.
21. Richardson, C.T., Walsh, J. and Hicks, M.I. (1976): The effect of cimetidine, a new histamine H$_2$-receptor antagonist, on meal-stimulated acid secretion, serum gastrin and gastric emptying in patients with duodenal ulcer. *Gastroenterology 71*, 19-23.
22. Longstreth, G.F., Go, V.L.W. and Malagelada, J.-R. (1977): Postprandial gastric, pancreatic and biliary response to histamine H$_2$-receptor antagonists in active duodenal ulcer. *Gastroenterology 72*, 9-13.
23. Heading, R.C., Logan, R.F.A., McLoughlin, G.P., Lidgard, G.E. and Forrest, J.A.H. (1977): Effect of cimetidine on gastric emptying. In: *Cimetidine: Proceedings of the second International Symposium on histamine H$_2$-receptor antagonists*, pp. 145-152. Editors: W.L. Burland and M.A. Simkins. Excerpta Medica, Amsterdam-Oxford-Princeton.
24. Sewing, K.F., Hagie, L., Ippoliti, A.F., Isenberg, J.I., Samloff, I.M. and Sturdevant, R.A.L. (1978): Effect of one-month treatment with cimetidine on gastric secretion and serum gastrin and pepsinogen levels. *Gastroenterology 74*, 376.
25. Arnold, R. and Creutzfeldt, W. (1978): Basal and meal-stimulated serum gastrin, antral G-cells and gastrin concentration during cimetidine therapy. In: *Cimetidine: Proceedings of an International Symposium on histamine H$_2$-receptor antagonists*, pp. 87-89. Editor: W. Creutzfeldt. Excerpta Medica, Amsterdam-Oxford-Princeton.
26. Spence, R.W., Celestin, L.R., McCormick, D.A., Owens, C.J. and Oliver, J.M. (1978): The effect of long-term treatment with cimetidine on gastric acid secretion and gastric responses in man. In: *Cimetidine: Proceedings of an International Symposium on histamine H$_2$-receptor antagonists*, p. 116-135. Editor: W. Creutzfeldt. Excerpta Medica, Amsterdam-Oxford-Princeton.
27. Spence, R.W., McCormick, D.A., Oliver, J.M. and Celestin, L.R. (1978): The effect on serum gastrin of withdrawal of cimetidine after one year's treatment. In: *Cimetidine: the*

Westminster Hospital Symposium, pp. 153-167. Editors: C. Wastell and P. Lance. Churchill Livingstone, Edinburgh.

28. Forrest, J.A.H., Fettes, M., McLoughlin, G. and Heading, R.C. (1979): Effect of long-term cimetidine on gastric acid secretion, serum gastrin and gastric emptying. *Gut 20,* 404-407.

29. Bodemar, G. and Walan, A. (1978): Maintenance treatment of recurrent peptic ulcer by cimetidine. *Lancet 1,* 403-407.

30. Bodemar, G., Walan, A. and Lundquist, G. (1978): Gastric concentrations at the end of and following long-term treatment with cimetidine and placebo. In: *Cimetidine: Proceedings of an International Symposium on histamine H_2-receptor antagonists,* pp. 233-235. Editor: W. Creutzfeldt. Excerpta Medica, Amsterdam-Oxford-Princeton.

31. Kennedy, T. (1978): Recurrent ulcer after vagotomy or gastrectomy treated with cimetidine. In: *Cimetidine: the Westminster Hospital Symposium,* pp. 79-83. Editors: C. Wastell and P. Lance. Churchill Livingstone, Edinburgh.

32. Barbezat, G.O. and Bank, S. (1978): Effect of prolonged cimetidine therapy on gastric acid secretion in man. *Gut 19,* 151-154.

33. Holden, R.J., Hearns, J.B., McKibben, B., Buchanan, K.B. and Crean, G.P. (1977): Long-term effects of cimetidine on gastric secretion. *Gut 18,* A949.

34. Holden, R.J., Weetch, M., Arachmandritis, N., Hearns, J. and Crean, G.P. (1978): Dose response of acid and pepsin secretion to pentagastrin infusion during treatment with cimetidine. *Gut 19,* A441.

35. Aadland, E. and Berstad, A. (1978): Effect of cimetidine on pentagastrin-stimulated acid and pepsin output before and after 6 weeks of cimetidine treatment. *Scand. J. Gastroenterol. 13,* 193-197.

36. Brown, P., Ceravolo, C. and Zambelli, A. (1978): Rebound rise in gastric acid secretion: study of cimetidine vs trithiozine: a preliminary report. *Curr. Ther. Res., Clin. Exp. 23,* 706-708.

37. Gray, G.R., Smith, I.S., Mackenzie, I. and Gillespie, G. (1978): Long-term cimetidine in the management of severe duodenal ulcer dyspepsia. *Gastroenterology 74,* 397-400.

38. Gudman-Hoyer, E., Jensen, K.B., Krag, E., Rask-Madsen, J., Rahbek, I., Rune, S.J. and Wulff, H.R. (1978): Prophylactic effect of cimetidine in duodenal ulcer disease. *Br. Med. J. 1,* 1095.

39. Bardhan, K.D., Saul, D.M., Edwards, J.L., Smith, P.M., Haggie, S.J., Wyllie, J.H., Duthie, H.L. and Fussey, I.V. (1979): Double-blind comparison of cimetidine and placebo in the maintenance treatment of healing chronic duodenal ulceration. *Gut 20,* 158-162.

40. Hansky, J., Korman, M.G., Hetzel, D.J. and Shearman, D.J.C. (1979): Relapse rate after cessation of 12 months cimetidine in duodenal ulcer. *Gastroenterology 76,* 1151.

41. Burland, W.L., Hawkins, B.W. and Beresford, J. (1979): Cimetidine treatment for the prevention of recurrence of duodenal ulcer: an international collaborative study. *Postgrad. Med. J.* (In press.)

42. Venables, C.W., Stephen, J.G., Blair, E.L., Reed, J.D. and Saunders, J.D. (1978): Cimetidine in the treatment of duodenal ulceration and the relationship of this therapy to surgical management. In: *Cimetidine: the Westminster Hospital Symposium,* pp. 13-27. Editors: C. Wastell and P. Lance. Churchill Livingstone, Edinburgh.

43. Blackwood, W.S. and Northfield, T.C. (1977): Nocturnal gastric acid secretion: effect of cimetidine and interaction with anticholinergics. In: *Cimetidine: Proceedings of the second International Symposium on histamine H_2-receptor antagonists,* pp. 124-130. Editors: W.L. Burland and M.A. Simkins. Excerpta Medica, Amsterdam-Oxford-Princeton.

44. Hetzel, D.J., Hansky, J., Shearman, D.J.C., Korman, M.G., Hecker, R., Taggart, G.J., Jackson, R. and Gabb, B.W. (1978): Cimetidine treatment of duodenal ulceration. Short-term clinical trial and maintenance study. *Gastroenterology 74,* 389-392.

45. Cargill, J.M., Peden, N., Saunders, J.H.B. and Wormsley, K.G. (1978): Very long-term treatment of peptic ulcer with cimetidine. *Lancet 2,* 1113-1115.

Discussion

Giacosa (Genoa): Starting from the speculative and experimental bases to which you referred at the beginning, and on the basis also of the animal studies previously reported, we performed a study some time ago on the behaviour of parietal cells in patients during cimetidine therapy. This study has shown that, at one month, after short-term therapy, there were no differences whatever; on the other hand, on subsequent evaluation at 9 months in patients healed at 28 days with 1 g and maintained on 400 mg in the evening, significant increases were found, not only in the parietal cell mass, which in vivo cannot be correctly demonstrated, but also in the parietal cell index, which was extrapolated by multiplying the number of cells per unit of surface area by the thickness of the glandular parenchyma.

We are now waiting to determine what happens after treatment is stopped. We are also in the process of assessing a group of patients treated with a lower dose. In Crean's study there was a very close relationship between the dose of the drug and the effect induced in the animal.

My question to Dr. Hunt is: in your opinion, what conclusions can be drawn?

Hunt: I am not sure that any conclusions can be drawn at this time. As I stressed in my presentation, the animal studies of Witzel and colleagues and Crean and colleagues used enormous doses of an H_2-receptor antagonist; such doses cannot be extrapolated to man, even though the pattern of gastric secretion in the rat may be similar. If Dr. Giacosa is trying to do a similar study in man, he will have great difficulty in controlling the experiment satisfactorily.

Baron (London): If my model is accepted, that there is a threshold for acid output below which duodenal ulcer does not occur, and if it is also accepted that those patients in whom the surgeon reduces acid output below this threshold with surgical vagotomy will not get a recurrence, then the medical model becomes entirely one of reducing acid output during cimetidine treatment to below this threshold. Dr. Hunt has shown, I think for the first time, that patients who do not heal with cimetidine are patients in whom overnight acid has not been abolished with a conventional dose of cimetidine. Could Dr. Hunt say whether this is because, while the pharmacokinetics in those patients is such that a satisfactory blood level of the drug is achieved, their parietal cells are resistant to that blood level, or because those patients did not achieve a satisfactory blood level with the standard dose of cimetidine?

Hunt: Dr. Baron has raised a number of important points. The first suggestion, that there might be some variability in response at night, was observed during the early studies with metiamide. This variability appeared to be related to gastric emptying. In fact, we do not have sufficient data on blood levels, because when this observation was originally made it was during our analysis of studies which had already been carried out. The data were being analysed from a variety of different angles, with the help of the statistician. The way in which these 2 groups were actually occurring was observed at that time. This is why it is not possible to say whether this is closely related to other factors, such as gastric emptying or gastrins, in these particular patients. These factors are now being studied prospectively.

Lorenz: It has been shown in man that cimetidine acts not only at H_2-receptors, but also that it influences histamine metabolism. This has been confirmed by 2 groups, ourselves and Wormsley and Thjodleifsson. We have set up a trial to determine whether there are patients with an abnormal histamine metabolism in their gastric mucosa. Do those non-responders reported by Dr. Hunt have an abnormal histamine metabolism?

Hunt: I cannot answer that question.

Baron: The obvious conclusion of the data is that it is the night acid which is important, not the day acid, in whether someone has an ulcer and whether that ulcer heals. Are there any data from anywhere in the world in which patients with ulcers have been treated with cimetidine at night only, to try to heal those ulcers?

Hunt: That is an attractive idea, which we have discussed on a number of occasions. To my knowledge, this has not yet been done.

The local effects of cimetidine, carbenoxolone and acetylsalicylic acid on buccal mucosal potential difference

G.J. Huston
Department of Clinical Pharmacology, St. Bartholomew's Hospital, London, United Kingdom

Introduction

Cimetidine and carbenoxolone are drugs used in the treatment of ulceration of the gastrointestinal tract: cimetidine acts by H_2-receptor antagonism, which leads to a decrease in gastric acid secretion [1]; the mode of action of carbenoxolone is unknown, although effects on cell turnover [2], changes in the characteristics of gastric mucus [3], and an effect on stabilisation of biological membranes [4] have all been suggested.

Many mucosal effects have been interpreted in terms of a 'mucosal barrier' [5], which acts as a protector of gastric mucosa against peptic ulceration. This barrier, which has no definite morphological boundaries, is defined in terms of its physiological functions. Increased H^+ ion insorption or Na^+ efflux from the mucosa [6], or a positive shift in transmucosal or transmural potential difference [7], have both been interpreted as indicating damage to this barrier.

None of these physiological parameters is entirely satisfactory as an explanation of morphological mucosal damage, but a correlation between a positive shift in gastric mucosal potential difference and increasing mucosal damage as assessed by multiple biopsies has been demonstrated [8, 9].

As the release of mucosal histamine may be of importance in the pathophysiology of mucosal damage [10], the possibility that H_2-receptor antagonists may interfere directly with the mechanisms of mucosal damage has been considered [11]; the present study examines this possibility further. The local effects of carbenoxolone, which is used to treat buccal ulcers and, when combined with alginic acid, is of proven value in the treatment of oesophagitis [12], have also been examined. The physiological parameter of functional mucosal integrity measured in this study was buccal mucosal potential difference (b.p.d.), which responds in a quantitatively-similar fashion to gastric potential difference induced by mucosal damaging agents [7, 13], and is not affected by changes in salivary flow or mineralocorticoid activity.

The direct and modifying effects of cimetidine 25 mg and carbenoxolone 5 mg on potential difference induced by acetylsalicylic acid were also examined.

Materials and methods

Eight healthy volunteers (6 males, age range 30-52 years; 2 females, aged 23 and 26 years) were studied. Prior to entry, each volunteer was medically examined, blood and urine samples were obtained for laboratory analysis, and informed written consent was obtained.

The study was designed as a single-blind randomised crossover, comparing the effects of both single and multiple doses of 4 medications: cimetidine 25 mg, carbenoxolone 5 mg, cimetidine placebo and carbenoxolone placebo. Half of the subjects were treated on the right side of the mouth throughout the course of the study, and half were treated on the left side. The treatment effect of multiple dosing with each of the 4 medications was examined both before and after acetylsalicylic acid challenge.

The order of treatments was randomised according to a Latin Square design, with at least 1 week between treatment regimes. Each treatment lasted 4 days, with b.p.d. measurements taken on days 1 and 4.

B.p.d. was measured using a probe electrode constructed from a perspex tube with a silver-silver chloride saline agar junction [14], which was placed on the lower lip between lip and gum as described by Huston [13]. The reference electrode was strapped over a bleb raised on the forearm by intradermal injection of saline [15]. The potential difference was measured on an Orion pH/mV meter, examined and accepted as conforming to U.K. safety requirements by the Equipment Safety Officer at St. Bartholomew's Hospital, London.

On day 1, the subjects received a standard breakfast at 8 a.m. At 11 a.m., the baseline b.p.d. on the left and right sides of the lip between lip and gum was measured. Five minutes after baseline measurement, each subject received the allocated treatment, administered in tablet form; the treatment tablet was placed between the buccal mucosa and gum on the appropriate side. After complete dissolution of the tablet, all drug residue was washed away with 100 ml of deionised water; b.p.d. was measured 5, 10 and 15 minutes after the time of complete dissolution. The subjects then received further treatment doses, always on the same side of the mouth, at approximately 6-hour intervals for the remainder of study day 1, and throughout days 2 and 3.

On day 4, the subjects received a standard breakfast at 8 a.m. and treatment at 9 a.m. After b.p.d. measurement at 11 a.m., a second treatment dose was administered; following complete dissolution and washing away of drug residue with 100 ml of deionised water, b.p.d. was again measured. The subject then received 3 tablets of acetylsalicylic acid 300 mg, dissolved in 15 ml deionised water, which was held in the vestibule of the mouth between lip and gum for 3 minutes. Drug residue was washed away with 100 ml deionised water, and b.p.d. was measured 2 minutes later and at 3-minute intervals for the next 21 minutes.

Statistical methods

On day 1, the pretreatment b.p.d. was compared with the b.p.d. measurements taken 5, 10 and 15 minutes after dissolution of the administered drug. On day 4, comparisons were made between baseline b.p.d. and the least negative b.p.d. recorded after acetylsalicylic acid administration; the elapsed time from acetylsalicylic acid administration to least negative b.p.d. was also examined. Since there was no barrier to prevent drug diffusion away from the treated side of the mouth, the b.p.d. on the untreated side may also have been affected by the administered drug; therefore, the potential differences on the treated and untreated sides were considered separately, and a comparison of treated side b.p.d. versus untreated side b.p.d. was made as well, by subtracting the untreated side b.p.d. value from the treated side value.

Statistical analysis of these data was carried out, after inspection of the standard deviations indicated that there was a normal distribution. Analysis of variance was used to test for significant differences between the effects of cimetidine, cimetidine placebo, carbenoxolone and carbenoxolone placebo. Where differences occurred, further analysis was performed, using Student's *t* test. Since there was no statistically-significant difference between the 2 placebo groups, these 2 groups were combined.

Results

The data from the study are shown graphically in Figures 1 and 2.

On day 1, no significant difference between pretreatment b.p.d. and b.p.d. measured at 5, 10 or 15 minutes after administration of a single treatment dose was found when the treated and untreated sides were examined separately. However, when treated side minus untreated side values were examined, significant differences were found between carbenoxolone and the combined placebo group at 10 and 15 minutes ($p < 0.01$), and also between cimetidine and carbenoxolone at 10 and 15 minutes ($p < 0.05$). No significant difference was found between cimetidine and the combined placebo group.

These data suggest that, although some diffusion of carbenoxolone to the untreated side of the mouth may have occurred, the local effect of carbenoxolone on the treated side was much greater on the treated mucosa. The direct effect of cimetidine on the buccal mucosa appeared to be minimal.

On day 4, a comparison was made between baseline b.p.d. and the least negative b.p.d. measured after administration of acetylsalicylic acid. The b.p.d. after acetylsalicylic acid was found to be significantly less negative on both treated and

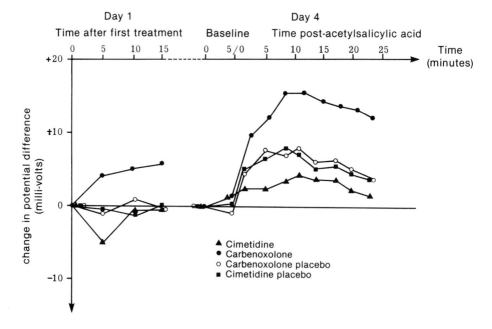

Fig. 1.   *Mean changes in potential difference on the treated side of the mouth.*

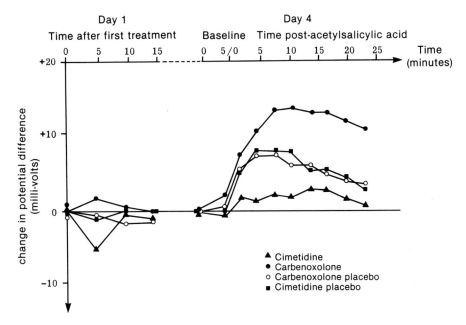

Fig. 2. *Mean changes in potential difference on the untreated side of the mouth.*

untreated sides of the mouth after carbenoxolone treatment than after either cimetidine or placebo ($p < 0.01$). When treated side minus untreated side values for carbenoxolone after acetylsalicylic acid were compared with those for placebo after acetylsalicylic acid, a significant difference was demonstrated for positive shift of b.p.d. ($p < 0.01$), suggesting that maximum potentiation of acetylsalicylic acid-induced b.p.d. change was occurring on the treated side, presumably due to a higher concentration of active agent on this side.

Analysis of the data from the treated mucosa alone showed no significant difference in acetylsalicylic acid-induced mucosal response between cimetidine and placebo. When a comparison of treated minus untreated sides was made, a significant difference between cimetidine and placebo *was* demonstrated ($p < 0.05$), suggesting that cimetidine may have a local concentration-dependent effect in attenuating acetylsalicylic acid-induced b.p.d. response.

A second comparison was made between baseline b.p.d. on day 1 and the least negative b.p.d. after administration of acetylsalicylic acid on day 4, in order to assess the maximum total change in b.p.d. over the 4-day period. After carbenoxolone treatment, b.p.d. was significantly less negative after acetylsalicylic acid on both treated ($p < 0.001$) and untreated ($p < 0.01$) sides of the mouth, when compared with placebo; when carbenoxolone was compared with cimetidine, there was a significant difference between the treated sides ($p < 0.001$), but no significant difference between the untreated sides. Using this maximum change measurement to compare treated minus untreated sides for the combined placebo group, a significant difference was demonstrated with carbenoxolone only ($p < 0.001$). No significant difference between most positive shift in b.p.d. over the 4-day period was found between cimetidine and placebo, or in the time taken to achieve least negative b.p.d. after acetylsalicylic acid for any treatment.

No adverse reactions or clinically-significant changes in laboratory tests were observed during the study.

Discussion

Most studies of mucosal damage and protection have been performed on gastric mucosa, and have involved either direct observation of mucosal ulceration [16, 17] or interpretation of physiological changes [6, 7]. The present study was based on this latter principle, which permits in vivo study without the necessity for mucosal destruction.

There has been some disagreement over the interpretation of mucosal physiological changes. Disruption of the gastric mucosal barrier was initially considered to be associated with the loss of luminal H^+ ions [6]. More recently, however, it has become apparent that H^+ loss may occur in the absence of mucosal injury, and that damage can occur at very low luminal concentrations of H^+ [18]; consequently, H^+ loss cannot be considered an absolute hallmark of mucosal damage.

There has been a similar controversy regarding the use of potential difference as an indicator of mucosal damage. It has been shown that local treatment with acetylsalicylic acid and ethanol causes a positive shift in mucosal potential difference [7, 13], and an association between a positive shift in gastric potential difference and gastric epithelial cell damage has been confirmed by biopsy experiments [9]. Before measured potential difference is accepted as an indicator of mucosal damage, sources of potential difference change *other* than interference with mucosal cell function should first be eliminated.

In the present study, the possible sources considered were: changes in the junction potentials caused by changes in the H^+ ion content of the solution bathing the probe electrodes, which we minimised by washing away drug residue from the buccal mucosa with deionised water before making potential difference measurements; mucosal/electrode pressure artifacts [13], eliminated as far as possible by avoiding mucosal distortion; diurnal potential difference changes produced by changes in autonomic activity [19], reduced by performing all experiments at the same time of day; and mineralocorticoid effects, which may produce large changes in potential difference in the large gut, but have been shown not to affect buccal potential difference [13].

Because of the possibility that local mechanical trauma caused by the treatment tablets themselves might affect potential difference, it was considered essential that identical placebos were obtained for both active treatments. Because of the difficulty in matching the carbenoxolone and cimetidine placebos, however, separate placebos for each agent were ultimately used. As anticipated, neither placebo produced a change in measured potential difference. In view of this lack of difference between placebo effects, the 2 placebo groups were combined.

As no barrier to the diffusion of either active agent was included in this study, the untreated side of the mouth probably represented a mucosal surface treated with a low concentration of active agent. It was apparent that carbenoxolone decreased b.p.d. on both sides of the mouth and potentiated acetylsalicylic acid-induced changes in potential difference, in marked contrast to its lack of direct effect on gastric potential difference in normal subjects and its effect in inhibiting acetylsalicylic acid-induced change in patients with gastric ulcer [20]. This finding does not support the assumption that carbenoxolone protects the normal functioning of squamous epithelium.

The apparently adverse local effect of carbenoxolone has been demonstrated in the cotton pellet granuloma test in rats [21] and, though low (10^{-5} M) concentrations of carbenoxolone have been shown to produce a 12-22% stabilisation of liposomal membranes, high concentrations (10^{-3} M) produce a marked lytic effect [4]. This latter observation may be particularly relevant, as it has been demonstrated that increased liposomal fragility is important in the genesis of drug-induced ulceration [22].

A combination of carbenoxolone and alginic acid has been shown to promote healing of ulcers and areas of oesophagitis in the lower oesophagus [12]. The mode of action here is not understood, but it is possible that this oesophageal effect is secondary to a qualitative alteration in the recurrently-refluxing gastric contents, and not to a direct effect on the squamous mucosa. The local mucosal concentrations generated by the 20 mg dose of carbenoxolone in this preparation are not known; however, they seem likely to be less than those produced by trapping a 5 mg carbenoxolone pellet in 1 position on the buccal mucosa.

In the present study, cimetidine treatment had an attenuating effect on acetylsalicylic acid-induced mucosal potential difference changes. This was in keeping with earlier findings that doses of cimetidine, insufficient to decrease acid secretion, decreased the incidence of mucosal lesions caused by local application of acetylsalicylic acid and hydrochloric acid in gastric mucosa in the rat [11]. This direct mucosal activity has been termed 'cytoprotection' and is possessed by some prostaglandins, probably through their ability to maintain the mucosal microcirculation [23]. It seems likely that cimetidine exerts a cytoprotective influence on the gastric [24] and buccal mucosa, possibly by antagonising local histamine effects, histamine being an important mediator in drug-induced mucosal damage [25].

Within the limitations of interpretation of physiological parameters already mentioned, it seems that cimetidine may have a protective effect against acetylsalicylic acid-induced impairment of buccal mucosal function, while carbenoxolone appears to potentiate acetylsalicylic acid-induced effects. It may be significant that there is no controlled evidence of benefit from carbenoxolone pellets in the treatment of buccal ulceration [26]; anecdotal reports of benefit mention 'Bioral gel' [27-28] in which the silicone gel base has a waterproofing and physically-protective effect, so that therapeutic efficacy may be due to the vehicle, rather than the active agent.

Further clinical or biopsy evidence of beneficial or deleterious effects on squamous mucosa is required for both cimetidine and carbenoxolone, as both have significant systemic effects which may affect their local activity [29, 30]. It is apparent from the present study that not all mucosal surfaces respond in the same fashion to 'barrier protectors'.

Acknowledgements

Cimetidine and cimetidine placebo were kindly supplied by Smith Kline & French Laboratories, and carbenoxolone and carbenoxolone placebo by Biorex Laboratories. The advice given by Dr R.J. Horton is gratefully acknowledged.

References

1. Henn, B.M., Isenberg, J.I., Maxwell, V. and Strudevant, R.A.L. (1975): Inhibition of gastric acid secretion by cimetidine in patients with duodenal ulcer. *N. Engl. J. Med. 293,* 371-375.
2. Lipkin, M. (1970): Carbenoxolone sodium and the rate of extrusion of gastric epithelial cells. In: *Carbenoxolone sodium,* pp. 11-15. Editors: F.M. Sullivan and J.H. Baron. Butterworths, London.
3. Johnston, B., Lindup, W.E., Shillingford, L.J.S., Smith, M. and Parke, D.V. (1975): The pharmacological biochemistry of carbenoxolone. Its effect on gastric mucosa. In: *Fourth symposium on carbenoxolone,* pp. 13-21. Editors: F. Avery-Jones and D.V. Parke. Butterworths, London.
4. Symons, A.M. (1976): The effect of sodium carbenoxolone on the permeability of phosphatidylcholine and phosphatidylcholine cholesterol liposomes. *Biochem. Pharmacol. 25,* 1545-1547.
5. Hollander, F. (1954): Two-component mucosal barrier: its activity in protecting gastroduodenal mucosa against peptic ulceration. *Arch. Intern. Med. 93,* 107-129.
6. Davenport, H.W. (1967): Salicylate damage to the gastric mucosal barrier. *N. Engl. J. Med. 276,* 1307-1312.
7. Murray, H.S., Strottman, M.P. and Cooke, A.R. (1974): Effect of several drugs on gastric potential difference in man. *Br. Med. J. 1,* 19-21.
8. Eastwood, G.L. and Erdman, K.R. (1978): Effect of ethanol on canine gastric epithelial ultrastructure and transmucosal potential difference. *Am. J. Dig. Dis. 23,* 429-435.
9. MacKercher, P.A., Ivey, K.J., Baskin, N.N. and Krause, W.J. (1977): Protective effect of cimetidine on aspirin-induced gastric mucosal damage. *Ann. Intern. Med. 87,* 676-679.
10. Johnson, L.R. (1968): Source of the histamine released during damage to the gastric mucosa by acetic acid. *Gastroenterology 54,* 8-15.
11. Guth, P.H., Aures, D. and Paulsen, G. (1979): Topical aspirin plus HCl gastric lesions in the rat. Cytoprotective effect of prostaglandin, cimetidine and probanthine. *Gastroenterology 76,* 88-93.
12. Reed, P.I. and Davies, W.A. (1978): Controlled trial of carbenoxolone/alginate antacid combination in reflux oesophagitis. *Curr. Med. Res. Opin. 5,* 637-644.
13. Huston, G.J. (1978): The effects of aspirin, ethanol, indomethacin and 9α-fludrocortisone on buccal mucosal potential difference. *Br. J. Clin. Pharmacol. 5,* 155-160.
14. Edmonds, C.J. and Cronquist, A. (1970): A simple millivoltmeter and electrodes for measurement of rectal electrical potential in man. *Med. Biol. Eng. Comput. 8,* 409-410.
15. Archampong, E.G. and Edmonds, C.J. (1972): Effect of luminal ions on the transepithelial electrical potential difference of human rectum. *Gut 13,* 559-569.
16. Douthwaite, A.H. and Lintott, G.A.M. (1938): Gastroscopic observation of effect of aspirin and certain other substances on the stomach. *Lancet 2,* 1222-1225.
17. Muir, A. and Cassar, I.A. (1955): Aspirin and ulcer. *Br. Med. J. 2,* 7-12.
18. Silen, W. (1977): New concepts of the gastric mucosal barrier. *Am. J. Surg. 133,* 8-12.
19. Skrabal, F., Aubock, J., Edwards, C.R.W. and Braunsteiner, H. (1978): Subtraction potential difference in vivo assay for mineralocorticoid activity. *Lancet 1,* 298-302.
20. Hossenbocus, A. and Colin-Jones, D.G. (1975): Protection of the human gastric mucosa from aspirin by carbenoxolone. In: *Fourth symposium on carbenoxolone,* pp. 91-102. Editors: F. Avery-Jones and D.V. Parke. Butterworth, London.
21. Finney, R.S.H. and Tarnoky, A.L. (1960): The pharmacological properties of glycyrrhetinic acid hydrogen succinate (di-sodium salt). *J. Pharm. Pharmacol. 12,* 49-56.
22. Ferguson, W.W., Edmonds, A.W., Starling, J.R. and Wangensteen, S.L. (1973): Protective effect of prostaglandin E₁ (PgE₁) on liposomal enzyme release in serotonin-induced gastric ulceration. *Ann. Surg. 177,* 648-654.
23. Robert, A., Nezamis, J.E. and Lancaster, C. (1977): The cytoprotective property of

prostaglandins. *Gastroenterology 72,* 1121.

24. Okabe, S., Takeuchi, K., Urushidani, I. and Takagi, K. (1971): Effect of cimetidine, a histamine H$_2$-receptor antagonist, on various experimental gastric and duodenal ulcers. *Am. J. Dig. Dis. 22,* 677-684.

25. Johnson, L.R. (1966): Histamine liberation by gastric mucosa of pylorus-ligated rats damaged by acetic or salicylic acids. *Proc. Soc. Exp. Biol. Med. 121,* 384-386.

26. MacPhee, I.T., Sircus, W., Farmer, E.D., Harkness, R.A. and Cowley, G.C. (1968): Use of steroids in treatment of aphthous ulceration. *Br. Med. J. 2,* 147-149.

27. Bank, S. (1971): Carbenoxolone sodium gel in the treatment of herpes febrilis. *S. Afr. Med. J. 45,* 596.

28. Samuel, O.W. (1967): Periadenitis mucosa necrotica recurrens treated with topical carbenoxolone gel. *Practitioner 199,* 220-222.

29. Tomkins, A.M. and Edmonds, C.J. (1975): Electrical potential difference, sodium absorption and potassium secretion by the human rectum during carbenoxolone therapy. *Gut 16,* 277-284.

30. Leslie, G.B. and Walker, T.F. (1977): A toxicological profile of cimetidine. In: *Proceedings of the second International Symposium on histamine H$_2$-receptor antagonists,* p. 24. Editors: W.L. Burland and M.A. Simkins. Excerpta Medica, Amsterdam-Oxford-Princeton.

Discussion

Pallone (Rome): I would like to report data obtained in the course of a trial taking place in our Unit, regarding the effects of cimetidine upon the histology of the gastric mucosa. It was confirmed that there is a type B gastritis (as described by the classification of Strickland and Mackay) in a very high proportion of cases. We found that the inflammation of the antral mucosa does not seem to be much influenced by treatment with cimetidine, whether the ulcer heals or not. However, in contrast with our finding in patients treated with placebo, those treated with cimetidine (irrespective of the dose used) had, after 8 weeks' treatment, a significantly higher incidence of inflammatory changes in biopsies from the body of the stomach. If patients with duodenal ulcers treated with cimetidine are divided into 2 groups, those healed and those not healed, it can be seen that the proportion of abnormal biopsies in the fundus in healed patients is significantly higher than before treatment, whereas non-healers behave exactly like those on placebo.

This is a result which can be interpreted in various ways.

Molinari (Genoa): In the first place, I want to express my doubts about what has been said of the effects of carbenoxolone and cimetidine upon the oral mucosa. I am not a physiologist, but there seem to me to be 2 experimental models which are extremely different if we look at them in relation to the stomach, where we have hydrogen ions and thus a possibility of back-diffusion, whereas the oral mucosa is structurally different from the gastric mucosa and thus has a physiological picture which differs very greatly from that of the stomach. I tend to think that the changes described by our colleague may be due to a local action of the 2 drugs rather than to a change in a mucosal barrier, whose existence is open to question.

Lorenz: We should discuss first the carbenoxolone results and the question of the model, and then discuss the gastritis problem.

In the sequence of events which occurs in mucosal permeability changes, which include not only histamine release but also kinin formation which is achieved by pepsin, does Dr. Huston think that some of the differences observed result from the secondary effects which occur in the 2 models? It is known that pepsin is an excellent kinin-forming enzyme.

Huston: Yes, I am certain that that could be so. Referring to the local effects, I had hoped that local physical effects had been eliminated by using a double placebo — that is, placebos which were physically exactly the same, apart from containing the drug. It would be a mistake, obviously, to say that this is analogous to a stomach model; it is not, it is an experimental system. There is much more to mucosal damage than the local effect. For instance, it is known that indometacin produces very little local effect, but it is a potent gastric irritant, perhaps through producing local ischaemia and/or through decreasing local hydrogen ion secretion, which has been shown recently.

The model is very limited. It should not be compared to the stomach. It was simply being used to look for an inhibitory effect of cimetidine. We were looking at histamine, but clearly there is no way of eliminating the possibility of secondary messengers.

Lorenz: If cimetidine is so effective within this model, have histamine concentrations been studied? Is it possible to take a biopsy, or to do something similar?

Huston: We are very tempted to take biopsies, but human studies would be precluded and it would have to be animal studies. We have not done that yet.

Effects of cimetidine on pancreatic function and disease

G. Dobrilla, M.C. Bonoldi, F. Chilovi and G. Bertaccini
Division of Gastroenterology and Service of Endoscopy and Digestive Physiopathology, General Regional Hospital, Bolzano; and Institute of Pharmacology, University of Parma, Parma, Italy

Introduction

The question of whether or not H_2-antagonists interfere with pancreatic function has a double justification. First, it is impossible to exclude a direct effect of H_2-antagonists on the exocrine pancreas, because the presence of H_2-receptors in this organ has not been studied sufficiently. Second, compounds which so markedly inhibit gastric acid secretion could theoretically have an indirect influence on pancreatic secretion through decreased release of endogenous secretin. However, when the pancreas is diseased, inhibition of gastric function by the H_2-receptor antagonists may, paradoxically, improve pancreatic function. This point will be discussed below.

Effects of H_2-antagonists on pancreatic secretion

Studies in animals

The effect of metiamide on pancreatic secretion was studied in cats both after intravenous infusion of 2.0 U/kg/hour of secretin, which produces near-maximal bicarbonate secretion in these animals, and after intraduodenal instillation of 1 mEq/hour of acid, which causes endogenous secretin release [1]. Infusion of metiamide 12 μmol/kg/hour failed to significantly modify the pancreatic output of either bicarbonate or enzymes in response to both these types of stimulation (Fig. 1).

In our experiments in anesthetized dogs with cannulation of the pancreatic duct, the effect of both metiamide and cimetidine on pancreatic secretion stimulated by intravenous injection of cholecystokinin-pancreozymin (CCK-Pz) octapeptide was studied (Fig. 1). After intravenous administration of metiamide 10 mg/kg, pancreatic secretion was partially inhibited, but a further injection of CCK-Pz octapeptide 20 ng/kg restored the secretory response of the pancreas to initial values (Fig. 2). A larger dose of metiamide (50 mg/kg) increased the degree of the secretory inhibition and also rendered the inhibition irreversible, notwithstanding very large doses of octapeptide (320 ng/kg) (Fig. 3). When cimetidine was used in doses ranging from 10-30 mg/kg, the resulting secretory inhibition was scanty and transient (Fig. 4). Only very high doses of cimetidine (50 mg/kg) reduced pancreatic secretion appreciably, but this inhibition was reversed by further stimulation with CCK-Pz octapeptide (Fig. 5). The highest doses of the H_2-blockers used in the dog (50 mg/kg) caused a transient but remarkable hypotension (40-80 mm Hg). However, it

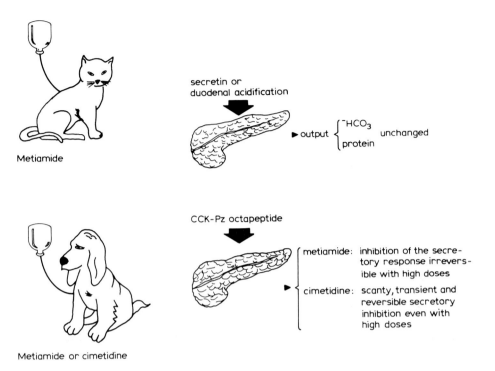

secretin or
duodenal acidification

output $\left\{ \begin{array}{l} ^-HCO_3 \\ protein \end{array} \right.$ unchanged

Metiamide

CCK-Pz octapeptide

metiamide: inhibition of the secretory response irrevers-
ible with high doses

cimetidine: scanty, transient and
reversible secretory
inhibition even with
high doses

Metiamide or cimetidine

Fig. 1. Effects of H_2-antagonists on pancreatic secretion in the cat [1] and the dog.

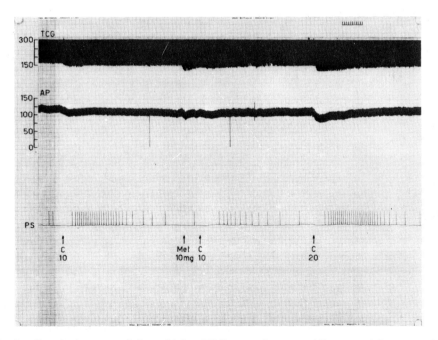

Fig. 2. Results in mongrel dogs, 22 kg. TCG = tachogram; AP = arterial pressure (mm Hg); PS = pancreatic secretion from the Wirsung duct. C = cholecystokinin-pancreozymin octapeptide (ng/kg); Met = metiamide (mg/kg).

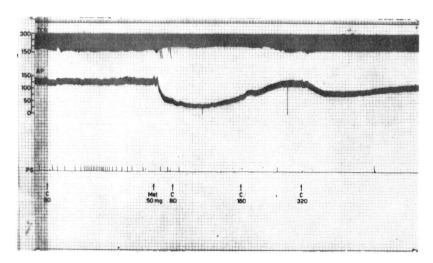

Fig. 3.   Results in a mongrel dog, 14 kg. For further details, see legend to Figure 2.

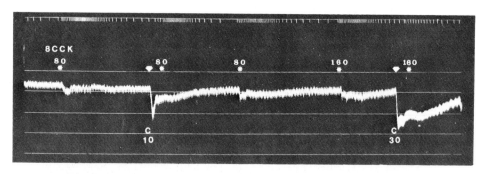

Fig. 4.   Results in a mongrel dog, 15 kg. Top: each stroke in the record of the drop counter represents 1 drop of pancreatic secretion. Bottom: the distance between 2 parallel lines is 40 mm Hg arterial pressure (mean basal pressure = 130 mm Hg). 8CCK = cholecystokinin-pancreozymin octapeptide (ng/kg); C = cimetidine (mg/kg).

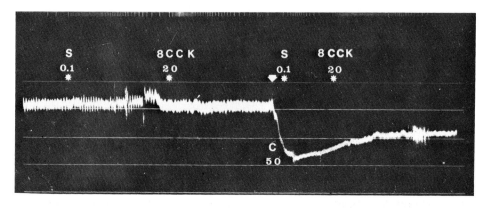

Fig. 5.   Results in a mongrel dog, 19 kg. S = secretin (U/kg). For further details, see legend to Figure 4.

is not probable that this effect is responsible for the inhibition of pancreatic secretory response to CCK-Pz octapeptide, since it has been observed [2] that, during the hypotension induced by peptides of the tachykinin family [3], the pancreatic exocrine secretion can actually be increased.

Our experiments so far have not allowed us to establish whether or not H_2-receptors are involved in pancreatic secretion. Only the accurate use of H_2-receptor selective agonists (like dimaprit or impromidine), which would have an effect opposite to that of H_2-blockers and would be competitively inhibited by them, will provide direct evidence for or against a role of H_2-receptors in the pancreas. This kind of study is now in progress in our laboratories.

Studies in man

From 1976 to 1979, 7 studies of the effects of H_2-antagonists on pancreatic secretion have been reported on a total of 79 subjects, of whom 48 were duodenal ulcer patients, 25 were healthy volunteers, and 6, although not well-defined, were probably also healthy subjects; the organization and results of these studies are compared in Table I. Except for the Dobrilla et al. study [9] (Fig. 6), pancreatic stimulation was carried out by intravenous infusion of hormones.

During the infusion of metiamide, significant inhibition of the enzyme-secretory response to sustained stimulation with exogenous secretin plus CCK-Pz was observed [4]. This inhibitory effect of metiamide in man seems to agree with our observations in anesthetized dogs. However, the hormone-stimulated pancreatic secretion of enzymes is not affected by either acute or prolonged administration of cimetidine; here again the results in man are in agreement with our experimental

Table I. Effects of H_2-antagonists on pancreatic secretion in man.

Study	Subjects	Stimulus	H_2-antagonist	Results
[4]○	8 DU patients	S + CCK-Pz	intravenous metiamide	-HCO₃ unchanged; Try decreased
[5]●	12 DU patients	S or S + CCK-Pz	oral cimetidine	-HCO₃, Am, Try and Ch-Try unchanged
[6]○	6 not well-defined subjects	S + CCK-Pz	oral cimetidine	-HCO₃, Am and Lip unchanged
[7]○	10 DU patients	meal	oral cimetidine	Lip and Try unchanged
[8]●	10 DU patients	S + C	oral cimetidine	-HCO₃, Lip and Ch-Try unchanged
[9]○	25 normal volunteers	S + CCK-Pz	oral cimetidine	-HCO₃, Lip, Try and Ch-Try unchanged
[10]●○	8 DU patients	meal	oral cimetidine	Try unchanged

○ = secretory study during H_2-antagonist administration; ● = secretory study after short-term treatment with H_2-antagonist. DU = duodenal ulcer. S = secretin; CCK-Pz = cholecystokinin-pancreozymin; C = ceruletide. Try = trypsin; Am = amylase; Ch-Try = chymotrypsin; Lip = lipase.

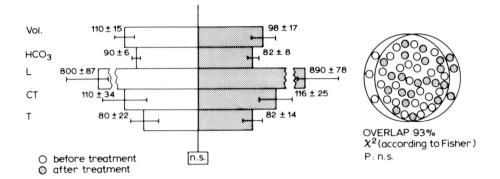

Fig. 6.   Pancreatic secretion in 25 normal volunteers before and after treatment with oral cimetidine 400 mg. Hormonal stimulation with 1 CU GIH secretin and 1 Ivy U GIH cholecystokinin-pancreozymin was given by rapid intravenous injection 90 minutes after the administration of cimetidine. Bicarbonate, lipase (L), chymotrypsin (CT) and trypsin (T) are expressed as concentrations (mean ± SEM). Statistical comparison was carried out by Student's paired t test and cluster analysis. Right: a schematic representation of the cluster analysis results; S.CCK.Pz test does not allow any separation in 2 population groups. n.s. = not significant.

data. Secretion of water and electrolytes was not affected by either metiamide or cimetidine.

The lack of significant effects of cimetidine on electrolyte and enzymatic pancreatic secretion was also observable in meal-stimulated subjects. The strong inhibition of gastric acid secretion without interference with pancreatic secretion is peculiar to cimetidine. In fact, other antisecretory compounds, such as anticholinergics, inhibit the secretory response of the stomach less, but decrease pancreatic flow and enzyme secretion both under basal conditions and during secretin stimulation [11].

Effects of cimetidine on pancreatic disease

Cimetidine and acute pancreatitis

Two observations, 1 in man [12], and the other in animals [13], suggested the possibility that oral administration of cimetidine might be followed by acute pancreatitis. The clinical case involved a 78-year-old patient suffering from parkinsonism and congestive failure, who was being treated with potassium salts, levodopa and furosemide, with its previously-reported potentially-toxic effect on the pancreas. Nevertheless, the investigators ruled out the possibility of the acute pancreatitis having been caused by this diuretic, because the patient was treated with furosemide during and after this disease without detectable adverse effects. However, the fact that this patient had been taking furosemide for some time without suffering from abdominal pain does not exclude its toxic action on the pancreas. Likewise, alcohol, cholelithiasis and hyperparathyroidism do not always cause pancreatitis. Moreover, stasis in the splanchnic area resulting from congestive heart failure could contribute to causing acute damage of the pancreas, whose susceptibility to ischemic injury has been recently reported [14].

Experimental acute hemorrhagic and necrotizing pancreatitis was described in rats given cimetidine and very large doses of pentagastrin and carbachol [13]. However, other experiments on cimetidine-treated rats with mercaptamine-induced duodenal ulcer have shown that cimetidine does not aggravate the interstitial pancreatitis and/or peripancreatitis often observed in association with this type of ulcer [15]. Moreover, in 2,182 patients receiving cimetidine for 4-8 weeks, acute pancreatitis and/or an increase in serum or urinary amylase was not observed, nor has any case of acute pancreatitis been reported in 121 patients undergoing treatment with full therapeutic doses lasting up to 1 year [16]. In 174 duodenal ulcer patients treated with cimetidine in controlled endoscopic trials [17-19], clinical and laboratory data never suggested acute pancreatic damage.

The effect of cimetidine on acute pancreatitis and on the acute phase of chronic relapsing pancreatitis

In patients with acute pancreatitis, gastric and pancreatic function should be reduced. Theoretically, cimetidine, which strongly inhibits basal and food-stimulated gastric acid output and has no apparent effect on the human exocrine pancreas, might be a suitable therapeutic agent. A therapeutic role of cimetidine would be valuable in view of the presently-unsatisfactory options for treatment of acute pancreatitis [20, 21]. However, there have been few studies reported on the use of cimetidine in acute pancreatitis.

In 1 study, 11 patients with alcoholic pancreatitis in its acute clinical phase (7 males and 4 females aged 20-63 years) were treated with a continuous infusion of cimetidine 800 mg/day, in addition to analgesics, nasogastric suction and fluid replacement [22]. No deterioration in their clinical course was observed; there was a rapid fall in serum amylase (Fig. 7), and the intragastric pH remained at or above

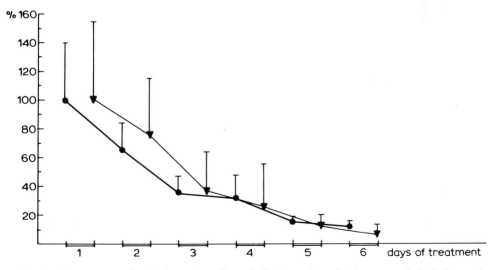

Fig. 7. Percentage of variation of amylasemia in 16 patients in the acute clinical phase of chronic relapsing pancreatitis treated with a continuous intravenous infusion of cimetidine 1200 mg/24 hours (●—●) [23], and in 11 patients receiving continuous intravenous infusion of cimetidine 800 mg/24 hours (▼—▼) [22]. 100% = maximal increase of amylasemia.

pH 7. In another series of 16 patients with chronic pancreatitis treated with cimetidine, no adverse effect was observed and there was a prompt reduction in serum amylase (Fig. 7); all patients became painfree within 24 hours of commencing treatment [23]. Unfortunately, because of the uncontrolled nature of this study no reliable conclusion can be drawn as to the value of intravenous cimetidine in the treatment of acute pancreatitis.

Moreover, the only double-blind controlled study comparing cimetidine and saline suggests that cimetidine administered intravenously in 6-hourly doses of 300 mg is not superior to placebo in cases of mild or moderately-severe alcoholic pancreatitis [24]. However, the number of patients in this study (13 in the cimetidine group and 11 in the placebo group) was too small to draw definite conclusions as to the value of cimetidine. A better distinction between patients with acute pancreatitis is also required.

Studies in rats with trypsin-induced acute pancreatitis, using doses of cimetidine equivalent to those recommended in man, have failed to show any therapeutic effect [25], but it is difficult to extrapolate this finding from rat to man.

The effect of cimetidine on chronic pancreatitis

Maldigestion and then malabsorption occur in chronic pancreatitis only when pancreatic function (i.e. pancreatic enzyme output) is reduced by 90% or more [26, 27]. At this stage, oral pancreatic extracts are routinely employed [28-32]. However, even if clinically useful, these preparations rarely abolish steatorrhea [33, 34]. This is principally due to the irreversible inactivation of the pancreatic enzymes by gastric juice when intraluminal pH decreases to less than 4.0 [34-36]. Various methods to prevent gastric inactivation of pancreatic extracts have been proposed, notably antacids, anticholinergics, enteric-coated tablets, and H_2-antagonists.

Antacids may reduce intragastric acidity and therefore partially prevent the destruction of ingested enzymes, but the increased volume of gastric secretion, due to the loss of pH-related gastric secretory inhibition, causes dilution of the enzyme activity in the duodenum. Consequently, the concentration of pancreatic enzymes in the duodenum is inadequate [37]. Anticholinergics cannot be used as an adjunctive protective measure because only large doses, inevitably associated with side-effects, significantly reduce gastric acid secretion [38]. Enteric-coated tablets have been found ineffective in some clinical trials [39, 40].

From a theoretical point of view, a drug such as cimetidine, capable of reducing both the output of acid and volume of gastric secretion, might reduce the inactivation of the pancreatic extracts in the stomach and duodenum [41] (Table II).

In practice, a comparison of the therapeutic responses of antacids, enteric-coated pancreatic enzymes and cimetidine to oral enzymes in severe pancreatic insufficiency has shown that cimetidine and pancreatin, administered orally, produce significantly higher postprandial duodenal recoveries and concentrations of trypsin and lipase than pancreatin alone; that neither enteric-coated enzymes nor neutralizing antacids were more effective than pancreatin alone in decreasing steatorrhea or improving duodenal enzyme delivery; and that steatorrhea is inversely related to duodenal lipase recovery [33].

Tables III and IV show the effects of cimetidine on steatorrhea due to pancreatic insufficiency in patients affected by chronic alcoholic pancreatitis and in patients with cystic fibrosis. In all 49 patients treated with the combination of pancreatic

Table II. Basis for the beneficial effect of cimetidine in pancreatic insufficiency.

Cimetidine effects	Consequence on the pancreatic enzymes	
Marked depression in meal-induced gastric secretory response	Intragastric destruction of pancreatic enzymes	↓
Decrease of intragastric activity	Intragastric destruction of pancreatic enzymes	↓
Great decrease of delivery of gastric acid in duodenum	Intraduodenal destruction of pancreatic enzymes	↓
Reduction of gastric secretory volume	Intraduodenal concentration of pancreatic enzymes	↑

Table III. The effect of cimetidine on pancreatic steatorrhea.

Study	Total number of patients	Patients with steatorrhea		Fecal fat (g/24 hours)	
		pe	pe + c	pe	pe + c
Mayo Clinic Group [33, 34]	6	6	2	27	11
Bianchi Porro et al. [42]	6	6	2	12	5.5
Dobrilla et al. [1978-9: unpublished data]	8	8	3	30	12

Fecal fat values are means. pe = after treatment with pancreatic extracts; pe + c = after treatment with pancreatic extracts and cimetidine.

Table IV. The effect of cimetidine on steatorrhea in cystic fibrosis patients.

Study	Total number of patients	Patients with steatorrhea		Fecal fat (g/24 hours)	
		pe	pe + c	pe	pe + c
Ahuja and Mann [43]	5	4	3	13	9
Cox et al. [44]	10	—	—	25	16
Hubbard et al. [46]	6	—	—	49	28
				Fecal weight (g/24 hours)	
Boyle et al. [45]	8	—	—	257	198

Fecal fat and weight values are means. pe = after treatment with pancreatic extracts; pe + c = after treatment with pancreatic extracts and cimetidine.

extracts and cimetidine, a decrease in fecal fat or fecal weight was observed. In chronic pancreatitis this decrease was greater than 50%, and steatorrhea disappeared in approximately two-thirds of the patients. Only 1 study reported steatorrhea in patients with cystic fibrosis [43]; it persisted in 4 of 5 patients when they were on replacement treatment with pancreatic extracts, and in 3 of 5 when they were given cimetidine.

While the combination of pancreatic extracts and cimetidine seems necessary for a more satisfactory correction of steatorrhea, resolution of azotorrhea occurs in most patients using other treatment groups as well, such as pancreatic enzymes alone or associated with antacids (aluminium magnesium hydroxide or sodium bicarbonate) and enteric-coated preparations [34, 47]. This is probably because lipase is more readily destroyed than proteolytic pancreatic enzymes; moreover, lipase needs additional factors such as colipase and bile acids for full enzymatic activity [48]. It has also been demonstrated that addition of antacids to H_2-antagonists and pancreatic extracts results in a further increase of enzymatic concentration in the intestine, due to a more prolonged stability of duodenal pH at an approximately neutral value [49].

Recent evidence shows that highly-concentrated pancreatic extracts given in a granulated form protected by an enteric coating induce significant increases in intraduodenal enzyme concentrations, and last longer in the duodenum than when given in a non-granulated form [50, 51]. Therefore, theoretically, the addition of cimetidine with or without antacids to such a granulated form might increase this effect even further. Also suggesting a possible therapeutical role of cimetidine are some preliminary unpublished data showing that an abnormal PABA test can be partially corrected by pancreatic extracts alone, and fully corrected by the further addition of cimetidine 2 hours before the meal (Fig. 8). If confirmed, this may be of interest as a guide in treatment.

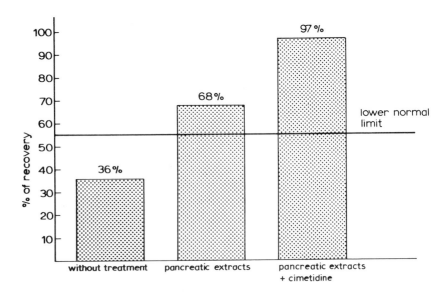

Fig. 8.   *Results of BzTyPABA test in a patient with marked pancreatic steatorrhea, before and after administration of pancreatic extracts (Pancrex V forte, 8 tablets with test meal) and cimetidine (600 mg, 120 minutes before PABA test).*

Conclusions

Cimetidine, given in the same dose and frequency as in the treatment of peptic ulcer, does not impair exocrine pancreatic function. Moreover, there is no evidence that cimetidine causes acute pancreatitis. Some open trials suggest that cimetidine is of value in the treatment of acute pancreatitis and the acute phase of chronic relapsing pancreatitis. This needs to be confirmed in double-blind controlled studies, even though some preliminary controlled data are not very encouraging.

When added to pancreatic extracts and administered to patients with severe pancreatic insufficiency, cimetidine, principally by preventing gastric inactivation of pancreatic enzymes, enhances their concentration in the duodenal lumen and consequently corrects maldigestion of fat and consequent steatorrhea. Therefore, in cases when steatorrhea is not corrected by conventional replacement treatment alone, it is useful to add cimetidine and to continue with this H_2-antagonist, particularly if clinical improvement is very marked. In fact, only this would justify the substantial cost of this treatment, which would surely be very prolonged.

Acknowledgments

The authors gratefully acknowledge the useful advice of Dr. K.G. Wormsley in preparing the text.

References

1. Konturek, S.J., Demitrescu, T., Radecki, T. and Dembinski, A. (1973): Effect of metiamide, a histamine H_2-receptor antagonist, on gastric and pancreatic secretion and peptic ulcers induced by histamine and pentagastrin in cats. In: *International Symposium on histamine H_2-receptor antagonists.* p. 247. Editors: C.J. Wood and M.A. Simkins. Smith Kline & French, Welwyn Garden City.
2. Bertaccini, G., De Caro, G. and Impicciatore, M. (1967): Effects of physalaemin on some exocrine secretions of dog and rats. *J. Physiol. (London) 193,* 497.
3. Bertaccini, G. (1976): Active polypeptides of nonmammalian origin. *Pharmacol. Rev. 28,* 127.
4. Thjodleifsson, B. and Wormsley, K.G. (1975): Effect of metiamide on the response to secretin and cholecystokinin in man. *Gut 16,* 33.
5. Domschke, W., Domschke, S. and Demling, L. (1977): A double-blind study of cimetidine in patients with duodenal ulceration: clinical, kinetic and gastric and pancreatic secretory data. In: *Cimetidine,* p. 217. Editors: W.L. Burland and M.A. Simkins. Excerpta Medica, Amsterdam-Oxford-Princeton.
6. Galmiche, J.P., Colin, R., Al-Saati, M.N. and Geffroy, Y. (1977): Effect of cimetidine on pancreatic exocrine secretion. *Lancet 1,* 647.
7. Longstreth, G.F., Go, V.L.W. and Malagelada, J.-R. (1977): Postprandial gastric, pancreatic and biliary response to histamine H_2-receptor antagonists in active duodenal ulcer. *Gastroenterology 72,* 9.
8. Cavallini, G., Vaona, B., Bovo, P., Mirachian, R., Angelini, G. and Scuro, L.A. (1978): Effect of histamine H_2-receptor antagonists on the exocrine pancreatic secretion. *Acta Hepato-gastroenterol. 25,* 388.
9. Dobrilla, G., Filippini, M., Valentini, M. and Bonoldi, M.C. (1978): Influenza della somministrazione acuta di cimetidina sulla secrezione pancreatica. In: *Cimetidina, farmacologia e clinica,* p. 249. Editor: P. Lucchelli. Smith Kline & French, Milan.
10. Maugdal, D.P., Lawrence, D., Sanderson, F.M. and Northfield, T.C. (1979): Cimetidine on pancreatic and biliary function in man. *Br. J. Clin. Pharmacol. 8,* 229.

11. Dreiling, D.A. and Janowitz, H.D. (1960): Inhibitory effect of a new anticholinergic on the basal and secretin stimulated pancreatic secretion in patients with and without pancreatic disease. Therapeutic and theoretic implications. *Am. J. Dig. Dis. 5,* 639.

12. Arnold, F., Dayle, P.J. and Bell, G. (1978): Acute pancreatitis in a patient treated with cimetidine. *Lancet 1,* 382.

13. Joffe, S.N. and Lee, F.D. (1978): Acute pancreatitis after cimetidine administration in experimental duodenal ulcers. *Lancet 1,* 383.

14. Warshaw, A.L. and O'Hara, P.J. (1978): Susceptibility of the pancreas to ischaemic injury in shock: a newly recognized cause of pancreatitis. *Gastroenterology 74,* 1109.

15. Szabo, S. and Goldman, H. (1978): Cimetidine and pancreatitis: lesson from animal experiments. *Lancet 1,* 266.

16. Burland, W.L. (1978): Evidence for the safety of cimetidine in the treatment of peptic ulcer disease. In: *Cimetidine: Proceedings of an International Symposium on histamine H_2-receptor antagonists,* p. 238. Editor: W. Creutzfeldt. Excerpta Medica, Amsterdam-Oxford-Princeton.

17. Albano, O., Barbara, L., Miglioli, M., Bianchi Porro, G., Petrillo, M., Blasi, A., Marletta, F., Cheli, R., Molinari, F., Coltorti, M., Del Vecchio Blanco, C., Dobrilla, G., Valentini, M., Scuro, L.A., Cavallini, G., Verme, G. and Pera, A. (1978): Cimetidine in short-term medical treatment of active duodenal ulcer: a multicentre endoscopic double-blind study on 164 patients. *Ital. J. Gastroenterol. 10,* 247.

18. Dobrilla, G., Valentini, M., Filippini, M., Felder, M., Bonoldi, M.C. and Moroder, E. (1978): Therapie mit Cimetidin beim Ulcus duodeni. Klinisch-endoskopische Studie an 76 Patienten. *Münch. Med. Wochenschr. 120,* 24.

19. Bianchi Porro, G., Dobrilla, G., Verme, G., Gallo, M., Petrillo, M. and Valentini, M. (1979): Comparison of sulglicotide with cimetidine in short-term treatment of duodenal ulcer: double-blind controlled trial. *Br. Med. J. 2,* 17.

20. Soergel, K.H. (1978): Medical treatment of acute pancreatitis. What is the evidence? *Gastroenterology 74,* 620.

21. Filippini, M. and Dobrilla, G. (1979): Trasylol e pancreatite acuta. *Ital. J. Gastroenterol. 11,* 2s.

22. Dammann, H.G. and Augustin, H.J. (1978): Cimetidine and acute pancreatitis. *Lancet 1,* 66.

23. Dobrilla, G., Bonoldi, M.C. and Chilovi, F. (1979): Considerazioni sul trattamento degli attachi acuti di pancreatite. *Boll. Soc. Med. Chir. Bolzano.* (In press.)

24. Meshkinpur, H., Molinari, M.D., Gardner, L. and Noeler, F.K. (1979): Cimetidine in the treatment of acute alcoholic pancreatitis. *Gastroenterology 76,* 1201.

25. Evander, A. and Ihse, I. (1979): Influence of cimetidine on acute experimental pancreatitis. *Dan. Med. Bull. 26,* 13.

26. Di Magno, E.P., Go, V.L.W. and Summerskill, W.H.J. (1973): Relations between pancreatic enzyme outputs and malabsorption in severe pancreatic insufficiency. *N. Engl. J. Med. 288,* 813.

27. Di Magno, E.P., Malagelada, J.-R. and Go, V.L.W. (1975): Relationship between alcoholism and pancreatic insufficiency. *Ann. N.Y. Acad. Sci. 252,* 200.

28. Littmann, A. and Hanscon, H.D. (1969): Pancreatic extracts. *N. Engl. J. Med. 281,* 201.

29. Schneider, R., Sammons, H.G. and Beale, D.J. (1970): Pancreatic enzyme therapy. *Br. Med. J. 2,* 735.

30. Taubin, H.L. and Spiro, H.M. (1973): Nutritional aspects of chronic pancreatitis. *Am. J. Clin. Nutr. 26,* 367.

31. Saunders, J.H.B. and Wormsley, K.G. (1975): Pancreatic extracts in the treatment of pancreatic exocrine insufficiency. *Gut 16,* 157.

32. Dobrilla, G. (1978): Enzimi pancreatici: valutazione critica del loro ruolo terapeutico. *Ital. J. Gastroenterol. 10,* 21s.

33. Regan, P.T., Malagelada, J.-R., Di Magno, E.P., Glanzman, S.L. and Go, V.L.W. (1977): Comparative effects of antacids, cimetidine and enteric coating on the therapeutic

response to oral enzymes in severe pancreatic insufficiency. *N. Engl. J. Med. 297,* 854.

34. Di Magno, E.P., Malagelada, J.-R., Go, V.L.W. and Moertel, C.G. (1977): Fate of orally ingested enzymes in pancreatic insufficiency. Comparison of two dosage schedules. *N. Engl. J. Med. 296,* 1318.

35. Heizer, W.D., Claeveland, C.R. and Iber, F.L. (1965): Gastric inactivation of pancreatic supplements. *Johns Hopkins Med. J. 116,* 261.

36. Go, V.L.W., Poley, J.-R., Hoffmann, A.F. and Summerskill, W.H.J. (1970): Disturbances in fat digestion induced by acid jejunal pH due to gastric hypersecretion in man. *Gastroenterology 58,* 638.

37. Deering, T.B. and Malagelada, J.-R. (1977): Comparison of an H_2-receptor antagonist and a neutralizing antacid on postprandial acid delivery into the duodenum in patients with duodenal ulcer. *Gastroenterology 73,* 11.

38. Ivey, K.Y. (1975): Anticholinergics: do they work in peptic ulcer? *Gastroenterology 68,* 154.

39. Goodchild, M.C., Sagarò, E., Brown, G.A., Cruchley, P.M., Jukes, H.R. and Anderson, I.M. (1974): Comparative trial of Pancrex V forte and Nutrizym in treatment of malabsorption in cystic fibrosis. *Br. Med. J. 3,* 712.

40. Graham, D.Y. (1977): Enzyme replacement therapy of exocrine pancreatic insufficiency in man: relation between in vitro enzyme activities and in vivo patency in commercial pancreatic extracts. *N. Engl. J. Med. 296,* 1314.

41. Regan, P.T., Malagelada, J.R., Di Magno, E.P. and Go, V.L.W. (1978): Rationale for the use of cimetidine in pancreatic insufficiency. *Mayo Clin. Proc. 53,* 79.

42. Bianchi Porro, G., Dolcini, R., Grassi, E., Petrillo, M. and Prada, A. (1977): Cimetidine in treatment of pancreatic insufficiency. *Lancet 2,* 878.

43. Ahuja, A.S. and Mann, N.M. (1978): Cimetidine in cystic fibrosis. *Arch. Dis. Child. 53,* 766.

44. Cox, K.L., Isenberg, J.N., Osher, A.B. and Dooley, R.R. (1978): The effect of cimetidine on pancreatic replacement therapy in the maldigestion of cystic fibrosis. *Cystic Fibrosis Club abstracts and pediatric research 12,* 433.

45. Boyle, B.J., Long, W.B., Huang, N., Widzer, S.J. and Balistreri, W.F. (1979): Effect of cimetidine and pancreatic enzymes on serum and fecal bile acid and fat absorption in cystic fibrosis. *Clin. Res. 26,* 612.

46. Hubbard, V.S., Dunn, G.D., Lester, L.A. and di Sant'Agnese, P.A. (1979): Effectiveness of cimetidine in patients with cystic fibrosis. *Clin. Res. 72,* 552.

47. Regan, P.T., Malagelada, J.-R., Di Magno, E.P. and Go, V.L.W. (1978): Cimetidine as an adjunct to oral enzymes in the treatment of malabsorption due to pancreatic insufficiency. *Gastroenterology 74,* 468.

48. Hofmann, A.F. (1978): Lipase, colipase, amphipatic dietary proteins, and bile acids: new interactions at an old interface. *Gastroenterology 75,* 530.

49. Saunders, J.H.B., Drummond, S. and Wormsley, K.G. (1977): Inhibition of gastric secretion in the treatment of pancreatic insufficiency. *Br. Med. J. 1,* 418.

50. Worning, H. (1979): The effect of enzyme substitution in patients with pancreatic insufficiency. *Scand. J. Gastroenterol.* (Submitted.)

51. Ihse, I., Lilja, P. and Lundquist, I. (1980): Intestinal concentrations of pancreatic enzymes following pancreatic replacement therapy. *Scand. J. Gastroenterol.* (In press.)

Discussion

Bertaccini (Parma): One comment about Dr. Dobrilla's paper, regarding animal experiments: we must not think only of effects which may be of practical importance. The question concerning the possible role of H_2-receptors is more important, considering that both metiamide and cimetidine, at high doses, can block the exocrine secretion induced by cholecystokinin octapeptide or by secretin. The fundamental point is this: we have observed these reductions, irreversible in the case of metiamide, reversible in the case of cimetidine, but this does not imply that H_2-receptors are necessarily involved. The effects may be non-specific. It follows that the definitive test of the role of H_2-receptors will come if it can be confirmed that the selective agonists of the H_2-receptors have an effect opposite to that of the inhibitors (that is, a stimulant effect).

Lorenz: This subject has become increasingly important recently. Has Dr. Dobrilla any idea whether histamine has anything to do with pancreatitis, so that H_2-receptor antagonists could have some direct effect on this condition?

Dobrilla: I have no data on that.

Cavallini (Verona): I would like to stress one point. I think that in Copenhagen a study was described in a poster in which animals treated for experimental pancreatitis with cimetidine did worse than those treated with placebo.

Another comment: it may seem strange but, in our study, in which we are treating patients with chronic pancreatitis with or without pancreatic insufficiency with cimetidine or with nothing (i.e., only with antacids), despite a great reduction in steatorrhoea, the fecal weight was virtually unchanged and the gain in body weight was not as striking as was to be expected.

Recent results with cimetidine treatment (II)

Chairmen: A. Blasi *(Catania, Italy)*
R. Naccarato *(Padua, Italy)*

Prophylaxis of acute gastroduodenal mucosal lesions: a controlled trial*

V. Speranza, N. Basso, M. Bagarani, S. Fiorani°, E. Bianchi and A. Materia
VI Surgical Clinic and °Intensive Care Unit, University of Rome, Rome, Italy

Introduction

Acute gastroduodenal mucosal lesions, the so-called 'stress lesions', occur frequently in critically-ill, 'high-risk' patients [1-4]. Several trials have verified the efficacy of prophylactic measures — usually the administration of antacids — in the prevention of these lesions in certain restricted categories of high-risk patients [5-12]. At present, however, only preliminary data are available on cimetidine prophylaxis in high-risk patients [3, 6-13].

The present study was carried out to evaluate the respective efficacy of prophylactic cimetidine, of prophylactic antacids, and of no treatment in the prevention of stress lesions in high-risk patients.

Subjects and methods

From March 1978 to April 1979, 800 consecutive patients admitted to the Intensive Care Unit and the Departments of Neurosurgery and Plastic Surgery of the

Table I. Criteria for classification as 'high-risk'.

	Number of patients
Respiratory failure (endotracheal; $pCO_2 > 50$, $pO_2 < 60$)	82
Neurosurgery (midline lesions)	46
Sepsis (toxic shock; complicating major surgery)	31
Acute renal failure (oliguria < 500 ml/24 hours; anuria > 24 hours; BUN 0.8 gr% > 48 hours; creatinine 2 mg% > 48 hours)	23
Postoperative complications following major surgery	21
Hypotension (30-40 mm Hg drop from normal values, or 100 mm Hg drop in hypertensive patients, > 24 hours)	15
Burns (20% of total body surface or more)	13
Head injury (coma)	10
Politrauma	7

*This work was supported by grants 78.01.877.65 and 78.01.848.65 from the Consiglio Nazionale delle Richerche, Rome, Italy.

University of Rome and the Ospedali Riuniti of Rome were reviewed. Of these 800 patients, 168 were classified as high-risk, based on criteria established from a review of our hospital records and of the literature (see Table I), and were entered into the study.

Sixty patients received cimetidine 200 mg at 6-hourly intervals, either intravenously or by mouth, throughout the course of the study; 52 patients received an antacid (aluminum magnesium hydroxide) 10 ml/hour, either by nasogastric tube or by mouth; the remaining 56 patients received no treatment. During the study period, all patients were observed for the development of clinical signs indicating gastrointestinal hemorrhage, and all patients with suspected or proven upper gastrointestinal tract bleeding immediately underwent upper gastrointestinal panendoscopy.

Treatment lasted at least 10 days, and 137 patients completed the study. Of the remaining 31 patients, 16 died before the tenth day of the study (mean survival time of 4 days), 6 did not comply with the therapy and 9 were transferred to other institutions.

Results

Table II shows the distribution of patients in each treatment group by risk categories. Risk categories and risk factors in the 3 groups were comparable.

One patient in the antacid group, and no patients in the cimetidine group, presented with upper gastrointestinal bleeding; this difference is not statistically significant. However, there were 8 patients in the no treatment group with upper gastrointestinal bleeding: patients in this group with 1 risk factor had a 14% chance of bleeding, while those with 2 or more risk factors had a 25% chance of bleeding.

Discussion

The significant occurrence of upper gastrointestinal bleeding in critically-ill patients has been well-established [7-10, 13-18].

Table II.   Risk categories for each group.

	Cimetidine (%)	Antacid (%)	No treatment (%)
Respiratory failure	41	48	45
Neurosurgery	25	25	26
Sepsis	18	18	18
Acute renal failure	11	14	16
Postoperative complications	16	4	16
Hypotension	9	7	12
Burns	9	9	8
Head injury	7	2	8
Politrauma	9	7	0
Mean number of risk factors per patient	1.5	1.4	1.5

Although the pathophysiological mechanism involved in acute gastroduodenal mucosal lesions is not completely understood, it has become increasingly clear that prophylaxis may be successful in preventing these bleeding lesions. In our controlled and randomized trial, both cimetidine and antacid prophylaxis significantly diminished the occurrence of upper gastrointestinal bleeding, when compared with the occurrence of bleeding in patients receiving no treatment. The main advantages of cimetidine over antacids were: excellent patient compliance, simplicity of clinical administration, and lack of problems related to the route of administration.

The present study also revealed that it is possible to clearly differentiate, on the basis of precise criteria, between patients with a high risk of upper gastrointestinal bleeding due to stress and patients without such risk. Just over 20% of the 800 patients consecutively admitted to our intensive care unit were in the high-risk category. Of the remaining 80%, considered low-risk, not 1 presented with bleeding.

The results of this study suggest that prophylactic measures in a precisely-characterized group of high-risk patients are of significant benefit in the prevention of acute gastroduodenal mucosal lesions, and that the prophylactic administration of cimetidine may have significant advantages over antacids.

References

1. Beil, A.R., Mannix, J. and Beal, J.M. (1964): Massive upper gastrointestinal hemorrhage after operation. *Am. J. Surg. 108,* 324.
2. Czaja, A.J., McAlhany, J.C. and Pruitt, B.A. (1974): Acute gastroduodenal disease after thermal injury: an endoscopic evaluation of incidence and natural history. *N. Engl. J. Med. 291,* 925.
3. Fisher, M., Lorenz, W., Reimann, H.J., Troidl, H., Rhode, H., Schwarz, B. and Hamelmann, H. (1977): Cimetidine prophylaxis of acute gastroduodenal lesions in patients at risk. In: *Cimetidine,* p. 280. Editor: W. Creutzfeldt. Excerpta Medica, Amsterdam.
4. Stremple, J.F., Mori, H., Lev, R. and Glass, G.B. (1973): The stress ulcer syndrome. In: *Current problems in surgery.* Yearbook Medical Publishers, Chicago.
5. Chernov, M.S., Hale, H.W. and Wood, M.D. (1971): Prevention of stress ulcer. *Am. J. Surg. 122,* 674.
6. Hastings, P.R., Skillman, J.J., Bushnell, L.S. and Silen, W. (1978): Antacid titration in the prevention of acute gastrointestinal bleeding. A controlled, randomized trial in 100 critically-ill patients. *N. Engl. J. Med. 298,* 1041.
7. Jungers, P., Kleinknecht, D. and Barbanel, C. (1972): Les hémorragies digestives chez l'insuffisant rénal aigu. *Ann. Chir. 26,* 893.
8. Kamada, T., Fusamoto, H., Kawano, S., Noguchi, M., Hiramatsu, K., Masuzawa, M., Abe, H., Fujii, C. and Sugimoto, T. (1977): Gastrointestinal bleeding following head injury: a clinical study of 433 cases. *J. Trauma 17,* 44.
9. Lewis, E.A. (1973): Gastroduodenal ulceration and haemorrhage of neurogenic origin. *Br. J. Surg. 60,* 279.
10. Lucas, C.E., Sugawa, C., Riddle, J., Rector, F., Rosenberg, B. and Walt, A.J. (1971): Natural history and surgical dilemma of 'stress' gastric bleeding. *Arch. Surg. 102,* 266.
11. McAlhany, J.C., Czaja, A.J. and Pruitt, B.A. (1976): Antacid control of complications from acute gastroduodenal disease after burns. *J. Trauma 16,* 645.
12. McDougall, B.R.D., Bailey, R.J. and Williams, R. (1977): H$_2$-receptor antagonist and antacids in the prevention of acute gastrointestinal haemorrhage in fulminant hepatic failure: two controlled trials. *Lancet 1,* 617.
13. Fisher, R.P. and Streple, J.F. (1972): Stress ulcers in posttraumatic renal insufficiency in patients from Vietnam. *Surg. Gynecol. Obstet. 134,* 790.

14. Skillman, J.J., Bushnell, L.S., Goldman, H. and Silen, W. (1969): Respiratory failure, hypotension, sepsis, and jaundice: a clinical syndrome associated with lethal haemorrhage from acute stress ulceration of the stomach. *Ann. Surg. 172,* 564.

15. Bourgeois, P., Roge, J., Garaix, P., Martin, E. and De Roissard, M. (1964): Les hémorragies digestives au cours de la réanimation respiratoire. *Sem. Hop. 54,* 2931.

16. Czaja, A.J., McAlhany, J.C. and Pruitt, B.A. (1976): Gastric acid secretion and acute gastroduodenal disease after burns. *Arch. Surg. 111,* 243.

17. Voisin, C., Guerrin, F., Wattel, F. and Tonnel, A.B. (1970): Hémorragies et lésions gastroduodénales en cours de réanimation respiratoire. *Lille Med. 15,* 1140.

18. Norton, L., Greer, J. and Eiseman, B. (1970): Gastric secretory response to head injury. *Arch. Surg. 101,* 200.

Prophylactic treatment with cimetidine after renal transplantation

Y. Vanrenterghem, L. Roels and P. Michielsen
Academisch Ziekenhuis Sint-Rafaël, Leuven, Belgium

Peptic ulceration is a frequent complication after renal transplantation. In a study reported by Owens [1], it occurred in 18% of the patients in the study group, with a mortality rate of 43% when complicated by gastrointestinal hemorrhage or perforation.

In our own series of 80 patients, who underwent transplantation between 1963 and 1972, gastrointestinal bleeding was responsible for death in 6 cases. Selective vagotomy and pyloroplasty in high acid secretors, combined with routine intensive antacid treatment, decreased the mortality to 1 patient in our subsequent group of 95 patients, transplanted between 1973 and 1976 [2]. Since June 1977, no further prophylactic pyloroplasties have been performed, but all transplanted patients have been routinely maintained on cimetidine 1 g/day for 1 year after surgery. This dose was reduced if renal insufficiency occurred, and as soon as the steroid dose was decreased to below 30 mg/day, the cimetidine dose was reduced to 400 mg/day.

Prophylactic cimetidine administration after renal transplantation has been found highly efficient by some investigators [3, 4], but a recent report cited finding 3 ulcers in 24 patients treated with cimetidine and no ulcers in 182 patients treated with antacids [5].

On the other hand, cimetidine has been shown to increase the in vitro response of T cells to mitogens [6]. In general, administration of cimetidine appears to augment the delayed hypersensitivity responses [7]. In dogs receiving routine immunosuppressive drugs after renal transplantation, the onset of rejection occurred earlier in animals treated with cimetidine, and survival was considerably shortened [8].

As both the safety and the efficiency of cimetidine prophylaxis in renal transplant patients have been questioned, the present paper reports on a retrospective study of 42 consecutive patients who were treated with cimetidine and have completed a 1-year follow-up, compared with data from our earlier 1-year follow-up of 42 consecutive patients transplanted before June 1977 and not treated with cimetidine (control group).

All 84 patients were transplanted with cadaveric kidneys, without taking into account the results of typing for HLA transplantation antigens, and were then placed on the following immunosuppressive regime:

1. methylprednisolone sodium succinate 1 g at the moment of transplantation;

2. prednisone 100 mg/day for the first 2 days after surgery, followed by a reduction in dose of 10 mg every other day until a dose of 50 mg/day was reached, and then continued slow reduction to a dose of 20 mg/day at the end of the first year after surgery;

3. cyclophosphamide 300 mg/day, administered intravenuously for 2-3 days after transplantation;

4. azathioprine administered continuously, starting with 4 mg/kg/day and slowly decreasing to 2 mg/kg/day; and

5. antilymphocyte globulin 2.5 g on day 1, followed by 1.25 g/day for 9 days.

This treatment regime was administered to all patients, except that 13 patients in the cimetidine group received antilymphocyte globulin only for the first 2 days after transplantation, due to a temporary shortage of this product. Acute rejection crises were treated by increasing the prednisone dose to 200 mg/day, associated in some cases with intermittent bolus therapy with 1 g of methylprednisolone sodium succinate or cyclophosphamide, 300 mg intravenously.

As shown in Table I, the 2 groups were comparable with respect to those factors known to influence the risk of ulceration; there were, however, 5 duodenal ulcers and 1 bleeding esophagitis in the control group, and none in the cimetidine group.

The tolerance for cimetidine was excellent: its administration was discontinued in 3 patients with unexplained fever and serum creatinine increase, and in 8 other patients with leucopenia; retrospectively, though, there was no indication that these side-effects were attributable to cimetidine.

From these data, it can be concluded that prophylactic administration of cimetidine for 1 year after renal transplantation can prevent most acute gastrointestinal hemorrhages. Our data are in agreement with the experience of others [4], but do not agree with the results of Hussey and Belzer [5]. There is no obvious explanation for this discrepancy.

Although the effectiveness of 1 year of cimetidine treatment seems well-established, the optimum duration of cimetidine treatment after transplantation has yet to be determined. In the Rudge et al. study [4], treatment lasted only 4-6 weeks and excellent results were obtained. In our own patients, only 2 of the 6 gastrointestinal complications seen occurred before 6 weeks. This high incidence of late ulcers is probably due to our policy of long-term aggressive treatment in the presence of multiple episodes of graft rejection, which leads to prolonged administration of high doses of steroids (see Table II). Our data suggest that routine prophylaxis for 6 months would cover the main risk period; another alternative would be to give long-term treatment only to patients with a high peak acid excretion. For the normal acid producers, treatment could probably be limited to the period during which high steroid doses are given.

Table I. Clinical data.

	Cimetidine group	Control group
Number of patients	42	42
Sex (males/females)	(32/10)	(27/15)
Mean age (years)	32.9 ± 9.97	32.7 ± 10.63
Months on dialysis	15.14 ± 15.37	18.57 ± 17.69
Mean peak acid secretion before transplantation (mEq/half hour)	14.04 ± 8.89	9.56 ± 4.66
Duodenal ulcer	0	5 (4 with bleeding)
Bleeding gastroesophagitis	0	1

Table II. Steroid treatment in the cimetidine and control groups, expressed as mg of prednisone/day.

Days after transplantation		Cimetidine group	Control group
0- 15	mean ± SD	189.33 ± 83.90	182.57 ± 101.20
	median	197.60	176.00
16- 30	mean ± SD	125.90 ± 88.22	105.61 ± 75.37
	median	80.00	59.30
31- 90	mean ± SD	64.68 ± 30.60	75.67 ± 52.78
	median	49.50	61.00
91-180	mean ± SD	39.63 ± 7.38	42.32 ± 19.60
	median	38.20	36.70
181-365	mean ± SD	36.90 ± 15.54	32.21 ± 16.76
	median	27.30	27.10

Gastrointestinal hemorrhages occurred in the control group on days 20, 39, 58, 61, 110 and 288.

Table III. Immunological comparison of cimetidine and control groups.

	Cimetidine group	Control group
Nontransfused patients	1	7
Preformed HLA antibodies	4	5
Number of HLA compatibilities for A and B locus	1.5 ± 1.2	1.8 ± 1.0
Phytohemagglutinin*	284.4 ± 259.0	171.4 ± 123.0
Mixed lymphocyte cultures	11.9 ± 18.7	9.21 ± 13.8
Patient survival at 1 year	94.83%	94.87%
Graft survival at 1 year	83.33%	80.95%

*The difference between cimetidine and control groups was statistically significant: $0.01 < p < 0.02$.

In most studies of cimetidine administration in transplant patients, the drug has been administered for a short period of time [3, 9]. Since, in the present study, cimetidine was administered continuously for 1 year, a possible harmful effect on graft tolerance was more likely to become apparent. Before transplantation, the cimetidine and control groups were comparable from the immunological point of view (Table III). Only the response to phytohemagglutinin stimulation was significantly stronger in the cimetidine group. Patient and graft survival at 1 year were almost identical in the 2 groups.

Sixty-seven rejection crises occurred in the cimetidine group, compared with 71 in the control group (Table IV). The number of crises per patient and the severity of individual crises were not significantly different between the groups. There was a slight tendency for rejection crises to occur somewhat earlier in the cimetidine group, although the total dose of steroids administered was not significantly different during any time period (Table II).

We were unable to demonstrate any influence of cimetidine administration on

Table IV.   Rejection crises in the cimetidine and control groups.

		Cimetidine group	Control group
Number of crises per patient	0	3	7
	1	18	15
	2	15	10
	3	5	5
	4	1	4
	5	0	1
Grade*	0	9	3
	1	37	40
	2	14	15
	3	3	5
	4	0	2
	5	4	6
Day of occurrence	< 30	45	41
	31-60	6	14
	61-90	6	5
	91-180	2	4
	181-365	8	7

*Grade 0: rejection without serum creatinine increase
Grade 1: rejection with serum creatinine increase < 1 mg %
Grade 2: rejection with serum creatinine increase > 1 mg %
Grade 3: rejection with serum creatinine increase > 1 mg % for > 30 days
Grade 4: rejection with temporary hemodialysis
Grade 5: rejection with kidney destruction or death of the patient

graft tolerance. In evaluating the significance of this finding, the relatively high standard immunosuppressive regime administered should be taken into account. It may not be justified to extrapolate our results to groups receiving less aggressive immunosuppressive therapy and lower steroid doses.

A discrepancy between our results in humans and results previously reported in dogs [8] could be explained by the high doses of cimetidine ($\pm$ 30 mg/kg) administered to the group of animals showing a significant earlier rejection and decreased survival. In rats [6] and mice [10], an unexpected prolongation of skin graft survival following cimetidine treatment has been reported. Species and organ influences may perhaps explain these surprising results.

In conclusion, although in vitro and in vivo tests have demonstrated that cimetidine can increase delayed hypersensitivity reactions and lymphocyte response to mitogens, our data show no significant influence on kidney graft tolerance in patients receiving prophylactic cimetidine for 1 year. The incidence of duodenal ulcer and gastrointestinal hemorrhage, however, decreased significantly. Routine prophylactic cimetidine therapy seems efficient and safe in renal transplant patients.

References

1. Owens, M.L., Passaro, E., Wilson, S.E. and Gordon, E. (1977): Treatment of peptic ulcer

disease in the renal transplant patient. *Ann. Surg. 186,* 17.

2. Michielsen, P., Hauglustaine, D., Roels, L., Van Boven, W. and Waer, M. (1977): Evaluation of the clinical risk in renal transplantation. In: *Transplantation and clinical immunology, International Congress Series 423,* p. 221. Editors: J.L. Touraine, J. Traeger and R. Triau. Excerpta Medica, Amsterdam-Oxford-Princeton.

3. Jones, R.H., Rudge, C.J., Bewick, M., Parsons, V. and Weston, M.J. (1978): Cimetidine: prophylaxis against upper gastrointestinal haemorrhages after renal transplantation. *Br. Med. J. 1,* 398.

4. Rudge, C.J., Jones, R.H., Bewick, M., Weston, M.J. and Parsons, V. (1979): Peptic ulcer after renal transplantation. *Lancet 1,* 562.

5. Hussey, J.L. and Belzer, F.O. (1979): Cimetidine in renal transplant recipients. *Lancet 1,* 1089.

6. Smith, M.D., Couhig, E., Miller, J.S. and Salaman, J.R. (1979): Cimetidine and the immune response. *Lancet 1,* 1406.

7. Avella, J., Madsen, J.E., Binder, H.J. and Askenase, P.W. (1978): Effect of histamine H_2-receptor antagonists on delayed hypersensitivity. *Lancet 1,* 624.

8. Zammit, M. and Toledo-Pereyra, L.H. (1979): Increased rejection after cimetidine treatment in kidney transplants. *Transplantation 27,* 358.

9. Charpentier, B. and Fries, D. (1978): Cimetidine and renal-allograft rejection. *Lancet 1,* 1265.

10. Goodwin, J.S., Goldberg, E.M. and Williams, R.C. (1979): Prevention of skin graft rejection in mice treated with cimetidine. *Clin. Res. 27,* 37A.

Double-blind controlled trial of cimetidine in bleeding peptic ulcer

J.P. Galmiche, R. Colin, M. Veyrac, P. Hecketsweiler, D. Ouvry, P. Tenière* and P. Ducrotté
*Department of Gastroenterology and *Surgical Clinic, Hôpital Charles Nicolle, Rouen, France*

Introduction

Cimetidine, a histamine H_2-receptor antagonist, has been shown to be an effective treatment for peptic ulcer healing. An additional apparent benefit of this drug — effectiveness in controlling acute upper gastrointestinal bleeding — was reported in preliminary uncontrolled studies [1-4]; however, further double-blind trials failed to show any effect of cimetidine on continued bleeding or rebleeding [5-7]. Our own interim results [8] were in agreement with these latter studies, but as the cimetidine-treated patients in our trial were significantly older than those who received placebo and, moreover, as we observed that the duration of hemorrhage and the volume of blood replacement were significantly reduced by cimetidine treatment in patients who stopped bleeding during the trial [8, 9], we decided to continue our study in the hope of identifying 1 or more subgroups of patients in which cimetidine may be effective in controlling acute upper gastrointestinal bleeding from peptic ulcers. In this paper, we present results of our double-blind randomized trial, which was conducted in accordance with the principles of the Helsinki Declaration.

Subjects and methods

Ninety-six patients with acute upper gastrointestinal bleeding and endoscopically-proven gastric and/or duodenal ulceration entered the trial. All entering patients presented with hematemesis occurring in the 24 hours prior to endoscopy, with fresh blood in the gastric or duodenal lumen at endoscopic assessment, or with both of these signs of acute bleeding. Patients with obvious arterial bleeding at endoscopy were excluded from the study, as were patients with known blood dyscrasias, bleeding abnormalities (e.g. anticoagulant treatment), significant renal insufficiency (serum creatinine > 30 mg/l), stress ulcers, Mallory Weiss syndrome or portal hypertension (esophageal varices). Patients with malignant gastric ulceration were also excluded; if gastric biopsies at the end of the study revealed a previously unsuspected malignancy, they were excluded at that time.

After admission to the hospital, patients received standard blood replacement therapy and endoscopy was performed within 12 hours. The study period started at the time of endoscopy and lasted 7 ± 1 days. Patients who fulfilled the criteria for admission to the trial were randomized either to the cimetidine or the placebo group according to a predetermined randomized prescription list. Cimetidine 1.6 g/day or placebo was administered in 1 liter of a 5% glucose solution intravenously at a constant rate of infusion for 3 days. Thereafter, the treatment was administered orally: cimetidine or matched placebo 3 times a day after meals and 400 mg at bedtime for 4 days.

During the first 48 hours, all patients received an intragastric instillation of 2 liters of a standard antacid mixture (aluminium magnesium hydroxide, aminocaproic acid, thrombin, glucids and water).

Blood loss was replaced up to a hematocrit of at least 35%.

Pulse rate and blood pressure were checked 3-hourly and hematocrit was measured twice daily throughout the trial. During the first 2 days, samples of gastric juice were aspirated every 6 hours and their appearance was recorded, with particular reference to the presence or absence of fresh blood. Blood samples for routine laboratory analysis (WBC, platelets, glycemia, creatinine, SGOT and SGPT) were taken before treatment on day 3, and again at the end of the trial.

When the patient did not rebleed, endoscopy was repeated at the end of the trial; biopsies were systematically taken in cases of gastric ulcers. When patients did not respond to treatment, their study period was considered as completed and an emergency endoscopy was performed to confirm recurrent or persistent bleeding. Criteria for treatment failure were defined as follows: persistent bleeding (i.e., bleeding requiring more than 8 blood units in addition to the initial blood replacement to recover a hematocrit equal to or higher than 35%), or recurrent bleeding after the initial hemorrhage had ceased completely for at least 24 hours.

Study of gastric pH

In order to assess the respective effects of antacid mixture and cimetidine, the gastric pH of 2 patients (1 with gastric ulcer and 1 with duodenal ulcer) was continuously monitored under the 4 following conditions: control period (no treatment), intragastric antacid instillation, cimetidine alone, and cimetidine plus antacid instillation.

After an overnight fast, each of these 2 patients swallowed a Beckman Cecar electrode (sensitivity ± 0.03 pH) attached to the nasogastric tube used for intragastric instillation. The distance from the open tip of the nasogastric tube to the distal end of the pH probe was 10 cm. The pH probe was connected to a Beckman pH meter and the gastric pH was recorded on graph paper at a speed of 2.5 mm/minute. After an equilibration period of 1 hour, the 4 therapeutic regimens being tested were administered successively, in random order, with each 6-hour period of monitoring separated from the next by a 2-hour wash-out. The doses of antacid mixture (0.5 1/6 hours) and of cimetidine (0.4 g/6 hours, infused intravenously) were the same as those administered in the trial. Before and after each experiment, the pH electrode was standardized at 2 different buffers (pH 1 and pH 7). The recorded tracings were analyzed, and the results were expressed as the percentage of time below each pH interval.

Statistics

For statistical analysis, χ^2 and Fisher's exact tests were used.

Results

Ninety-six patients completed the trial; 2 of these were excluded when gastric biopsies at the end of the study period revealed malignant gastric ulceration. A third patient, who rebled on day 3 from a Mallory Weiss syndrome, was also excluded. Of the remaining 93 patients, 47 had received placebo and 46 had received cimetidine treatment. These 2 groups were well-matched for age, sex, past history of peptic ulcer disease, duration of dyspepsia, incidence of previous gastroduodenal bleeding,

Table I.   Comparison of the trial groups.

	Placebo group (n = 47)	Cimetidine group (n = 46)	p
Age (mean ± SEM)	54.6 ± 2.6	57.4 ± 2.3	NS
Sex	31 male	28 male	NS
	16 female	18 female	
History of peptic ulcer disease	21	24	NS
Duration of dyspepsia (years, mean ± SEM)	10.16 ± 3.13	9.97 ± 2.15	NS
Previous gastrointestinal hemorrhage	8	12	NS
Anti-inflammatory drug users	28	24	NS
Hematocrit (%) on admission (mean ± SEM)	31.4 ± 0.7	32.4 ± 0.9	NS

NS = not significant.

Table II.   Site of lesions in trial groups.

	Placebo group	Cimetidine group
Gastric ulcer	24	24
Duodenal ulcer	11	12
Multiple gastric and/or duodenal ulcers	11	9
Anastomotic ulcer	1	1
Total patients in group	47	46

Table III.   Treatment failure, according to site of ulceration. Total number of patients in each subgroup who completed the trial is given in parentheses.

	Placebo group	Cimetidine group	p
Gastric ulcer	5 (24)	0 (24)	< 0.05
Duodenal ulcer	1 (11)	2 (12)	NS
Multiple ulcers	5 (11)	3 (9)	NS
Anastomotic ulcer	1 (1)	0 (1)	—
All patients	12 (47)	5 (46)	< 0.10

NS = not significant.

Table IV. Outcome of bleeding, according to age.

Age	Treatment group	No rebleeding	Treatment failure	Significance level
< 50 years	Placebo	17	0	NS
	Cimetidine	12	1	$p < 0.005$
≥ 50 years	Placebo	18	12	$p < 0.02$
	Cimetidine	29	4	

NS = not significant.

Table V. Duration of hemorrhage and blood replacement in patients who did not rebleed during course of study.

	Placebo group (n = 35)	Cimetidine group (n = 41)	Significance
Duration of hemorrhage			
less than 2 days	21	36	$p < 0.01$
more than 2 days	14	5	
Number of blood units* required (mean ± SEM)	3.31 ± 0.38	1.87 ± 0.25	$p < 0.01$

*Variations in hematocrit during the study were not significantly different in cimetidine and placebo groups. Cimetidine: 6.4 ± 1.2 (mean ± SEM); placebo: 8.0 ± 0.9 (mean ± SEM).

Table VI. Comparison of the present study with 3 controlled trials of cimetidine in upper gastrointestinal bleeding.

Trial	Dosage (mg/24 hours)	Route of administration	Results
LaBrooy et al. [6]	1600	Orally (4 × 400 mg)	Negative
Pickard et al. [7]	1000	Intravenous bolus (4 × 250 mg)	Negative
Dykes et al. [10]	1200	Intravenous infusion (discontinuous)	Positive in patients over 65 years old, and in those with gastric ulcers
Present study	1600	Intravenous infusion (continuous)	Positive in patients over 50 years old, and in those with gastric ulcers

and mean hematocrit value on admission to the trial (Table I), and also for site of bleeding ulcer (Table II). More than half of the patients who bled had received anti-inflammatory drugs (acetylsalicylic acid in about two-thirds of these cases) immediately before their hemorrhage.

The outcome of bleeding according to endoscopic findings is presented in Table III. In the placebo group, 12 patients (26%) were classified as treatment failures, while only 5 (11%) of the cimetidine-treated patients failed to stop bleeding; this difference just fails to reach a 5% level of significance. No treatment failure at all was observed in the subgroup of gastric ulcer patients treated with cimetidine, a statistically-significant difference from the 5 failures in the subgroup of gastric ulcer patients on placebo ($p < 0.05$).

Since the incidence of failure was significantly higher among patients in the placebo group who were older than 50 years, we examined this factor separately (Table IV) and found a significant difference between placebo and cimetidine in older patients ($p < 0.02$).

Of the 52 patients who had taken anti-inflammatory drugs prior to hemorrhage, 8 of the 28 who received placebo rebled, compared with only 1 of the 24 treated with cimetidine ($p < 0.05$).

Seventeen patients were classified as treatment failures and withdrawn from the trial: 5 from the cimetidine group and 12 from the placebo group. All 5 of the patients who failed on cimetidine were operated; 2 of these 5 died post-operatively. Surgery was indicated in 6 of the 12 patients who failed on placebo; 1 of these died pre-operatively, 2 during the operation and 1 post-operatively. In the other 6 placebo failures, cimetidine therapy was substituted for placebo following withdrawal from the trial; bleeding stopped quickly in 5 of the 6, and the sixth, who was 91 years old, refused surgery and died.

In the patients who did not rebleed during the course of the study, the duration of the hemorrhage period and the blood replacement requirements were significantly lowered by cimetidine, as compared with placebo (Table V).

The results of gastric pH monitoring in 2 patients under 4 different treatment conditions are shown in the Figure.

No side effects were observed in any patients during the trial.

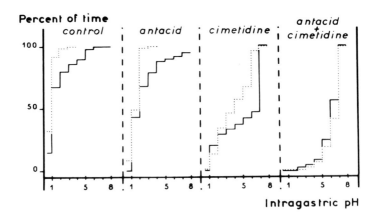

Figure   Intragastric pH monitoring in 2 patients with bleeding peptic ulcers, under 4 different therapeutic regimes. Solid line = patient with gastric ulcer; dotted line = patient with duodenal ulcer. Results are expressed as percent of time below each corresponding pH interval.

Discussion

The results of the present study indicate that cimetidine therapy significantly benefits patients with bleeding gastric ulcers, but not those with duodenal or multiple ulceration.

The effectiveness of cimetidine in older patients and in patients who took anti-inflammatory drugs prior to hemorrhage may have been related to the site of ulceration in these patients, as those with gastric ulcers tended to be older, and used gastrotoxic drugs more frequently, than other patients. However, there was no statistical difference in age or consumption of gastrotoxic drugs between gastric ulcer patients treated with cimetidine and those who were given placebo.

A comparison of the present trial with 3 previously-published studies shows important differences in methodology and conflicting results (Table VI). In 2 of these 3 studies [7, 10], entering patients presented with a wider range of causes of gastrointestinal bleeding (i.e., Mallory Weiss syndrome, hemorrhagic gastritis, esophagitis, bleeding from unknown etiology). In the Dykes et al. study [10], cimetidine and placebo groups were not comparable with respect to site of bleeding, since 9 out of 25 patients with gastric ulcers received cimetidine (36%), compared with 18 out of 29 patients with duodenal ulcers (72%). Moreover, the dosage and route of administration of cimetidine varied considerably between trials. It is interesting to note that only the 2 trials in which high doses of cimetidine were administered by intravenous infusion gave positive results, and then in older patients and/or those with gastric ulcers in both cases.

Control of acidopeptic mucosal injury is a major aim in the treatment of acute gastroduodenal bleeding [11]. In duodenal ulcer patients, Barbezat and Bank [12] showed that, following an oral dose of cimetidine 200 mg, all subjects were achlorhydric for 1.82 ± 0.39 (mean $\pm$ SEM) hours. After oral cimetidine 400 mg, achlorhydria lasted 2.75 ± 0.35 (mean $\pm$ SEM) hours. In seriously-ill patients [13], gastric pH fell to 1.9 about 5 hours after an intravenous injection of cimetidine 300 mg, while after an intravenous dose of 400 mg it was still at the baseline level of 5.9 after 4.5 hours, but had fallen to 3.0 after 6 hours.

Our results in patients with bleeding peptic ulcers showed that, even with a high dose (400 mg, intravenously infused), cimetidine alone failed to control gastric pH above 5 (see Figure). Although antacid mixture alone was less effective than cimetidine, the combination of these treatments reduced to almost zero the time of exposure of the gastric mucosa to low pH. These results suggest that the failure to demonstrate the effectiveness of cimetidine in 2 previously-reported double-blind trials [6, 7] could be a consequence of either insufficient doses or of inadequate route of administration. Cimetidine plus antacids may represent a useful alternative in the treatment of gastrointestinal bleeding.

The mechanism of action of cimetidine in the treatment of bleeding gastric ulcers remains unclear. It is highly unlikely that the healing effect of cimetidine in peptic ulcer plays an important part since the patients stopped bleeding very shortly after the treatment was initiated. Furthermore, endoscopy performed at completion of the trial did not reveal any major change in the size or appearance of ulcerations except that they had stopped bleeding. The significant decrease in blood replacement requirements in patients who stopped bleeding after cimetidine therapy suggests that this drug might alter gastric mucosal blood flow. This effect of cimetidine on blood requirements does not seem to be the result of excessive transfusion in patients who received placebo, since the mean variation in hematocrit value during the trial was similar in placebo and treated groups (Table V). However, in spite of some evidence for H_2-receptors in the gastromesenteric circulation [14, 15], no definite information is yet available on the actual effect of cimetidine in pathological conditions of therapeutic use in man [16, 17]. Recently, Dykes et al. [10] suggested that cimetidine could prevent acid proteolytic digestion of a fresh clot attached to an eroded vessel. In vitro studies [18, 19] have shown that both soluble coagulation and platelet function are extremely sensitive to a minor decrease in pH level, and that pepsin enhances platelet disaggregation.

Conclusions

Further controlled trials are still necessary to investigate specific aspects of cimetidine therapy in gastrointestinal bleeding, such as bleeding erosive gastritis and esophagitis. At this time, though, and in view of the results reported in this paper, we recommend the routine use of intravenous cimetidine 1600 mg/day in patients with bleeding gastric ulcer and in the high-risk group, especially in older patients and those with a history of anti-inflammatory drug ingestion.

References

1. Burland, W.L. and Parr, S.N. (1977): Experiences with cimetidine in the treatment of seriously-ill patients. In: *Cimetidine: Proceedings of the second International Symposium on histamine H_2-receptor antagonists,* p. 345. Editors: W.L. Burland and M.A. Simkins. Excerpta Medica, Amsterdam-Oxford-Princeton.
2. Bubrick, M.P., Wetherille, R.E., Onstadt, G.R., Andersen, R.C. and Hitchcock, C.R. (1978): Control of acute gastroduodenal hemorrhage with cimetidine. *Surgery 84,* 510.
3. Dunn, D.H., Silvis, S., Onstadt, G., Fischer, R., Howard, R.D. and Delaney, J.P. (1977): The treatment of hemorrhagic gastritis with the H_2-blocking antihistamine cimetidine. *Gastroenterology 72,* 1053.
4. MacDonald, A.S., Steele, B.J. and Bottomley, M.C. (1976): Treatment of stress-induced upper gastrointestinal haemorrhage with metiamide. *Lancet 1,* 68.
5. Eden, K. and Kern, K. Jr. (1978): Current status of cimetidine in upper gastrointestinal bleeding. *Gastroenterology 74,* 446.
6. LaBrooy, S.J., Misiewicz, J.J., Edwards, J., Smith, P.M., Haggie, S.J., Libman, L., Sarner, M., Wyllie, J.H., Croker, J. and Cotton, P. (1979): Controlled trial of cimetidine in upper gastrointestinal haemorrhage. *Gut 20,* 892.
7. Pickard, R.G., Sanderson, I., South, M., Kirkham, J.S. and Northfield, T.C. (1979): Controlled trial of cimetidine in acute upper gastrointestinal bleeding. *Br. Med. J. 1,* 661.
8. Galmiche, J.P., Colin, R., Hecketsweiler, P., Le Grix, A., Metayer, P., Le Bihan, M., Tenière, P. and Geffroy, Y. (1978): Traitement des hémorragies digestives ulcéreuses par la Cimétidine. Résultats d'une étude contrôlée en double aveugle. *Gastroenterol. Clin. Biol. 2,* 771.
9. Galmiche, J.P., Colin, R., Hecketsweiler, P., Metayer, P., Tenière, P., Le Grix, A. and Geffroy, Y. (1980): Traitement par la Cimétidine des hémorragies ulcéreuses gastroduodénales. Résultats d'une étude contrôlée en double aveugle. In: *Proceedings of the VIth World Congress of Gastroenterology, Madrid.* (In press.)
10. Dykes, P.W., Hoare, A.M., Hawkins, C.F. and Kang, J.Y. (1978): The treatment of upper gastrointestinal haemorrhage with cimetidine. In: *Cimetidine: the Westminster Hospital Symposium,* p. 337. Editors: C. Wastell and P. Lance. Churchill Livingstone, Edinburgh.
11. Simonian, S.J. and Curtis, L.E. (1976): Treatment of hemorrhagic gastritis by antacid. *Ann. Surg. 184,* 429.

12. Barbezat, G.O. and Bank, S. (1977): Basal acid output response to cimetidine in man. In: *Cimetidine: Proceedings of the second International Symposium on histamine H$_2$-receptor antagonists,* p. 110. Editors: W.L.Burland and M.A. Simkins. Excerpta Medica, Amsterdam-Oxford-Princeton.
13. Nagler, J. (1978): Cimetidine and gastric pH. *Gastroenterology 4,* 770.
14. Guth, P.H. and Smith, E. (1978): Histamine receptors in the gastric microcirculation. *Gut 19,* 1059.
15. Owen, D.A.A., Flynn, S.B., Harvey, C.A., Johnson, B.M., Farrington, H.C. and Shaw, K.D. (1978): The evidence for histamine receptors in the gastromesenteric circulation. In: *Cimetidine: the Westminster Hospital Symposium,* p. 207. Editors: C. Wastell and P. Lance. Churchill Livingstone, Edinburgh.
16. Delaney, J.P., Michel, H.M. and Bond, J. (1978): Cimetidine and gastric blood flow. *Surgery 84,* 190.
17. Levine, B.A., Schwesinger, W.H., Sirinck, K.R., Jones, D. and Pruitt, B.A. (1978): Cimetidine prevents reduction in gastric mucosal blood flow during shock. *Surgery 84,* 113.
18. Green, F.W., Kaplan, M.M., Curtis, L.E. and Levine, P.H. (1978): Effect of acid and pepsin on blood coagulation and platelet aggregation: a possible contributor to prolonged gastroduodenal mucosal haemorrhage. *Gastroenterology 74,* 38.
19. Djaldetti, M., Fishman, P., Bessler, H. and Chaimoff, C. (1979): pH-induced platelet ultrastructural alterations. A possible mechanism for unpaired platelet aggregation. *Arch. Surg. 114,* 707.

Discussion

Pio (Fermo): I would like to ask whether, in Professor Speranza's study, the 9 patients who bled were later treated with cimetidine and, if so, what the results were.

Basso: All the patients who bled were later treated with cimetidine, intravenously or orally. Of these, none was operated on; one died from a cardiac infarct after bleeding had ended. Clearly, we can draw no conclusions from this.

Ciammaichella (Rome): In the Head Injury Division of the San Giovanni Hospital, we have studied 10 cases with 3 features in common: second-degree coma, tracheostomy for respiratory difficulties, and cerebral angiography, which showed only contusions, without intracranial haematomata. Serum gastrin was measured radioimmunologically in all 10 patients and the response was very characteristic: peak gastrin level was found at 24 hours, after which it fell slowly. After the fourth day following the head injury, gastrin was returning towards normal, but remained slightly above control levels. Thus, the maximum blood gastrin in patients with head injuries occurred in the first day and then fell until the fourth day.

Bianchi (Milan): I want to ask a rather general question, possibly a naive one, to Professor Speranza. When we speak of the stress ulcer syndrome, generally we mean a gastric lesion, as he himself has shown. But from his series, and also from my own experience, I have found that the lesions in general are in the duodenum, with only about 1 in 8 affecting the stomach. These duodenal lesions are mostly revealed by endoscopy, and are being found to be present much more frequently than was thought to be the case. Would Professor Speranza comment on this?

Speranza: I have never said, nor do I think that anyone has said, that stress lesions are gastric and not duodenal. Included in the stress ulcer syndrome, that is to say acute gastroduodenal lesions, are all ulcers affecting alkaline mucosa, gastric as well as duodenal, because this ulceration occurs only in alkaline mucosa — even chronic peptic ulcers arise in alkaline mucosa or at the border between alkaline and acid mucosa, whereas erosions affect mainly the mucosa of the fundus. As the fundus and the body are in the stomach and not in the duodenum, it is rare to find erosions with those characteristics in the duodenum, except during the phase preceding acute ulceration. However, under conditions of stress there may be either a gastric ulcer or a duodenal ulcer, just as in conditions of stress we know that there may be an exacerbation of a chronic gastric or duodenal ulcer. When a patient has a simple operation, a cholecystectomy, but also has a duodenal ulcer which does not require surgery, we use prophylaxis to prevent post-operation bleeding from that ulcer.

So, we have this concept of acute stress ulcer, which means that during stress — including hypercapnia, hypovolaemia, hypoxaemia, head injury, respiratory failure, or any gross disturbance of homeostasis — when a certain stage is reached, adrenergic mechanisms may cause splanchnic vasoconstriction and back-diffusion or, alternatively, an increase in histamine and alterations in mucus and other components of mucosal defences, resulting in ulceration or erosion.

Forestieri (Naples): I have 2 questions for Professor Speranza. First, in haemorrhagic gastric erosions, the role of the microcirculation is very important in influencing the flow-retrodiffusion relationship. Matsumoto has shown that pharmacological doses of corticosteroids are effective in the prevention and treatment of haemorrhagic gastric erosions. What is your experience?

Secondly: I see that you used 10 ml/hour of antacids. Do you think that that dose is sufficient, given that Lucas and others, for example, have demonstrated that, in general, the optimal dose is 30 ml/hour? Is that dose fixed, or is it modified in accordance with the pH of the gastric juice?

Speranza: I can answer the first question very quickly, as it is slightly outside the scope of the problem. The use of corticosteroids in pharmacological doses is intended for the treatment of shock, which some of these patients may present.

As regards antacid: in practice, aluminium magnesium hydroxide 10 ml/hour instilled into the stomach is, of course, not a large dose. We did not measure the pH to see whether it was, in fact, significantly augmented. Thirty ml/hour certainly could be appropriate, even though I do not believe that it is the amount of antacid instilled which influences the problem.

Festen (Nijmegen): I think that Dr. Michielsen should be congratulated on his study. As far as I am aware, the data on renal allograft rejection are the first to be presented. I know what a great amount of work is involved in compiling these data, but the problem with them is that they are, of course, retrospective. Can Dr. Michielsen tell us whether or not the selection of the grafts, with regard to the histocompatibility in the patients, changed during the 2 years of the study? If it has changed, that could be significant.

Michielsen: With regard to whether the 2 groups were comparable as far as HLA compatibility is concerned, this was not taken into account in the selection of the recipients, as only local donors were used and we did not join either Eurotransplant or any similar organisation. Without taking HLA compatibility into account, we have graft survivals with cadaver kidneys close to 80% overall, and in both of these groups there were identical 85% survivals.

Looking retrospectively at the data, the mean number of compatibilities was identical in both groups, but this happened purely by chance; it was not taken into account in the selection.

Turpini (Pavia): Dr. Michielsen, did cimetidine effectively control the haemorrhagic diathesis associated with renal insufficiency?

Michielsen: Cimetidine was given only after transplantation, and coagulation disorders disappear after transplantation in any case.

Effect of cimetidine in reducing intragastric acidity in patients undergoing elective caesarean section

J.P. Howe, J. Moore, W. McCaughey and J.W. Dundee
Department of Anaesthetics, The Queen's University of Belfast, Belfast, United Kingdom

Introduction

Mendelson's syndrome — the pulmonary acid aspiration syndrome — is an infrequent but dreaded complication of obstetrical anaesthesia [1]. It is a specific form of aspiration pneumonia caused by the inhalation of acid gastric contents into the lungs of the parturient patient at any time during the peri-operative period. Classically, however, it occurs during the induction of anaesthesia for emergency caesarean section [2].

The clinical presentation is that of severe respiratory distress, characterised by intense bronchospasm, cyanosis and tachypnoea [1], followed by progressive hypoxia [3], systemic hypotension [4] and pulmonary oedema [5].

Moderate to severe consolidation is visible on radiological examination [6], and death frequently ensues 5-10 days postoperatively. The pathological process is that of a chemical pneumonitis, which has been likened to a burn injury to the lung parenchyma [4].

When, in 1946, Mendelson first described the condition which now bears his name, he postulated that it was caused by the acid content of the inhaled vomitus and reproduced it in rabbits by instilling 0.1 N hydrochloric acid into the trachea [1].

Subsequent workers confirmed this finding [4, 7-11], and also found that, when the pH of the gastric contents was below a certain level, aspiration into the lungs invariably resulted in chemical pneumonitis. Elevation of the pH above this level (usually 1.5-2.0) resulted in less severe pulmonary damage, or even no damage at all.

No equivalent work has been done on human subjects, but it is generally accepted that, for man, the critical pH level is 2.5 [12-14]. To avoid the consequences of acid aspiration, gastric pH must be maintained above this value.

Mortality due to Mendelson's syndrome is recorded triennially in the *Report on Confidential Enquiries into Maternal Deaths in England and Wales.* Examination of the last 5 reports reveals that pulmonary aspiration is consistently responsible for approximately 40-50% of anaesthetic-related maternal mortality, and for about 5% of total maternal mortality. From 1973-5, the last reported triennium, 13 patients died of pulmonary aspiration out of a total anaesthetic mortality of 31 [15].

It is not surprising that a wide variety of prophylactic measures have been advocated for the prevention of Mendelson's syndrome [16, 17], with the primary objective of reducing the acidity and volume of the gastric contents and the secondary objective of blocking the access of the gastric contents to the

Table I. Methods of prophylaxis against the pulmonary acid aspiration syndrome.

Reduction of acidity and volume of gastric contents before operation:
— fasting throughout labour
— antacid therapy during labour
— gastric evacuation by wide-bore tube
— apomorphine-induced vomiting
— metoclopramide before induction of anaesthesia

Prevention of regurgitation during intubation:
— 'awake intubation'
— oesophageal blockers
— patient lying on side
— tilting patient head-up or head-down
— cricoid pressure

---

tracheobronchial tree, should vomiting or regurgitation occur (Table I). It is the first of these 2 objectives which is most relevant to the present study.

The value of fasting throughout labour is self-evident [1]. Other measures, such as gastric evacuation by wide-bore tube [18, 19], apomorphine-induced vomiting [20, 21], and intravenous metoclopramide [22-24] have all been used prior to anaesthesia.

The most widely-advocated practice is that of administering oral antacid therapy during labour, and several agents and treatment regimens have been recommended [11, 13, 25-30]. These have the advantages of therapeutic efficacy in a high proportion of patients [28], ease of administration, and safety to the infant.

Antacids also have disadvantages, however, in that they cause frequent maternal nausea and vomiting [31]; occasional patients are not protected by antacid treatment, probably due to inadequate mixing of the antacid with an unknown volume of highly-acidic stomach contents [26, 32]. Furthermore, it has been suggested that antacids themselves may cause chemical pneumonitis if inhaled into the lungs in undiluted form [33-35], and 2 previously-reported animal experiments support this suggestion [11, 36]. The *Report on Confidential Enquiries into Maternal Deaths in England and Wales* for the years 1973-5 notes that 8 of the 9 patients who died from Mendelson's syndrome during that period (88.9%) had in fact received adequate antacid therapy [15].

A new approach to the problem may be the use of cimetidine, an H_2-receptor antagonist [37], whose effectiveness in elevating gastric pH is well-documented [38-40] and whose efficacy in the treatment of various acid-peptic disorders has been well established [41].

The aims of the present study were: to examine the effectiveness of an intravenous dose of cimetidine 200 mg in reducing gastric acidity and volume in patients undergoing elective caesarean section, to determine the optimum timing of cimetidine administration, and to assess its effects on both mother and fetus.

Because of the widespread distribution of H_2-receptors throughout the body [42-44], a preliminary study of 20 patients in normal labour was undertaken [45], and showed that cimetidine 200 mg intravenously, administered during the first stage of labour, does not affect uterine tone, nor does it affect the rate or rhythm of the fetal heart.

Patients and methods

We studied 45 healthy mothers-to-be, at or about term and scheduled for elective caesarean section. They were expected to deliver normal, healthy infants of equivalent gestational developments. Informed verbal consent was obtained from each patient, and the study was approved by the hospital's Ethical Committee.

Patients were randomly allocated either to a control group of 15 patients, who received neither cimetidine nor antacids, or a cimetidine group of 30 patients, who received cimetidine 200 mg intravenously approximately 60 minutes (10 patients), 90 minutes (10 patients), or 120 minutes (10 patients) prior to anaesthesia.

The 2 groups were comparable with regard to age, weight, height and haemoglobin concentration. The majority of patients (31 of the 45) were of parity 1 or 2, and the most common indication for surgery was previous caesarean section with cephalopelvic disproportion (80%).

A widely-accepted anaesthetic technique was employed [46], and all patients in the control group were anaesthetised by consultant obstetrical anaesthetists.

Following the induction of anaesthesia and tracheal intubation, a double-lumen Salem Sump tube was introduced, per oram, into the stomach of all patients. Its presence was confirmed, and the gastric contents were evacuated. This procedure was repeated at the conclusion of anaesthesia, prior to extubation of the trachea. The volume of both aspirates was noted, and pH was determined with a Corning 113 pH meter.

At delivery, 20 ml of maternal venous blood and 20 ml of blood from the umbilical cord of the delivered placenta were withdrawn. These samples were assayed for maternal and cord concentrations of cimetidine, gastrin and glucose.

Results were analyzed for significance, using Student's t test for unpaired samples.

Results

Gastric pH at intubation

At intubation, gastric aspirates and, therefore, pH values were obtained from 44 of the 45 patients (Fig. 1). Patients in the cimetidine group showed a significantly higher pH than those in the control group ($p < 0.001$ in the 60-minute subgroup, $p < 0.01$ in the 90-minute subgroup, and $p < 0.05$ in the 120-minute subgroup).

The mean [47] pH of patients in the control group was 2.1, while in the cimetidine-treated patients it was 5.1 (60 minutes), 4.5 (90 minutes), and 3.7 (120 minutes). Twelve of the 14 control patients had pH values less than 2.5, and were therefore 'at risk' of developing acid aspiration; in the cimetidine group, the number of patients at risk was 0 of 10 (60 minutes), 3 of 10 (90 minutes), and 4 of 10 (120 minutes).

Thus, at intubation, those patients given cimetidine 60 minutes before anaesthesia had the highest mean pH (5.1), and none of them had a pH below the critical level of 2.5.

Gastric pH at extubation

At extubation, gastric aspirates were obtained from 34 of the 45 patients (Fig. 2).

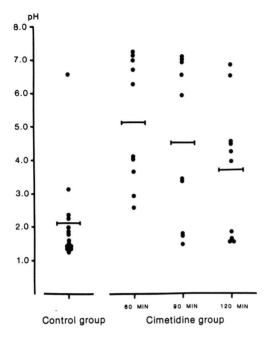

Fig. 1. Individual (•) and mean (⊢—⊣) pH of maternal gastric contents at intubation. Patients were either untreated (control group), or treated with cimetidine 200 mg intravenously at 60, 90 or 120 minutes prior to elective caesarean section.

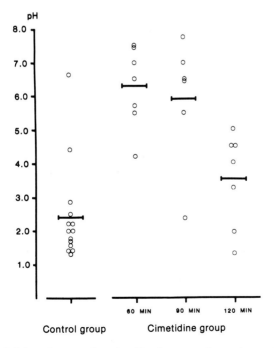

Fig. 2. Individual (○) and mean (⊢—⊣) pH of maternal gastric contents at extubation. Patients were either untreated (control group), or treated with cimetidine 200 mg intravenously at 60, 90 or 120 minutes prior to elective caesarean section.

Compared with the control group, significantly higher pH values were found in the cimetidine 60-minute and 90-minute subgroups ($p < 0.001$), but not in the 120-minute subgroup.

The mean pH in the control group was 2.4, and in the 3 cimetidine subgroups it was 6.3 (60 minutes), 5.9 (90 minutes), and 3.5 (120 minutes). Ten of the 14 control patients had pH values less than 2.5 and were therefore to be considered at risk of acid aspiration; in the cimetidine group, the number of patients at risk was 0 of 7 (60 minutes), 1 of 6 (90 minutes), and 2 of 7 (120 minutes).

Therefore, at extubation as at intubation, the patients given cimetidine 60 minutes before anaesthesia had the highest mean pH (6.3), and none of them had a pH below 2.5.

pH change during the course of operation (all patients)

The mean pH values noted at the beginning and end of anaesthesia reveal that the control group showed a rise in pH during the course of operation from 2.1 to 2.4 (Fig. 3), a finding which agrees with previously reported data [48]. In the cimetidine group, the 60-minute subgroup had the highest mean pH values at both intubation and extubation, and mean pH rose during the course of operation from 5.1 to 6.3. Although the mean pH values of the 90-minute subgroup rose from 4.5 at intubation to 5.9 at extubation, there were 4 patients in this subgroup with individual pH values of less than 2.5.

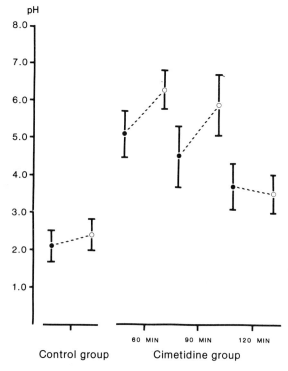

Fig. 3.   *Mean pH of maternal gastric contents at intubation (•) and extubation (○). Patients were either untreated (control group), or treated with cimetidine 200 mg intravenously at 60, 90 or 120 minutes prior to elective caesarean section.*

The mean pH of the 120-minute subgroup *fell* during the course of operation, from 3.7 to 3.5; presumably, the maximum therapeutic effect of cimetidine had passed by the time operation began.

pH change during the course of operation (60-minute subgroup)

A comparison of control patients with those given cimetidine 60 minutes before anaesthesia shows a marked contrast between these 2 groups (Fig. 4). Six of the 7 cimetidine-treated patients from whom both intubation and extubation samples were obtained showed rises in gastric pH intraoperatively. The 1 patient whose pH fell showed a decrease from 6.7 to 6.5.

However, 2 of these 6 patients had pH values only marginally above the critical level of 2.5 at intubation (2.52 in 1 case, 2.9 in the other). This illustrates a disadvantage of cimetidine as compared with the use of conventional antacids: cimetidine has no effect on the acidity of gastric contents already present at the time of its administration. (By extubation, the pH values of these 2 patients had risen to 4.20 and 5.50, respectively.)

Patients at risk

As shown in Table II, a large proportion of the patients in the control group were in this category, with pH levels below 2.5: 12 of the 14 patients at intubation (85.8%)

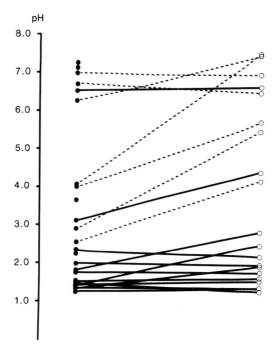

Fig. 4.   Individual pH of maternal gastric contents at intubation (•) and extubation (o). Patients were either untreated (——), or treated with cimetidine 200 mg intravenously at 60 minutes prior to elective caesarean section (----).

Table II.   Number of patients in the control and cimetidine groups with gastric contents pH levels of less than 2.5 at intubation and extubation. (Numbers in parentheses indicate the total number of aspirates obtained.)

	Control group	Cimetidine group		
		60 minutes	90 minutes	120 minutes
Intubation	12 (14)	0 (10)*	3 (10)*	4 (10)
Extubation	10 (14)	0 (7)*	1 (6)	2 (7)

*$p < 0.05$.

Table III.   Mean volume (and range) of maternal gastric contents in patients in the control and cimetidine groups. The unit of measurement for all volumes is milliliters.

	Control group	Cimetidine group		
		60 minutes	90 minutes	120 minutes
Intubation	20 (0-52)	14 (4-28)	10 (4-40)	15 (3-56)
Extubation	12 (0-48)	3 (0- 8)	2 (0- 8)*	7 (0-41)

*$p < 0.05$.

and 10 of the 14 at extubation (71.5%). On the other hand, there were *no* patients at risk in the 60-minute cimetidine subgroup; the difference with the control group is highly significant ($p < 0.001$ at intubation, $p < 0.01$ at extubation; χ^2 test). When cimetidine was administered 90 minutes before anaesthesia, a significantly smaller percentage of patients at risk was found only at intubation ($p < 0.02$), but the difference with the control group at extubation was not significant. No statistically-significant difference was found between control patients and those to whom cimetidine was given 120 minutes prior to anaesthesia, either at intubation or extubation.

Volumes

The aspirated volumes obtained were low in all patients, rarely exceeding 50 ml (Table III). This reflects the fasting state of the patients, the fact that they were not in active labour, and the absence of opiate analgesia [49].

While the mean volumes of the cimetidine-treated patients were generally lower, only those obtained at extubation from the 90-minute subgroup were statistically significant when compared with those of the control patients ($p < 0.05$) [50].

No correlation could be demonstrated between pH and volume of individual samples in either group. This appears to be the case whether patients are untreated, treated with cimetidine [51], or treated with antacids [26].

Maternal and umbilical blood cimetidine levels

Maternal venous blood and umbilical cord blood concentrations of cimetidine at delivery showed a significant degree of placental transfer of cimetidine (Fig. 5). The mean fetal to maternal ratio in the 30 patients treated with cimetidine was 0.75. This closely approximates the ratios as calculated separately for each of the 3 subgroups, tending to indicate that mother and fetus handle this drug similarly during the first 2 hours following injection. However, our preliminary study [45] showed that the fetal/maternal ratio rises at later sampling times. It also showed that cimetidine could not be detected in 7 out of 9 samples of infant 'heel prick' blood when it had been administered to the mother more than 8 hours prior to anaesthesia [McGowan, personal communication]. Although no correlation between individual drug concentrations and gastric pH and volumes was found, the 60-minute subgroup reflected an overall trend, in that 10 out of 10 mothers had a gastric pH greater than 2.5, and 9 of them had blood cimetidine concentrations greater than 0.5 μg/ml [38, 52].

Infant monitoring

Because of the placental transfer of cimetidine, it was obviously desirable to look at its effects in the infant. The parameters we examined were: Apgar scores at 2 and 5 minutes after delivery [53], scored from 8 and excluding 'colour' [54]; gastric pH and volume at delivery and at 2 hours after delivery; blood glucose concentrations at

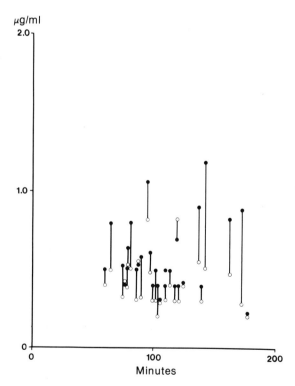

Fig. 5. Blood cimetidine concentrations (μg/ml) in mothers (•) and infants (o) at delivery. All mothers were treated with cimetidine 200 mg intravenously prior to elective caesarean section.

delivery and at 2 hours after delivery [55]; weight changes at 24 hours and at 8 days after delivery; and feeding progress.

There was no statistically-significant difference between the cimetidine and control groups for any of these parameters.

Conclusions

Cimetidine significantly reduces gastric acidity in the obstetrical patient, but gastric pH is only maintained above 2.5 during the course of operation when the drug is administered about 60 minutes prior to anaesthesia; this has no significant effect on the volume of gastric contents. Cimetidine is detectable in umbilical cord blood, but does not appear to produce any effect on the infant parameters studied.

Acknowledgements

Our grateful thanks are due to Dr M. Reid and Dr G. McClure, Consultant Neonatologists, Royal Maternity Hospital, Befast; Professor K. Buchanan, Department of Medicine, the Queen's University of Belfast; and the obstetrical and nursing staffs at Jubilee Maternity Hospital, Belfast, Craigavon Area Hospital, Craigavon, and Royal Maternity Hospital, Belfast.

References

1. Mendelson, C.L. (1946): The aspiration of stomach contents into the lungs during obstetric anesthesia. *Am. J. Obstet. Gynecol. 52,* 191.
2. Crawford, J.S. (1970): The anaesthetist's contribution to maternal mortality. *Br. J. Anaesth. 42,* 70.
3. Fisk, R.L., Symes, J.F., Aldridge, L.L. and Couves, C.M. (1970): The pathophysiology and experimental therapy of acid pneumonitis in ex vivo lungs. *Chest 57,* 364.
4. Awe, W.C., Fletcher, W.S. and Jacob, S.W. (1966): The pathophysiology of aspiration pneumonitis. *Surgery 60,* 232.
5. Alexander, I.G.S. (1968): The ultrastructure of the pulmonary alveolar vessels in Mendelson's (acid pulmonary aspiration) syndrome. *Br. J. Anaesth. 40,* 408.
6. Arms, R.A., Dines, D.E. and Tinstman, T.C. (1974): Aspiration pneumonia. *Chest 65,* 136.
7. Teabeaut, J.R. (1952): Aspiration of gastric contents. An experimental study. *Am. J. Path. 28,* 51.
8. Bannister, W.K., Sattilaro, A.J. and Otis, R.D. (1961): Therapeutic aspects of aspiration pneumonitis in experimental animals. *Anesthesiology 22,* 440.
9. Bosomworth, P.P. and Hamelberg, W. (1962): Etiologic and therapeutic aspects of aspiration pneumonitis. Experimental study. *Surg. Forum 13,* 158.
10. Hamelberg, W. and Bosomworth, P.P. (1964): Aspiration pneumonitis: experimental studies and clinical observations. *Anesth. Analg. (Cleveland) 43,* 669.
11. Taylor, G. and Pryse-Davies, J. (1966): The prophylactic use of antacids in the prevention of the acid pulmonary aspiration syndrome (Mendelson's syndrome). *Lancet 1,* 288.
12. Vandam, L.D. (1965): Aspiration of gastric contents in the operative period. *N. Engl. J. Med. 273,* 1206.
13. Roberts, R.B. and Shirley, M.A. (1974): Reducing the risk of acid aspiration during Caesarean section. *Anesth. Analg. (Cleveland) 53,* 859.
14. Editorial (1977): White-lipped anaesthesia. *Lancet 2,* 123.
15. Department of Health and Social Security (1979): *Report on Confidential Enquiries into Maternal Deaths in England and Wales, 1973-1975.* Editors: J. Tomkinson, A. Turnbull,

G. Robson, E. Cloake, A.M. Adelstein and J. Weatherall. H.M.S.O., London.

16. Crawford, J.S. (1978): Caesarean section. In: *Principles and practice of obstetric anaesthesia*, 4th edition, pp. 272-277. Blackwell Scientific Publications, London.

17. Moir, D.D. (1976): General anaesthesia. In: *Obstetric anaesthesia and analgesia*, pp. 131-141. Bailliere Tindall, London.

18. Doughty, A. (1972): Anaesthesia for operative obstetrics and gynaecology. In: *A practice of anaesthesia*, p. 1448. Editors: W.D. Wylie and H.C. Churchill-Davidson. Lloyd-Luke, London.

19. Hohmann, J.E. (1979): Routine gastric aspiration. *Anesthesiology 50,* 170.

20. Holdsworth, J.D., Furness, R.M.B. and Roulston, R.G. (1974): A comparison of apomorphine and stomach tubes for emptying the stomach before general anaesthesia in obstetrics. *Br. J. Anaesth. 46,* 526.

21. Holdsworth, J.D. (1978): The place of apomorphine prior to obstetric analgesia. *J. Int. Med. Res. 6,* 26.

22. Jacoby, H.I. and Brodie, D.A. (1967): Gastrointestinal actions of metoclopramide. An experimental study. *Gastroenterology 52,* 676.

23. Howells, T.H., Khanam, T., Kreel, L., Seymour, C., Oliver, B. and Davies, J.A.H. (1971): Pharmacological emptying of the stomach with metoclopramide. *Br. Med. J. 2,* 558.

24. Howard, F.A. and Sharp, D.S. (1973): Effects of metoclopramide on gastric emptying time during labour. *Br. Med. J. 1,* 446.

25. Williams, M. and Crawford, J.S. (1971): Titration of magnesium trisilicate mixture against gastric acid secretion. *Br. J. Anaesth. 43,* 783.

26. Peskett, W.G.H. (1973): Antacids before obstetric anaesthesia. *Anaesthesia 28,* 509.

27. Lahiri, S.K., Thomas, T.A. and Hodgson, R.M.H. (1973): Single dose antacid therapy for the prevention of Mendelson's syndrome. *Br. J. Anaesth. 45,* 1143.

28. Hutchinson, B.R. and Newson, A.J. (1975): Preoperative neutralization of gastric acidity. *Anaesth. Intensive Care 3,* 198.

29. Hester, J.B. and Heath, M.L. (1977): Pulmonary acid aspiration syndrome: should prophylaxis be routine. *Br. J. Anaesth. 49,* 595.

30. Holdsworth, J.D. (1978): A fresh look at magnesium trisilicate. *J. Int. Med. Res. 6,* 70.

31. Murphy, J.E. (1974): An Andrusil acceptability study. *J. Int. Med. Res. 2,* 19.

32. Robinson, J.S. and Thompson, J.M. (1979): Fatal aspiration (Mendelson's) syndrome despite antacids and cricoid pressure. *Lancet 1,* 228.

33. Scott, D.B. (1978): Mendelson's syndrome. *Br. J. Anaesth. 50,* 977. (Editorial.)

34. Moir, D.D. (1978): The contribution of anaesthesia to maternal mortality. *J. Int. Med. Res. 6,* 40.

35. Heaney, G.A.H. and Jones, H.D. (1979): Aspiration syndromes in pregnancy. *Br. J. Anaesth. 51,* 266.

36. Wheatley, R.G., Kallus, F.T., Reynolds, R.C. and Giesecke, A.H. (1979): Milk of magnesia is an effective preinduction antacid in obstetric anesthesia. *Anesthesiology 50,* 514.

37. Black, J.W., Duncan, W.A.M., Durant, C.J., Ganellin, C.R. and Parsons, E.M. (1972): Definition and antagonism of histamine H_2-receptors. *Nature 236,* 385.

38. Burland, W.L., Duncan, W.A.M., Hesselbo, T., Mills, J.G. and Sharpe, P.C. (1975): Pharmacological evaluation of cimetidine. A new histamine H_2-receptor antagonist in healthy man. *Br. J. Clin. Pharmacol. 2,* 481.

39. Henn, R.M., Isenberg, J.E., Maxwell, V. and Sturdevant, R.A.L. (1975): Inhibition of gastric acid secretion by cimetidine in patients with duodenal ulcer. *N. Engl. J. Med. 293,* 371.

40. Parsons, E.M. (1977): The antagonism of histamine H_2-receptors in vitro and in vivo, with particular reference to the actions of cimetidine. In: *Cimetidine: Proceedings of the second International Symposium on histamine H_2-receptor antagonists*, pp. 13-23. Editors: W.L. Burland and M.A. Simkins. Excerpta Medica, Amsterdam-Oxford-Princeton.

41. Bardhan, K.D. (1978): Cimetidine in duodenal ulceration. In: *Cimetidine: the West-minster Hospital Symposium,* pp. 31-56. Editors: C. Wastell and P. Lance. Churchill Livingstone, Edinburgh.
42. Ash, A.S.F. and Schild, H.O. (1966): Receptors mediating some actions of histamine. *Br. J. Pharmacol. Chemother. 27,* 427.
43. Chand, N. and Eyre, P. (1975): Classification and biological distribution of histamine receptor sub-types. *Agents Actions 5,* 277.
44. Blyth, D.I. (1973): Some effects of histamine in the depolarised rat uterus. *Br. J. Pharmacol. 49,* 445.
45. Dundee, J.W., McGowan, W.A.W. and Moore, J. (1979): Cimetidine in the first stage of labour. Preliminary results. *Anaesthesia 34,* 118.
46. Moir, D.D. (1976): General anaesthesia. In: *Obstetric anaesthesia and analgesia,* pp. 129-156. Bailliere Tindall, London.
47. Feinstein, A.R. (1978): Central tendency and the meaning of pH values. *Anesth. Analg. (Cleveland) 58,* 1. (Editorial.)
48. Christensen, V. and Skovsted, P. (1975): Effects of general anaesthetics on the pH of gastric contents in man during surgery. A survey of halothane, flurothane and cyclopropane. *Acta Anaesthesiol. Scand. 19,* 49.
49. Nimmo, W.S., Wilson, J. and Prescott, L.F. (1975): Narcotic analgesics and delayed gastric emptying during labour. *Lancet 1,* 890.
50. Stoeling, R.K. (1978): Gastric fluid pH in patients receiving cimetidine. *Anesth. Analg. (Cleveland) 57,* 675.
51. Dobb, G. (1978): Pulmonary acid aspiration syndrome: prophylaxis with cimetidine. In: *Cimetidine: the Westminster Hospital Symposium,* p. 240. Editors: C. Wastell and P. Lance. Churchill Livingstone, Edinburgh.
52. Pounder, R.E., Williams, J.G., Russell, R.C.G., Milton-Thompson, G.J. and Misiewicz, J.J. (1976): Inhibition of food stimulated gastric acid secretion by cimetidine. *Gut 17,* 161.
53. Apgar, V. (1953): Proposal for new method of evaluation of new-born infants. *Curr. Res. Anaesth. 32,* 360.
54. Crawford, J.S., Davies, P. and Pearson, J.F. (1973): Significance of the individual components of the Apgar score. *Br. J. Anaesth. 45,* 148.
55. Jefferys, D.B. and Vale, J.A. (1978): Effect of cimetidine on glucose handling. *Lancet 1,* 383.

Effect of intravenous cimetidine on intragastric pH at caesarean section

J. Wilson
Simpson Memorial Maternity Pavilion, Royal Infirmary, Edinburgh, United Kingdom

Introduction

The acidity of gastric contents in pregnant patients in labour has been recognised as a problem at least since Mendelson described the acid aspiration syndrome in 1946 [1]. Various measures have been suggested to prevent acidic material from reaching the lungs, such as emptying the stomach before anaesthesia or obstructing the oesophagus at anaesthesia [2]. The pH of the gastric contents is of the greatest importance in these patients, since the pathological response in the tracheo-bronchial tree is directly proportional to acidity [3]; the danger is greatest if the pH is less than a critical level of 2.5. Antacid therapy reduces the risk, and if magnesium trisilicate B.P.C. is given 2-hourly during labour, the population at risk decreases from 50% to 20% [4, 5]. The acid aspiration syndrome has, however, been reported in cases with a pH as high as 3.5 [6]. Recent work by Holdsworth may explain this enigma: it is possible for aliquots of magnesium trisilicate B.P.C. mixture to be regularly added to simulated gastric juice without properly mixing, resulting in islands of alkali in a sea of acid [7]. This occurrence of acidic (low pH) material is not restricted to emergency patients; we have seen a case of acid aspiration syndrome in an elective patient resulting from regurgitation of less than 5 ml of stomach contents.

In 1977, Baraka et al. investigated an anticholinergic drug, glycopyrronium bromide, and found that it reduced the incidence of pH levels below 2.5 from 66% in control unmedicated patients to 34% in those receiving it before anaesthesia [8].

Cimetidine appears to offer further help in dealing with this problem, and several recent investigations have looked at its use in both elective and emergency surgical patients [9-12]. In Belfast, Howe et al. have examined the problem of gastric acidity in cases presenting for elective caesarean section [13]. All of these authors have described some benefit from the use of cimetidine in this pre-operative situation.

The present study was designed to discover if a single 200 mg intravenous dose of cimetidine, given prior to anaesthesia for emergency obstetric surgery, would effect a beneficial change in the pH of the gastric contents of treated patients. In addition, we examined the maternal, placental and fetal distribution of this dose of the drug.

Method

For this double-blind study, patients were randomly allocated to either a cimetidine group, which received cimetidine 200 mg intravenously at the decision to operate, or a placebo group, which received intravenous saline. There were 20 patients in each group, but 3 of the cimetidine patients were later discounted. Informed consent was obtained from all patients in both study groups.

Immediately following induction of anaesthesia by thiopental sodium, suxamethonium chloride and intubation, a nasogastric tube was passed. A double-lumen tube was found to be most reliable and was ultimately adopted, the projecting small-bore tube being trimmed flush with the main tube. The stomach was then emptied by aspiration, using a 20 ml syringe, and the volume obtained was noted. Aspiration was repeated throughout anaesthesia at approximately 15-minute intervals, and the samples obtained were marked accordingly and stored at –4°C; pH was read when a sufficient number of samples had accumulated. On recovery from anaesthesia, the nasogastric tube was removed and the stomach emptied.

Prior to incision of the uterus, liquor amnii was aspirated through the uterine wall by the surgeon. On delivery of the neonate, the umbilical cord was double-clamped and samples of venous and arterial blood were obtained from the piece of cord thus isolated; a sample of maternal venous blood was also taken, and all blood and liquor samples were stored at –20°C.

The Apgar scores of all neonates, their general state and any need for intubation and/or intermittent positive pressure ventilation were noted at delivery. All neonates were cared for in the routine hospital manner, receiving daily examinations by paediatricians until discharge from hospital. All case records were studied by the author, and the babies' conditions up to and at the time of discharge were noted.

Early in the series it became apparent that, in obstetric emergencies, there would not necessarily be sufficient time to allow proper organisation of each case. Elective patients were therefore introduced into the trial at this stage.

Results

A scattergram of the pHs of initial samples of gastric contents shows a fairly

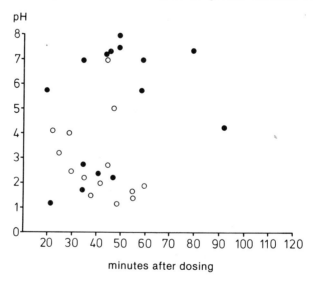

Fig. 1. Scattergram of pH levels of the initial aspirates in the cimetidine group (•) and the placebo group (○).

definite pattern, with most of the patients in the cimetidine group appearing in the higher pH area and most of those in the placebo group in the critical pH area (Fig. 1); 26.6% of the cimetidine group had pHs less than 2.5, compared with 57.1% of the placebo group.

The mean pH of the cimetidine group was 5.12, and that of the placebo group was 3.12; this difference is statistically significant ($p < 0.01$). Analysis of these results using the Mann Whitney U test shows that cimetidine treatment has a significant effect on pH. In addition, the probability that the pH levels would be higher than 2.5 in the first aspirate is higher for the cimetidine group than for the placebo group.

No treatment effect was observed on initial aspirate volumes, which ranged from 0.1 to 100 ml in the placebo group (mean: 7.68 ml), and from 0.25 to 50 ml in the cimetidine group (mean: 7.78 ml).

Samples taken subsequently and up to recovery showed a wide scattering of both pH levels and aspirate volumes. There was, however, a significant difference between the cimetidine and placebo groups: the mean pH levels for the placebo group were much nearer to the critital pH of 2.5 than were those of the cimetidine group and, in fact, mean pH of the placebo group was often *below* 2.5 (Fig. 2). Only 50% of the placebo group had pH levels higher than 2.5, compared with 91.6% of the cimetidine group.

All 4 specimens of blood and liquor (maternal venous, umbilical venous and arterial, and liquor amnii) were successfully collected in 9 of the patients on cimetidine; these results, together with figures for 2 other patients, are shown in the Table. There was a wide range of elapsed times between dosing and sampling in these patients, and this may help to account for the wide-ranging cimetidine levels observed. No significant relationship was found between the time elapsed between dosing and sampling and the resulting blood or liquor cimetidine levels. As expected, there was a gradient from maternal venous to liquor amnii levels; the ratio of mean umbilical venous to mean maternal venous cimetidine levels was approximately 1:2.

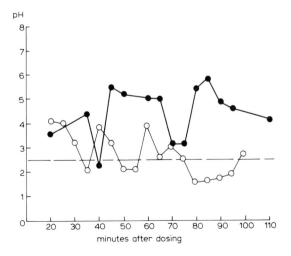

Fig. 2. Mean pH levels of the subsequent aspirates in the cimetidine group (•) and the placebo group (o).

Table.   Maternal and umbilical blood and liquor amnii cimetidine levels.

Patient	Minutes after dosing	Maternal venous (mg/l)	Umbilical		Liquor amnii (mg/l)
			venous (mg/l)	arterial (mg/l)	
1	45	1.02	0.63	—	0.4
2	30	1.01	0.74	—	—
3	37	1.55	0.79	0.32	0.2
4	30	1.17	0.73	0.20	0.5
5	45	1.32	ND	0.51	0.13
6	47	1.34	0.57	0.34	ND
7	35	1.12	0.61	0.22	ND
8	32	2.18	0.78	0.84	ND
9	38	0.85	0.26	0.29	0.14
10	58	0.64	0.46	0.13	0.27
11	68	0.36	0.32	0.15	0.42
Mean	42.27	1.05	0.51	0.33	0.21
SD	12.05	0.56	0.26	0.22	0.19

ND = cimetidine not detectable (less than 0.05 mg/l).

When discussing the neonatal data, it is important to remember that both elective and emergency operations were carried out. In the cimetidine group, 2 babies were born with Apgar scores of less than 4; both of these births involved elective surgery. One of these neonates reached a score of 10 at 5 minutes after birth, the other took 10 minutes to reach a score of 8. Two other babies in the cimetidine group had scores of less than 7 at 1 minute: 1 of them reached 9 at 5 minutes, the other reached the same score at 10 minutes. In the placebo group, 6 babies had Apgar scores of less than 4 at 1 minute; 3 of these were elective and 3 were emergency. Only 2 failed to reach a score of 7 at 10 minutes, and 1 of these suffered from severe congenital heart disease and died a few days later.

All babies received 2 or more full general examinations and at least 1 thorough neurological examination while in hospital. There were 7 cases of jaundice (5 in the cimetidine group and 2 in the placebo group) which required close supervision or ultraviolet-light therapy. There was no evidence to suggest a pharmacological cause, and all these cases were normal on discharge from hospital. All of the babies, including those with jaundice, were seen on discharge, usually 14 days after delivery; some were also seen at follow-up clinics at various times after discharge. There was only 1 further complication of early life: 1 baby in the placebo group required inguinal herniorrhaphy.

Discussion

To date, most investigations of the use of cimetidine pre-operatively have been on elective or emergency surgical patients [9-12, 14]; only Howe et al. have studied the problem in obstetrics, where the difficulties of this type of investigation are so much greater [13].

The present trial was designed to study the effects of cimetidine on the pH and volume of gastric contents of obstetric patients requiring surgery, and also to gain some knowledge of the placental passage of the drug. The results obtained show that the use of cimetidine had no significant effect on either the initial, subsequent or total volumes of gastric aspirate. This agreed with the results of Keating, Black and Watson [14], but was contrary to those of Coombs, Hooper and Colton [9], which showed significant volume changes when cimetidine was administered at least 45 minutes before gastric aspiration at anaesthetic induction. We did not do a time/volume relationship study as a part of the present trial, because of the relative lack of advance knowledge of the operation and the consequent unpredictability of induction time.

Our results showed that cimetidine does have a significant ability to raise the pH of gastric contents at induction of anaesthesia; this finding it is most important, as the majority of acid aspiration syndromes occur at this stage of anaesthesia. The subsequent state of gastric acidity is also of some importance, as aspiration may occur at any time in the course of the anaesthetic, but it is most likely to occur again at extubation. Our results showed that cimetidine does in fact raise pH levels throughout anaesthesia. Wide swings of pH do occur, but statistical analysis shows that the minimum value of the pH of cimetidine-treated patients is significantly higher than that of patients in the placebo group, and that the pH of cimetidine-treated patients is more likely to be above 2.5 than that of those on placebo.

The results of our maternal blood, umbilical blood and liquor amnii cimetidine measurements show that cimetidine crosses to the fetal circulation fairly rapidly and is excreted by the fetus, at least partially unaltered, into the liquor amnii. The cimetidine level in the fetal blood is significantly lower than in the maternal blood, which suggests some form of protein or fat binding on the maternal side, or some degree of disproportionate binding to maternal and fetal plasma proteins.

There was no evidence from the infants' Apgar scores or general condition at birth that cimetidine had any deleterious effect at that stage. Similarly, follow-up of the neonates showed no evidence of drug-induced pathology at discharge or, in some cases, even months later. The present study is the first to present any information on the neonate; our conclusion is that there is no significant pharmacological risk from the use of a 200 mg intravenous dose of cimetidine in pregnant patients shortly before delivery.

Since Teabeault's study in 1952 [3], it has been accepted that the critical pH level, below which the aspiration of gastric contents will cause Mendelson's syndrome, is 2.5. Teabeault's work was based on animal experimentation — for obvious reasons — but is accepted as being also relevant to humans. It follows, therefore, that the greater the pH is above 2.5 and the greater the proportion of the population with a pH of more than 2.5, the smaller the risk of acid aspiration occurring in that population. The present study seems to confirm that cimetidine has a part to play in the prophylaxis of this condition.

At present, our treatment options are starvation, antacid therapy, mechanical obstruction of the oesophagus and emptying of the stomach. We know that none of these methods is infallible, and it would therefore not seem unreasonable to propose the introduction of cimetidine treatment to increase the effectiveness of prophylactic therapy. It might at this stage be worthwhile to investigate the use of oral cimetidine prophylaxis both with and without antacids.

The use of a single 200 mg dose of cimetidine would appear from this trial to be harmless to the fetus and neonate, and it is unlikely that fetal cimetidine levels would be higher with, for example, prophylactic doses of 400 mg given orally every 6 hours to patients in labour.

References

1. Mendelson, C.L. (1946): The aspiration of stomach contents into the lungs during obstetric anesthesia. *Am. J. Obstet. Gynecol. 52,* 191.
2. Sellick, B.A. (1961): Cricoid pressure to control regurgitation of stomach contents during induction of anaesthesia. *Lancet 2,* 404.
3. Teabeault, J.R. (1952): Aspiration of gastric contents: an experimental study. *Am. J. Pathol. 28,* 51.
4. Taylor, G. and Pryse Davies, J. (1966): The prophylactic use of antacids in the prevention of the acid pulmonary aspiration syndrome. *Lancet 1,* 288.
5. White, W.D., Clark, T.M. and Stanley-Jones, G.H.M. (1976): The efficacy of antacid therapy. *Br. J. Anaesth. 48,* 1117.
6. Taylor, G. (1975): Acid pulmonary aspiration syndrome after antacids: a case report. *Br. J. Anaesth. 47,* 615.
7. Holdsworth, J.D., Johnson, K.R. and Mascall, D. (1978): A fresh look at magnesium trisilicate. In: *Proceedings of the obstetric anaesthetists' association, Edinburgh.*
8. Baraka, A., Saab, M., Salem, M.R. and Winnie, A.P. (1977): Control of gastric acidity by glycopyrrolate premedication in the parturient. *Anesth. Analg. (Cleveland) 56,* 642.
9. Coombs, D.W., Hooper, D. and Colton, T. (1979): Pre-anesthetic cimetidine alteration of gastric fluid volume and pH. *Anesth. Analg. (Cleveland) 58,* 183.
10. Dobb, G. (1978): Pulmonary acid aspiration syndrome: prophylaxis with cimetidine. In: *Cimetidine, the Westminster Hospital Symposium,* p. 235. Editors: C. Wastell and P. Lance. Churchill Livingstone, Edinburgh.
11. Jones, H.D., Bond, R.A., Harris, D.W. and Tomlin, P.J. (1978): Cimetidine prophylaxis against acid aspiration syndrome. In: *Proceedings of Anaesthetic Research Society, Belfast, 1970.*
12. Husemyer, R.P., Davenport, H.T. and Rajasekaran, T. (1978): Cimetidine for reducing acidity of gastric contents in elective surgery. *Br. J. Anaesth. 50,* 1080P.
13. Howe, F.P., Dundee, J.W., Moore, E.J. and McCaughey, W. (1979): *Presented at the British Pharmacological Society Meeting, Dublin, 1979.*
14. Keating, P.J., Black, J.F. and Watson, D.W. (1978): Effects of glycopyrrolate and cimetidine on gastric volumes and acidity in patients awaiting surgery. *Br. J. Anaesth. 50,* 1247.

Discussion

Baron (London): Could Dr. Howe and Dr. Wilson say again whether they had any cases of Mendelson's syndrome in their control patients, whether they predict that raising intragastric pH will prevent it, and whether they have made a policy decision in their obstetric units about how subsequent patients will be managed, as a result of the conclusions of their trials?

Howe: First, this was a small and tightly controlled study, the results of which apply only to elective patients. Certainly, however, these results are most hopeful. In view of the fact that antacids are unsuccessful, it is foreseeable in the not-too-distant future that cimetidine — quite likely in oral form — will be used on a broader basis clinically. Before this could take place, it will be necessary to organise a much larger trial in the clinical field, using oral cimetidine. The results of such a trial will have to be awaited before offering any firm conclusions.

Wilson: I entirely agree with Dr. Howe about this. A much larger trial is required. Probably the use of the oral form of cimetidine would be something for the future.

The effect of oral cimetidine on the basal and stimulated values of prolactin, thyroid stimulating hormone, follicle stimulating hormone and luteinizing hormone

G.F. Nelis
Department of Internal Medicine, Sophia Ziekenhuis, Zwolle, The Netherlands

Introduction

The advent of cimetidine therapy in 1976 was one of the major therapeutic break-throughs of this decade. Its effectiveness in lowering basal and stimulated gastric acid output has been documented. It is an effective treatment for peptic ulcer, peptic esophagitis and the Zollinger-Ellison syndrome. Its use has deepened our understanding of gastric physiology and pathophysiology. It has been reported to be safe and, apart from minor subjective complaints and minor elevations of serum creatinine, most of which are transient, no definite side-effects have been documented [1].

Hall has drawn attention to the development of gynecomastia in 2 male patients during cimetidine treatment [2], while Delle Fave et al. reported elevated plasma prolactin concentrations in each of 6 patients on oral cimetidine maintenance [3].

At the time we started our own investigations, the only definite study of the effect of cimetidine on prolactin reported a significant increase in plasma prolactin concentration after acute intravenous administration of cimetidine [4]. Since then, several reports have been published in which no increase after a single dose or regular maintenance dosage of oral cimetidine was found [5-7], while a significant rise after intravenous administration has been confirmed [5, 8, 9].

The aim of the present study was to investigate whether oral cimetidine treatment has an effect on basal levels of prolactin (PRL), thyroid stimulating hormone (TSH), follicle stimulating hormone (FSH) and luteinizing hormone (LH), and/or on the response after stimulation with thyrotropin (TRH) and luteinizing hormone releasing hormone (LHRH).

Subjects and methods

Thirteen male patients with duodenal and/or gastric ulcers and 15 healthy male volunteers were entered into the study. Active peptic ulceration in the patients was proven by endoscopy either 1 or 3 days prior to entry; most of them had a barium meal as well. In all patients with gastric ulcers, repeat endoscopy was performed; in patients with duodenal ulcers, this was only done if considered necessary.

Patients and volunteers were excluded from the study for use of hormone-containing drugs or drugs known to be associated with hyperprolactinemia [10], for Zollinger-Ellison syndrome, and for disorders or prior surgery of the hypothalanus, pituitary, thyroid or gonads. One patient with choriocarcinoma of the testis was entered into the TSH study only.

All patients were given oral cimetidine 1 g daily (200 mg at each of 3 meals and 400 mg at bedtime), from day 1 until day 28 of the study inclusively. Volunteers also received oral cimetidine 1 g daily, for 7 days; administration of the drug began at 1 p.m. on day 1. The difference in treatment regime between patients and volunteers is explained in the Discussion section of this paper.

Informed consent was obtained from all patients and volunteers, and the study was conducted in accordance with the principles of the Declaration of Helsinki.

On days 1-5, 8 and 15, blood samples were withdrawn from all volunteers, between 11 a.m. and 1 p.m., and were used to measure PRL levels. Stimulation tests were performed on patients on days 0, 28 and 56: beginning between 11 a.m. and noon, plasma levels of PRL, TSH, FSH and LH were measured, first before and then 10, 20, 60 and 90 minutes after intravenous stimulation with 200 mcg TRH and 150 mcg LHRH. Sera were separated and stored at -20°C until assay. All of the samples from the volunteers were run in 1 assay, as were all samples from any given patient.

Serum PRL, TSH, FSH and LH were estimated by radioimmunoassay using CEA-IRE-SORIN (CIS) kits (Fleurus, Belgium) corresponding to the following standards: MRC 71/222 (PRL), MRC 68/38 (TSH), MRC 69/104 (FSH) and MRC 68/40 (LH).

For statistical evaluation, Student's t test for paired observations was used.

Results

In the patients, basal and stimulated values of PRL, TSH, FSH and LH before, during and after cimetidine treatment were compared, each patient serving as his own control. The results are shown in Tables I-IV. With 1 exception, the values of these hormones at any time after stimulation during (day 28) or after (day 56) cimetidine treatment were not significantly different from those observed before cimetidine (day 1).

The exception was FSH: FSH blood levels at 10 minutes after stimulation with LHRH were slightly, though significantly, higher at day 56 (3.38 ± 0.47) than at

Table I. Basal and stimulated PRL blood levels ($\mu U/ml$) after intravenous administration of TRH in 12 patients with peptic ulcers before, during and after cimetidine.

		Minutes after administration of TRH				
		0	10	20	60	90
Before cimetidine	mean	296.8	1201.1	1247.1	663.3	495.7
(day 1)	SEM	22.6	187.6	236.9	76.4	40.2
During cimetidine	mean	273.5	1080.0	1089.6	615.4	417.3
(day 28)	SEM	36.1	108.0	108.7	49.5	46.7
After cimetidine	mean	261.4	969.6	1015.8	613.8	434.5
(day 56)	SEM	32.4	97.9	112.1	60.5	47.1

Table II.   Basal and stimulated TSH blood levels (μU/ml) after intravenous administration of TRH in 13 patients with peptic ulcers before, during and after cimetidine.

| | | Minutes after administration of TRH | | | | |
		0	10	20	60	90
Before cimetidine	mean	5.87	10.38	12.99	10.02	8.41
(day 1)	SEM	0.31	0.82	1.20	0.78	0.62
During cimetidine	mean	6.35	10.24	12.45	9.99	8.28
(day 28)	SEM	0.37	0.89	1.09	0.84	0.56
After cimetidine	mean	6.59	12.53	13.20	10.71	9.04
(day 56)	SEM	0.39	1.25	1.30	1.08	0.83

Table III.   Basal and stimulated FSH blood levels (μg/l) after intravenous administration of LHRH in 12 patients with peptic ulcers before, during and after cimetidine. (1 μg/l = 4 U/l)

| | | Minutes after administration of LHRH | | | | |
		0	10	20	60	90
Before cimetidine	mean	2.39	3.00	3.88	4.35	4.20
(day 1)	SEM	0.29	0.36	0.49	0.52	0.50
During cimetidine	mean	2.35	2.87	3.61	4.33	4.28
(day 28)	SEM	0.29	0.40	0.54	0.69	0.73
After cimetidine	mean	2.63	3.38	4.36	4.73	4.44
(day 56)	SEM	0.33	0.47	0.66	0.74	0.68

Table IV.   Basal and stimulated LH blood levels (μg/l) after intravenous administration of LHRH in 12 patients with peptic ulcers before, during and after cimetidine. (1 μg/l = 3 U/l)

| | | Minutes after administration of LHRH | | | | |
		0	10	20	60	90
Before cimetidine	mean	2.24	6.81	10.22	10.18	8.21
(day 1)	SEM	0.16	0.66	1.14	1.17	0.98
During cimetidine	mean	2.18	6.63	10.19	10.56	8.63
(day 28)	SEM	0.17	0.65	1.38	1.54	0.97
After cimetidine	mean	2.56	7.34	11.70	11.00	8.82
(day 56)	SEM	0.20	0.68	1.42	1.34	0.92

Table V.   PRL blood levels (µU/ml) in healthy volunteers before (day 1), during (days 2-5 and 8), and after (day 15) cimetidine.

	day 1	day 2	day 3	day 4	day 5	day 8	day 15
Mean	384.4	350.5	360.7	323.9	417.9	320.0	339.2
SEM	73.7	67.4	64.8	58.8	94.9	90.2	78.1
Number of volunteers	15	14	14	15	12	14	12

either day 1 (3.00 ± 0.36) or day 28 (2.87 ± 0.40).

In the volunteers, no statistically significant difference was found between the PRL values on any day, before, during or after the administration of cimetidine (Table V).

Discussion

Prolactin release has been found to have a sleep-related circadian rhythm, with 1 or more peaks between 2 and 5 a.m. [11] and a stabilization for several hours after 10 a.m. [12]. Because of this observed rhythm, we decided to perform our testing between 11 a.m. and 1 p.m.

Maximal PRL values have previously been reported to occur 10-20 minutes after intravenous administration of TRH, and maximal TSH values after 20 minutes [13, 14]; in these studies, the maximal PRL response was obtained with a TRH dose between 100 and 400 mcg. Our own standard TRH dose for testing in thyroid disease is 200 mcg; therefore, we chose to use a dosage of 200 mcg TRH in the present study, with sampling times after 10 and 20 minutes.

Our results indicate that oral cimetidine treatment does not influence the basal or stimulated values of PRL, TSH, FSH and LH after intravenous TRH and LHRH. (With a 95% confidence limit, 2 abnormal results were to be expected in the total of 40 comparisons we made; we have therefore concluded that the significantly higher FSH blood level observed in patients at 10 minutes after stimulation on day 56, 4 weeks after they had stopped receiving cimetidine, was probably a chance result.) Since the observed hormone values were not significantly different at any time after stimulation, we conclude that neither the initial nor the delayed response to TRH and LHRH changed during or after cimetidine.

Comparison of the stimulated values of PRL, TSH, FSH and LH obtained in the present study with earlier results is not possible, as we are not aware of any similar studies which have been previously reported; however, comparison of the basal values of PRL obtained in our study with results reported by several others after single-dose or maintenance cimetidine treatment is possible, and shows that our results are in accordance with those previously reported [5-7]. A recent study suggesting a diminished LH responsiveness [15] was not confirmed by our study.

The rise in PRL after oral cimetidine reported by Delle Fave et al. [3] remains unconfirmed, and is not satisfactorily explained by the higher dose or the longer period of administration used in their study; we did not find any rise in PRL during an 8-week regime of treatment with cimetidine 1.6 g daily in esophagitis patients [unpublished trial]. Whether the Delle Fave et al. results were affected by the circadian rhythm of PRL secretion remains speculative.

Since we could not exclude the possibility of our having missed a peak in PRL during the initial treatment phase, and since all of our patients were treated on an out-patient basis and their daily return to the laboratory was impractical, we also decided to study the short-term effect of cimetidine on basal PRL values in healthy volunteers. As is shown in Table V, we failed to show any effect of cimetidine on PRL.

In accordance with the results of other published studies [4, 5, 8, 9], we did find high PRL levels after intravenous administration of cimetidine, reaching a mean of 1,480 μU/ml $\pm$ 112.3 SEM in 8 patients.

It is possible that Arakelian and Libertun's study of histamine H_1- and H_2-receptor participation in the brain control of PRL secretion in lactating rats reveals a link between intravenous cimetidine and hyperprolactinemia [16]. Though interesting from a physiological point of view, major clinical consequences do not seem to rise from this observation.

As cimetidine does penetrate into the pituitary, but not into the brain [17], dopamine antagonism at the pituitary receptor site is an alternate possibility.

During the final preparation of the present paper, Funder and Mercer reported experimental evidence suggesting the competitive binding of cimetidine to androgen receptors, which could provide an explanation for cimetidine-associated gynecomastia [18].

Acknowledgments

We kindly acknowledge the technical assistance by Miss N. Holtslag and the critical review of the manuscript by Professor H. Doorenbos and Dr. W.D. Reitsma, Department of Medicine, State University, Groningen, The Netherlands.

References

1. Burland, W.L. and Simkins, M.A. (1977): *Cimetidine: Proceedings of the Second International Symposium on histamine H_2-receptor antagonists.* Excerpta Medica, Amsterdam-Oxford-Princeton.
2. Hall, W.H. (1976): Breast changes in males on cimetidine. *N. Engl. J. Med. 295,* 841.
3. Delle Fave, G.F., Tamburrano, G., De Magistris, L., Natoli, C., Santoro, M.L., Carratu, R. and Torsoli, A. (1977): Gynaecomastia with cimetidine. *Lancet 1,* 1319.
4. Carlson, H.E. and Ippoliti, A.F. (1977): Cimetidine, an H_2-antihistamine, stimulates prolactin secretion in man. *J. Clin. Endocrinol. Metab. 45,* 367.
5. Rowley-Jones, D. (1978): Cimetidine and serum prolactin. *Lancet 2,* 635.
6. Spiegel, A.M., Lepatin, R., Peikin, S. and McCarthy, D. (1978): Serum prolactin in patients receiving chronic oral cimetidine. *Lancet 1,* 881.
7. Valcavi, R., Bedogni, G., Dall'Asta, A., Dotti, C. and Portioli, I. (1978): Single oral dose of cimetidine and prolactin. *Lancet 2,* 528.
8. Cavallini, G., Lo Cascio, V., Angelini, G., Bovo, P., Vaona, B., Adami, S., Zuniga, G., Galvanini, G., Manfrini, C. and Scuro, A. (1978): Effect of acute and chronic cimetidine administration on human serum prolactin. In: *Abstracts of the VIth World Congress of Gastroenterology, Madrid,* p. 18. Editorial Garsi, London.
9. Daubresse, J.C., Meunier, J.C. and Ligny, G. (1978): Plasma prolactin and cimetidine. *Lancet 1,* 99.
10. Lamberts, S.W.J., Klijn, J.G.M. and Birkenhäger, J.C. (1978): Prolactine. *Ned. Tijdschr. Geneeskd. 122,* 1327.

11. Parker, D.C., Rossma, L.G. and Vanderlaan, E.F. (1973): Sleep-related nyctohemeral and briefly episodic variation in human plasma prolactin concentration. *J. Clin. Endocrinol. Metab. 36,* 1119.

12. Finkelstein, J.W., Kapen, S., Weitzman, E.D., Hellman, L. and Boyar, R.M. (1978): Twenty-four-hour plasma prolactin patterns in prepubertal and adolescent boys. *J. Clin. Endocrinol. Metab. 47,* 1123.

13. Jacobs, L.S., Snijder, P.J., Wilber, J.F., Utiger, R.D. and Daughaday, W.H. (1971): Increased serum prolactin after administration of synthetic thyrotropin releasing hormone (TRH) in man. *J. Clin. Endocrinol. Metab. 33,* 996.

14. Jacobs, L.S., Snijder, P.J., Utiger, R.D. and Daughaday, W.H. (1973): Prolactin response to thyrotropin-releasing hormone in normal subjects. *J. Clin. Endocrinol. Metab. 36,* 1069.

15. Van Thiel, D.H., Gavaler, J.S., Smith, W.I. and Paul, G. (1979): Hypothalamic-pituitary-gonadal dysfunction in men using cimetidine. *N. Engl. J. Med. 300,* 1012-1015.

16. Arakelian, M.C. and Libertun, C. (1977): H_1- and H_2-histamine receptor participation in the brain control of prolactin secretion in lactating rats. *Endocrinology 100,* 890.

17. Cross, S.A.M. (1977): The localisation of metiamide and cimetidine using autoradiographical techniques. In: *Proceedings of the European Society of Toxicologists,* pp. 288-290. Editors: W.A.M. Duncan and B.J. Leonard. Excerpta Medica, Amsterdam-Oxford-Princeton.

18. Funder, J.W. and Mercer, J.E. (1979): Cimetidine, a histamine H_2-receptor antagonist, occupies androgen receptors. *J. Clin. Endocrinol. Metab. 48,* 189.

Discussion

Portaleone (Turin): I am not entirely in agreement with the conclusions drawn by Professor Nelis, inasmuch as the secretion of prolactin is controlled by many other factors which were not considered in his study. The principal factor which may operate at the level of the hypothalamus and through a neuronal channel is vasopressin, which is available insofar as it derives from the neurohypophysis and so may mediate effects on either side of the blood-brain barrier. Thus the neuroendocrine effects obtained with intravenous cimetidine could be produced through an action mediated by vasopressin. It is only when very high plasma levels of cimetidine are reached, even after oral administration, that the same effect on the receptors of the posterior pituitary could be obtained, with a feed-back effect upon the hypothalamus leading to alterations in secretion of prolactin, TSH, LH and FSH, all hormones which are influenced by stimulation or blockade of H_1- and H_2-receptors in the hypothalamus.

Nelis: Of course, many other factors affect prolactin secretion. We standardised as much as we could, avoiding emergency patients as far as possible, and all of us included only patients with proven peptic ulcer in a stable state. None of the patients was heavily stressed, as heavy stress might also have influenced prolactin secretion. What was going to happen was very carefully explained to them. Before the test was started, saline was given and blood taken for other parameters, in order to acquaint the patients with the injection and the taking of blood.

Secondly, H_2-receptors are present in the hypothalamus, and I would expect that H_2-receptor blockers would act on them, but the main purpose of our study was to investigate whether oral cimetidine has any effect on them. I agree with Dr. Portaleone — we did some other studies with intravenous cimetidine, and in all those patients there was stimulation of prolactin secretion. This did not, however, happen with oral cimetidine.

Bianchi (Milan): As has been reported, gynaecomastia with high prolactin levels has occurred in some cases of Zollinger-Ellison syndrome. As I pointed out in my paper earlier in this symposium, we observed gynaecomastia with high prolactin levels in 2 of 6 Zollinger-Ellison cases, but this condition preceded the administration of cimetidine in both cases. In assessing the number of Zollinger-Ellison syndrome patients with this condition, perhaps the possibility that it existed prior to cimetidine treatment should be taken into account.

Nelis: As far as I remember, in cases in which gynaecomastia was found and in which prolactin was measured, only Bateson found a high prolactin level, and that was only in one patient. Hall, for instance, who first described this condition in 2 patients, estimated prolactin in one of them and found that it was normal. In those patients we have seen with breast soreness on cimetidine, the prolactin level has always been normal. It is the experience of most authors that the prolactin level is not raised in those patients with gynaecomastia or breast soreness. I think that gynaecomastia is unrelated to prolactin secretion.

Bianchi Porro (Milan): We have recently seen a patient on long-term cimetidine treatment, 400 mg at night, in whom gynaecomastia developed and who had completely normal plasma prolactin levels. This patient, who was aged 63 years, was taking only oral cimetidine. I do not yet know the blood cimetidine levels. How would Dr. Nelis interpret this finding?

Nelis: This is also our experience, that gynaecomastia is not only seen with very high doses of cimetidine. Some patients on a maintenance dose of 400 mg complained of gynaecomastia but, again, prolactin was normal in all of them, as in Dr. Bianchi Porro's patient.

Psychomotor and psychological effects of cimetidine after single and multiple oral doses in healthy students

E. Nuotto, M.J. Mattila, T. Ranta*, T. Seppälä and L. Tuomisto

*Departments of Pharmacology and *Gynecology, University of Helsinki, Helsinki, Finland*

Introduction

On the basis of autoradiographic studies performed in the rat, it has been concluded that cimetidine penetrates poorly to the brain [1]. There are, however, clinical reports which suggest that cimetidine can cause cerebral toxicity in children [2] and in elderly patients [3-5] treated with regular doses for various gastroenterological disorders. The main effects observed in adults have been restlessness, drowsiness and confusion, rather than sedation. Slurred speech, agitation, high pulse rate and a sluggish light reflex have been reported after an alleged intake of 12 g of cimetidine [6].

Moderate or high levels of blood cimetidine have been associated with these confusion states [3], and an abnormal blood/brain barrier due to renal or hepatic failure may have facilitated the entry of the drug into the central nervous system or otherwise modified its effects; physostigmine may partly counteract this cimetidine-induced confusion [7].

The present study was conducted in order to ascertain whether or not orally administered cimetidine in therapeutic doses might cause measurable psychomotor and/or psychological effects in healthy subjects. Since high doses of cimetidine elevate serum prolactin levels [8], we assayed blood samples for this hormone as well as for cimetidine.

Subjects and methods

Twelve healthy male medical students, aged 19-23 years and weighing 72.4 ± 9.0 (SD) kg, served as paid volunteers. They did not use medicines regularly or alcohol excessively, and the consumption of alcohol was prohibited during the course of the trial. Each subject was fully informed of the nature of the study.

Subjects were randomized, double-blind, to receive either cimetidine 400 mg 4 times daily or matching placebo tablets, and each subject was trained to master the psychomotor tests to be administered during the study (Table I).

The initial treatment period lasted 48 hours: testing began at 4 p.m. on day 1, and tests were administered before the first treatment dose and both 60 and 120 minutes after it. At each test time, subjects were also asked to indicate their feelings subjectively by marking a position between 2 extreme alternatives on a 10 cm horizontal line (visual analogue scale). The pairs of alternatives presented were: alert/sleepy, calm/nervous, bright/'slow brain', kind/hostile, interested/bored, gay/sad, skill-

Table I. Psychomotor skills, and the tests used to evaluate them.

Reactive skills were measured by recording reaction errors and cumulative reaction times in a choice reaction test.

Coordinative skills were measured by means of a tracking test driven at a fixed speed.

Discrimination of the fusion of flickering light was measured at a distance of 100 cm by wearing spectacles which eliminated eventual changes in pupillary diameter.

Speed anticipation was measured by having subjects assess the time after which a horizontal moving light would have reached a target had it continued at a constant rate instead of disappearing [9].

Body sway was recorded on an electronic device [10] recording deviations in lateral and in anteroposterior directions; the length of the recorded line in a time unit was measured and used for analysis.

Hand steadiness was measured by leading 10 unsharpened pencils through a tight hole in 2 opposite directions and measuring the cumulative time [11].

These tests have proven sensitive enough to detect drug-induced impairment after diazepam 10 mg or alcohol 0.8-1.0 g/kg; the speed anticipation test is somewhat less sensitive than the others, but does discriminate the interaction of diazepam 10 mg and alcohol 0.8 g/kg [9, 12].

ful/clumsy, active/passive, hungry/satisfied, contented/discontented, talkative/quiet and good performance/bad performance.

After day 1 testing, all subjects went home, continued treatment according to a regular schedule, and returned for a second round of testing before and 60 and 120 minutes after taking the final dose of the initial treatment phase on day 3. After completing the last test of this series, subjects received amfepramone 50 mg for a positive control, and tests were repeated 45 and 90 minutes later (Fig. 1).

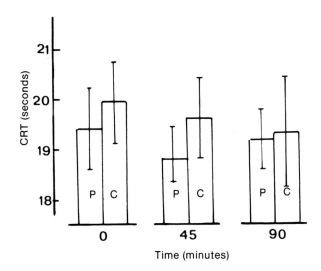

Fig. 1. Effect of amfepramone on cumulative choice reaction time (CRT), after placebo (P) and cimetidine (C). Time 0 refers to the 120-minute test on day 3, after which amfepramone 50 mg was administered. The differences P_0-P_{45} and C_0-C_{90} are statistically significant ($p < 0.02$).

Blood samples were taken in lithium heparin tubes for the chemical assay of cimetidine from the whole blood and for the radioimmunoassay of serum prolactin [13], and samples were stored at −20°C until assay.

Two-way analysis of variance and Student's *t* test for paired samples were used in the handling of the psychomotor data, both raw data and changes from zero performance. Data from the visual analogue scale were subjected to 2-way analysis of variance only. The ratios of original assessment to subsequent assessment were calculated, and analyzed with the paired *t* test.

Results

Blood cimetidine levels

Cimetidine concentrations in the whole blood after the first dose (Table II) approached those reported in previous absorption studies [14] and from the clinic [3]. On the average, the concentrations on day 3 were slightly higher than those found on day 1; due to a considerable deviation, though, this difference was not statistically significant.

Psychomotor skills

On the whole, the performance of the subjects remained fairly stable throughout the test sessions, and the performances on day 3 were rarely significantly different from those recorded on day 1 (Table III). The control values for different parameters were similar to those previously measured in many instances where diazepam and/or alcohol have impaired performance.

Table II.   Blood cimetidine levels in 12 subjects receiving cimetidine 400 mg 4 times daily. All day 1 measurements were made 2 hours after the first dose of the trial. All day 3 measurements were made 2 hours after the eighth dose of the trial.

Subject	Blood cimetidine (μg/ml)	
	Day 1	Day 3
1	1.49	2.15
2	1.43	0.98
3	1.21	2.35
4	1.16	2.16
5	1.58	3.03
6	1.39	1.61
7	1.04	3.07
8	1.14	1.87
9	1.08	1.67
10	1.29	1.31
11	1.26	1.64
12	1.12	1.32
Mean ± SD	1.27 ± 0.58	1.93 ± 0.65

Table III.   Effects of cimetidine and placebo on psychomotor performance. All data (from test times 0, 60 and 120 minutes on days 1 and 3) have been subjected to 2-way analysis of variance.

Parameter	Between drugs		Between test times	
	F	P	F	P
Coordination (errors)	0.506	0.478	0.519	0.761
Coordination (error %)	0.361	0.549	1.195	0.315
Reaction times	0.686	0.409	0.759	0.581
Reaction errors	0.024	0.878	0.497	0.778
Flicker fusion (Hz)	0.026	0.871	0.596	0.703
Body sway				
ap, eyes open	0.112	0.738	2.349*	0.044*
ap, eyes closed	0.025	0.874	1.674	0.145
lat, eyes open	0.167	0.684	1.407	0.226
lat, eyes closed	0.943	0.333	0.510	0.768
Speed anticipation				
mean	0.043	0.835	0.123	0.987
SD	0.980	0.324	0.680	0.639
Hand steadiness	2.089	0.151	1.878	0.102

ap = anteroposterior; lat = lateral; *$p < 0.05$.

When raw data were tested by 2-way analysis of variance, no drug-related impairment or improvement of performance was found (Table III). When changes from zero values were analyzed with the same test, 1 significant difference was detected: in the *hand steadiness* test, the performance after cimetidine improved significantly more than after placebo (F = 3.821; $p < 0.01$). No objective evidence was found to indicate a cimetidine-induced impairment of psychomotor skills.

When amfepramone was given after the 120-minute test on day 3, it tended to stimulate the subjects, as indicated by shortened reaction times (Fig. 1) and significantly less coordination errors ($p < 0.02$). The responses to amfepramone were similar whether it was administered after cimetidine or placebo, thus indicating a lack of psychomotor interaction between these drugs.

Psychological effects

When the raw data were analyzed by 2-way analysis of variance, the subjects saw themselves generally more nervous (F = 6.95; $p < 0.01$), disinterested (F = 6.08; $p < 0.02$), sad (F = 5.02; $p < 0.05$), and hostile (F = 4.84; $p < 0.05$) on days when they were treated with cimetidine.

However, these results were largely due to differences in the assessments at zero time (Fig. 2). To reveal drug effects as a trend towards either end of the scale, a similar analysis was performed on changes from the zero assessment. These figures revealed that cimetidine resulted in the subjects perceiving themselves as more kind (F = 5.94; $p < 0.001$), bright (F = 2.95; $p < 0.02$), gay (F = 9.59; $p < 0.001$), and skillful (F = 2.82; $p < 0.02$).

Since the conventional statistical handling of visual analogue data is subject to

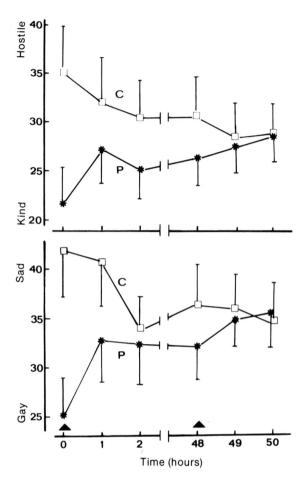

Fig. 2.   *Effect of cimetidine (C) and placebo (P) on the assessment of mood by visual analogue scales.* ▲ *indicates the administration of the first and eighth doses of cimetidine.*

criticism, we reanalyzed the data by calculating the ratio of initial value to treatment value for 2 hours on both day 1 and day 3. These ratios showed a rough Gaussian distribution [15]. When comparing cimetidine and placebo by paired t test for the parameters which showed significant differences when subjected to analysis of variance, cimetidine still rendered the subjects more kind ($t = 2.262; p < 0.05$) and gay ($t = 2.453; p < 0.05$) than placebo on day 1, but not on day 3. The other parameters (bright and skillful) lost their significance with this statistical treatment.

Since the psychological effects recorded were minimal, it is difficult to make a valid comparison between effects and cimetidine concentrations. When stratifying the whole material of cimetidine concentrations to the higher and lower halves separately for day 1 and day 3, the only statistically-significant finding was that high cimetidine levels indicated calmness at the base-line measurement on day 3 ($p < 0.05$). High cimetidine levels also indicated feeling gay and interested, but without reaching statistical significance. As a whole, no clear-cut correlation between psychological effects and cimetidine concentrations could be established.

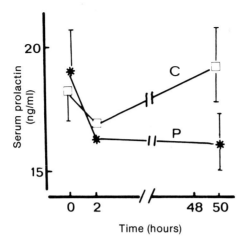

Fig. 3. Serum prolactin levels during subacute treatment with cimetidine 400 mg 4 times daily (C) or placebo (P).

Serum prolactin

As shown in Figure 3, serum prolactin levels tended to fall after the first dose of either cimetidine or placebo on day 1. On day 3, the cimetidine subjects had significantly higher prolactin levels than the placebo subjects ($p < 0.05$). No correlation between blood cimetidine and serum prolactin concentrations were seen in individual subjects.

Discussion

The present results demonstrate that single and multiple doses of cimetidine do not impair psychomotor responses in healthy volunteers. This finding does not support the view that cimetidine causes major cerebral toxicity, which has occasionally been reported [2-4, 7]. Since the blood cimetidine concentrations of the present study, in accord with those reported by Bodemar et al. [14], were not much lower than those reported by Schentag et al. [3] in confused patients, it seems reasonable to attribute the confusion state to complicating more or less severe diseases. It is possible that cimetidine could cause clear-cut side-effects even in healthy subjects after prolonged treatment. However, in our experience psychomotor performance usually recovers within 2 weeks after initial impairment by, for example, neuroleptics, antidepressants and benzodiazepines [9, 12]. The fact that cimetidine did not interact with amfepramone, a sympathomimetic stimulant, suggests that cimetidine effects were negligible in these circumstances.

The results from the subjective psychological assessments are not without interest, although the value of visual analogue scales continues to be a matter of debate [15]. In the present trial, some weak but positive mental effects were observed after cimetidine administration, which might suggest that central histaminergic mechanisms are involved with mood. H_1-antihistaminics are known to cause states of sedation and confusion, and H_2-agonists may do the same. Dimaprit, an H_2-agonist, causes drowsiness and sedation when given i.c.v. to goats [16].

The possibility that H_1-receptors mediate processes for mood improvement, while H_2-receptors mediate those for its impairment, awaits further experimentation.

Another remaining possibility is that clinically-reported central side-effects of cimetidine may be due to causes other than H_2-blockade. Cimetidine exerts a weak α-receptor blocking effect against noradrenaline in isolated aortic spirals in the rabbit [Mattila, unpublished, 1977], in the concentration which was present in our study (10^{-5} M). Physostigmine has reversed cimetidine-induced confusion in complicated clinical cases [7]; because it may counteract, for example, barbiturate sedation, we consider this antagonism to be non-specific, rather than a specific cholinergic/anticholinergic interaction.

The effects of oral cimetidine on serum prolactin were mild in comparison with those caused by high intravenous doses of cimetidine [8]. A delay in the prolactin response suggests a mechanism other than direct dopamine antagonism, thus tallying with in vitro results in which a direct cimetidine-dopamine antagonism could not be established [17]. Cimetidine probably has other effects on the hypothalamic area as well, as it can cause fever and alter the secretion of sex hormones [18]. The significance of these findings remains, at this point, unclear.

Acknowledgment

Our thanks to Smith Kline & French for the cimetidine assays.

References

1. Cross, S.A.M. (1977): The localisation of metiamide and cimetidine using autoradiographical techniques. In: *Proceedings of the European Society of Toxicology,* Volume 18, p. 288. Editors: W.A.M. Duncan and B.J. Leonard. Excerpta Medica, Amsterdam-Oxford-Princeton.
2. Thompson, J. and Lilly, J. (1979): Cimetidine-induced cerebral toxicity in children. *Lancet 1,* 725.
3. Schentag, J.J., Calleri, G., Rose, J.Q., Cerra, F.B., DeGlopper, E. and Bernhard, H. (1979): Pharmacokinetic and clinical studies in patients with cimetidine-associated mental confusion. *Lancet 1,* 177.
4. Delaney, J.C. and Ravey, M. (1977): Cimetidine and mental confusion. *Lancet 2,* 512.
5. Wood, C.A., Isaacson, M.L. and Hibbs, M.S. (1978): Cimetidine and mental confusion. *J. Am. Med. Assoc. 239,* 2550.
6. Nelson, P.G. (1977): Cimetidine and mental confusion. *Lancet 2,* 928.
7. Mogelnicki, S.R., Waller, J.L. and Finlayson, D.C. (1979): Physostigmine reversal of cimetidine-induced mental confusion. *J. Am. Med. Assoc. 241,* 826.
8. Burland, W.L., Gleadle, R.I., Lee, M.R., Rowley-Jones, D. and Groom, G.V. (1979): Prolactin responses to cimetidine. *Br. J. Clin. Pharmacol. 7,* 19.
9. Seppälä, T., Palva, E., Mattila, M.J. and Korttila, K. (1980): Effect of diazepam and tofisopam, alone and in combination with alcohol, on psychomotor skills and memory in man. *Psychopharmacologia.* (In press.)
10. Savolainen, K. and Linnavuo, M. (1979): Effects of m-xylene on human equilibrium measured with a quantitative method. *Acta Pharmacol. Toxicol. 44,* 315.
11. Lahtinen, U., Lahtinen, A. and Pekkola, P. (1978): The effect of nitrazepam on manual skill, grip strength, and reaction time with special reference to subjective evaluation of effects on sleep. *Acta Pharmacol. Toxicol. 42,* 130.
12. Seppälä, T., Linnoila, M. and Mattila, M.J. (1979): Drugs, alcohol and driving. *Drugs 17,* 389.

13. Seppälä, M., Hirvonen, E., Ranta, T., Virkkunen, P. and Leppäluoto, J. (1975): Raised serum prolactin levels in amenorrhoea. *Br. Med. J. 2,* 305.

14. Bodemar, G., Norlander, B., Fransson, L. and Walan, A. (1979): The absorption of cimetidine before and during maintenance treatment with cimetidine and the influence of a meal on the absorption of cimetidine: studies in patients with peptic ulcer disease. *Br. J. Clin. Pharmacol. 7,* 23.

15. Stubbs, D.F. (1979): Visual analogue scales. *Br. J. Clin. Pharmacol. 7,* 124.

16. Tuomisto, L. and Eriksson, L. (1980): Cardiovascular and behavioural changes after i.c.v. infusions of histamine and agonists in conscious goat. *Agents Actions.* (In press.)

17. Delitala, G., Stubbs, W.A., Yeo, T., Jones, A. and Besser, G.M. (1979): Failure of cimetidine to antagonise dopamine-induced suppression of prolactin in vitro. *Br. J. Clin. Pharmacol. 7,* 117.

18. Van Thiel, D.H., Gavaler, J.S., Smith, W.I. Jr. and Gwendolyn, P. (1979): Hypothalamic-pituitary-gonadal dysfunction in men using cimetidine. *N. Engl. J. Med. 300,* 1012.

Discussion

Baron (London): Related to the clinical central side effects of cimetidine, both in open series and in controlled trials, patients complain of a 'muzzy' head and of dizziness. These are subjective statements, but did Dr. Mattila ask his volunteers specifically whether they had any of these subjective symptoms?

Mattila: Unfortunately, we did not. We thought that our battery of visual analogue scale tests, which contain about 12 different items, might have covered that subject, but dizziness was not asked for specifically.

The safety of cimetidine: a continuing assessment

A.C. Flind, D. Rowley-Jones and Jane N. Backhouse
Smith Kline & French Laboratories, Welwyn Garden City, United Kingdom

Introduction

If the definition of 'safety' as 'freedom from danger or risks' is accepted, it is axiomatic that no effective, pharmacologically active drug can be 'safe'. Every act of prescribing is, or should be, the result of weighing the expected benefits against the risks. Drugs are primarily selected for development because of the expected benefits; to clarify risks is much more difficult and uncertain, even if just as important to the patient.

Peptic ulcer seldom threatens life. However efficacious a drug is for the treatment of peptic ulcer, it will be suitable for most patients only if the risk is relatively low. We have therefore regarded it from the outset as extremely important to assess individually all reports, from any source, which might represent an adverse reaction to cimetidine, to relate these to the pattern of events already known to us, and to come, if possible, to a reasonable conclusion. This has then to be communicated to doctors to form part of their judgement of benefit and risk in treating individual patients.

Method

Information on possible adverse reactions may be obtained from various sources: clinical trials, clinical pharmacological studies, post-marketing surveillance schemes, published reports of adverse events, and spontaneous reports to the manufacturer and to governmental regulatory bodies.

None of these is perfect. The advantage of clinical trials is the scientific quality of the data and the presence of controls. The drawback is the relatively small number of patients studied, with the clinical restrictions necessary in controlled trials. Even in the large trial programme undertaken with cimetidine, the number of patients entered into clinical trials in the United Kingdom (U.K.), Continental Europe, Scandinavia and South Africa over the 2-year period prior to first marketing in November 1976, was only about 0.4% of the estimated number of patients treated in the U.K. alone during the same period after marketing. Clinical trials are therefore likely to reveal only common side-effects; for example in the case of cimetidine, the usually trivial, transient diarrhoea which was reported in 1-2% of patients.

Formal post-marketing surveillance studies also suffer from lack of numbers, although a considerably larger cohort is sought than is the case with clinical trials. An appropriate control population is, however, difficult to find, and it is not possible to collect reports in such detail as in clinical trials. Post-marketing surveillance programmes involving cimetidine are in progress in the United States (U.S.A.) and the U.K.; an interim report on the former being included in this volume. The U.K. scheme aims eventually to register 10,000 patients with a control population of approximately equivalent size, and will monitor adverse events serious enough to lead to hospital attendance. These 10,000 patients will, however, still represent only about 1% or less of the estimated number of patients in the U.K. who will have been treated with cimetidine by the time patient recruitment is completed.

Journals are another source of adverse event reports. These are usually uncontrolled and often anecdotal and should not be overvalued by virtue of publication. They should be judged on the facts presented, rather than the opinions stated by the authors, and also assessed in the context of experience in general. Communications to journals can have an important function in stimulating further reports of adverse events; it is, therefore, particularly reassuring when such a publication is not followed by a number of similar reports.

Lastly, by far the largest potential source of data is the patients who have been prescribed the drug in normal clinical usage. The scheme for voluntary reporting of adverse events to the Committee on Safety of Medicines (C.S.M.) in the U.K. is one of the best developed in the world. It is known however that even here there is serious under-reporting [1]. In the U.K. many events are also reported by doctors to the manufacturer of the drug. Within Smith Kline & French U.K., all reports of adverse events are assessed by a medically qualified person, and followed up by questionnaire, telephone call and/or personal visit to the reporting doctor. The information obtained is relayed to the C.S.M. and also to the Corporate headquarters of the company in Philadelphia, U.S.A., where it is added to the worldwide database. There is a free interchange of information between worldwide headquarters and the various country Medical Departments of Smith Kline & French, so that information generated locally can be considered in the context of worldwide experience. It is noteworthy that, in spite of the uncontrolled and anecdotal nature of most of the reports, all the changes made in the U.K. Data Sheet (Prescribing Information) for cimetidine since marketing in November 1976 have been stimulated by this voluntary reporting system. It is evidence of this kind which forms the basis of this paper. The voluntary reports have also led to clinical pharmacological and animal studies to clarify the mechanism of possible reactions, and these have themselves greatly extended knowledge of cimetidine.

Results and discussion

Up to February 1979 Smith Kline & French U.K. had received 801 reports of adverse events associated with cimetidine since marketing in November 1976. During the same period the C.S.M. had received 1,527 such reports (this figure including all the reports passed on to the C.S.M. by the company). The estimated number of patients treated during this period in the U.K. was nearly three-quarters of a million. This figure is a conservative estimate based on the results of a number of different market research surveys [Dr. P. Goddard, personal communication]. The number of reports is approximately doubled if those from the U.S.A. and the rest of the world are added [unpublished data] and includes a mass of anecdotes and isolated events, many of which appear to be irrelevant.

The information drawn from these reports is best summarised by describing examples of areas which have proved to be of interest. In some of these the spontaneous reports have confirmed statements in the Data Sheet which were originally based on clinical trial data. In other areas alterations and additions have been made, and in some there has not been sufficient evidence to merit inclusion. The latter is a very important point if the Data Sheet is to be maintained as a prescribing aid rather than a quasi-legal document to assist in the avoidance of product liability.

Examples of these clinical areas are discussed below.

Gynaecomastia

'Five patients, 3 with Zollinger-Ellison syndrome, developed mild unexplained gynaecomastia during treatment with Tagamet® [cimetidine]', was a statement in the first Data Sheet [2]. This was modified to 'Mild gynaecomastia appears to be a rare response' in the second [3], as the frequency of gynaecomastia in widespread clinical usage was estimated to be about 0.1%. A recent survey [Rowley-Jones, unpublished] of the 36 reports of gynaecomastia received by Smith Kline & French U.K. between November 1976 and December 1978, has shown that, of the 20 patients for whom sufficient data for assessment were available, gynaecomastia regressed or improved in 16 patients, despite continued cimetidine treatment in 3. Gynaecomastia persisted in 2 of the remaining patients, 1 and 4 months after cimetidine withdrawal, while the other 2 continued their treatment with no regression of their breast symptoms. Such prolactin estimations as were obtained were unhelpful in elucidating aetiology; there was no evidence of any cimetidine-induced abnormality. No other sign of feminisation was reported in any of these patients. Clinically it appeared that in the majority of instances the gynaecomastia was of nuisance value only, and some patients found the relief of their gastrointestinal symptoms of greater importance than the gynaecomastia.

Mental confusion

Clinical trials did not reveal any important cimetidine-related effects in the central nervous system (CNS). The only report of a confusional state occurring during clinical trials was in a 55-year-old male patient on chronic haemodialysis who sustained a myocardial infarction and subarachnoid haemorrhage from which he subsequently died. Indeed CNS effects were not to be expected on the basis of autoradiographic studies in the rat, where cimetidine was shown not to cross the blood-brain barrier [4]. We received during the early part of 1977, shortly after marketing in the U.K., occasional reports of patients becoming confused whilst receiving cimetidine. One of the first, a striking but not very well documented report concerning a man in a very responsible position, described symptoms (mind-racing, tension and disturbed sleep) with a temporal relationship to cimetidine in an otherwise uncomplicated setting.

During 1977 and 1978 sporadic reports of possible CNS effects appeared in the literature [5-18]. These reports assumed greater significance when we received data during the summer of 1978 suggesting that cimetidine had been assayed in significant concentrations in the cerebrospinal fluid in patients with uraemia, which is known to increase the permeability of the blood-brain barrier. These observations were subsequently confirmed in published studies [19, 20]. In the second half of 1978 Smith Kline & French worldwide data were reviewed, including not only individual reports of confusion but also of delirium, psychosis, hypomania, hallucination and agitation. Altogether there were 57 such reports at the time and of the 44 providing enough information, only 9 were under the age of 65, or were without serious concomitant illness or other therapy to account for their abnormal mental state. We also noted that in these cases the impaired mental state tended to improve when cimetidine was withdrawn. The statement 'Reversible confusional states can occur, usually in the elderly or very ill' was included in the U.K. Data Sheet. The emergence of these cases has also stimulated a number of research studies to look for any more subtle central effects.

Interstitial nephritis

It is vital in the assessment of adverse events to consider each individual report; it is not only the number which is important but their quality and possible attribution to the drug concerned. A statement was inserted in the U.K. Data Sheet in 1979 that 'Interstitial nephritis, reversed on withdrawal of Tagamet®, has been encountered very rarely'. During 1978, 5 reports of this complication were received in the U.S.A., including one which was particularly well documented. This was a report of a 64-year-old male receiving cimetidine, 300 mg at night, for reflux oesophagitis, who developed a fever and evidence of renal failure about 6-8 weeks after the start of treatment and in whom renal biopsy suggested interstitial nephritis. Cessation of treatment resulted in a return of normal renal function. Five months later the patient was rechallenged with cimetidine and within 72 hours developed a fever, casts and cells in his urine and biochemical evidence of impairment of renal function. These changes were again completely reversed following withdrawal of treatment. There seemed little doubt therefore that cimetidine was implicated in the development of renal failure in this patient. Although the other 4 reports were not as well documented, the inclusion of a statement in the Data Sheet was felt to be justified. The prescribing physician might otherwise continue treatment in a patient who happened to develop renal failure on cimetidine, in ignorance of the possibility that in rare instances this might be due to the drug and reversible on withdrawal.

Anticoagulants

A statement to the effect that cimetidine can prolong the prothrombin time in patients receiving oral anticoagulants has been included in the Data Sheet since January 1979. Again this was based on a qualitative rather than quantitive assessment of individual reports. During the first half of 1978, 15 reports of possible interactions between oral anticoagulants and cimetidine had been received worldwide by Smith Kline & French, and of these, 11 were reporting potentiation of the anticoagulant effect and 4 were of antagonism. Our own U.K. data were equivocal, in that there were 2 reports each of potentiation and antagonism. We then received preliminary results of a formal interaction study in normal subjects suggesting that cimetidine potentiated the effect of warfarin and, at roughly the same time, 5 well-documented case reports from one hospital where the addition of cimetidine in patients already on acenocoumarol produced in each a prolongation of the prothrombin time. These findings were of sufficient importance to justify rapid communication to the medical profession and this was done in simultaneous letters to the Lancet and British Medical Journal [21, 22]. The complete findings of the interaction study have now been published by Serlin and his colleagues [23], and their paper also contains confirmatory data in patients.

Ulcer perforation

There have been several occasions when considerable debate in journals and elsewhere has not led to any alteration in the Data Sheet. For example, at one time it was postulated that treatment with an H_2-receptor antagonist drug could theoretically lead to hypergastrinaemia, in turn leading to an increase in parietal cell mass, which could result in increased acid secretion. This could have 2 possible effects. Acid secretion could increase to such an extent that treatment would be ineffective and a loss of control would result in a severe recurrence of an ulcer during therapy. Alternatively, when treatment was discontinued acid secretion could be increased above pre-treatment levels, the so-called 'rebound hypersecretion' which could result in a more rapid and severe recurrence of ulceration.

For about 4 months during late 1977 and early 1978 there were a number of published reports of ulcer perforation occurring both during and following cimetidine treatment [24-28]. Spence and his colleagues [29], however, produced evidence suggesting that the pharmacological speculation of rebound hypersecretion had no foundation. In their study, 24 patients received cimetidine, 1.6 g/day, 23 of them for 1 year. Although the peak gastrin response to an Oxo test meal was significantly increased after 1 year, the peak acid output in response to maximal stimulation with histamine was unaffected by treatment. Since this latter parameter is considered to be an index of parietal cell mass, prolonged treatment with cimetidine did not appear to alter the acid secretory status of the patients. Examination of reports to Smith Kline & French U.K. has also suggested that this complication is no more frequent than would be expected by chance (Table).

These figures should be viewed in the context of the very large number of patients who have stopped taking cimetidine. As Alexander-Williams has said 'Everybody who has ever taken it has stopped except those who are still on it' [30]. Indeed Spence's data have now been confirmed by Gudmand-Hoyer and his colleagues [31] in a clinical study showing no difference in relapse rates between patients who were treated with cimetidine for 1 year and those who had received a short course of treatment or whose ulcer had healed spontaneously. It is also reassuring to note that the published reports of ulcer perforation in patients on cimetidine did not continue to accumulate and in fact very few cases have been reported in the literature since [32].

Table. Reports of ulcer perforation associated with cimetidine treatment, including published cases, received by Smith Kline & French U.K. between November 1976 and August 1979.

	During treatment	After treatment
Duodenal ulcer	6	8
Gastric ulcer	1	2
Oesophageal ulcer	0	1
Pyloric ulcer	0	1
Total	7	12

White blood cell disorders

Because of the development of reversible granulocytopenia in association with metiamide and the suggestion that there are H_2-receptors on marrow stem cells [33] we
have been especially vigilant in examining and recording individual reports of blood
dyscrasias. Indeed there has been considerable interest in the literature in possible
haematological effects of cimetidine [11, 34-48]. The white cell abnormalities seen
with metiamide were almost certainly the result of the presence of a thiourea group
in the molecule, whereas in cimetidine this has been replaced by a cyanoguanidine
radical. In animal toxicological studies there was no evidence of bone marrow
toxicity, nor is cimetidine concentrated in the bone marrow [4]. To date there have
been 19 U.K. reports of white blood cell disorders, of which 15 represented a fall in
neutrophil count. There have also been 3 reports of bone marrow depression. None
of these cases can be directly attributed to cimetidine. In all of them other factors
known to have a potential for affecting the bone marrow were present, whether
other drugs, diseases or irradiation. Assessment of those reports which provide
sufficient detail has not revealed any common pattern. About half of the cases were
considered to be the result of bone marrow suppression and half were attributed to
peripheral destruction of white blood cells. Experience in the U.S.A. has gathered a
rather larger number of reports, so that the worldwide total is over 100 [49]. In only
1 of these, however, was no other factor found which could have contributed to the
changes which occurred.

It is impossible under these circumstances to be certain about the role of a
particular drug in the development of a blood dyscrasia. The following example
illustrates that even when at first sight attribution is clear, caution should
predominate. We received during 1977 a report of a 54-year-old male who had
received cimetidine 1 g/day for about 6 weeks, because of a duodenal ulcer. The
patient took a maintenance dose of cimetidine intermittently for the next 6 months.
Because he developed aphthous ulcers in the mouth a blood count was performed
and he was found to have a neutrophil count of $0.6 \times 10^9/l$ with a total lymphocyte
count of $2.04 \times 10^9/l$. Cimetidine had been stopped coincidentally the day before
the blood count and a week later the neutrophil count had risen to $2.46 \times 10^9/l$. It
was then discovered that, in spite of medical advice, the patient had taken 2 or 3
tablets during that week. When his ulcer dyspepsia recurred 3 months later,
cimetidine was reintroduced with no effect on the white cell count. In retrospect it
was considered that the symptoms associated with the changes in white blood count
represented the response to a viral infection and were unrelated to cimetidine, as
they resolved spontaneously and did not recur on re-challenge.

Other areas

With such a widely used drug as cimetidine there inevitably remain areas where the
data from all sources are not sufficient, or are too confused, to warrant the drawing
of any conclusions. For example, the presence of histamine receptors in the cardiovascular system, which is discussed elsewhere in this volume, has led to particular
vigilance for relevant adverse reactions to cimetidine. Isolated instances of myocardial infarction have been reported, but there is no evidence to date that these cases
were other than coincidental. In addition, some cases of arrhythmia of diverse types
have been reported [50-56]. Some of these have recurred on rechallenge, but they do

not follow any discernable pattern.

The question of whether cimetidine has anti-androgenic effects when used at therapeutic doses in humans is afflicted as much by the confused nature of the evidence as by the lack of it. Up to September 1979, 20 reports of impotence and/or loss of libido had been received by Smith Kline & French U.K., which in the context of the number of patients treated since November 1976, press publicity, and the natural frequency of these complaints in the relevant age groups, does not seem alarming. Results of endocrinological investigation of subjects receiving therapeutic doses of cimetidine have been contradictory or at least lacking confirmation [57-60]. No evidence of infertility has been reported.

Recently several cases of gastric cancer have been reported in patients who have been treated with cimetidine, and an aetiological link postulated with the hypothetical formation of nitrosamines in the stomach [61-65]. Facts are still few in this area. Spontaneous U.K. reports of gastric cancer occurring in patients who have had cimetidine amounted to 14 (including published cases) by September 1979. It is known, however, that cimetidine can mask the symptoms of gastric cancer [66-69] and that it may, therefore, be useful in treating terminal cases. The temporal associations of the reported cases are unconvincing. A great deal of investigative work remains to be done.

Conclusions

Events recorded in the initial clinical trial programme for cimetidine did not suggest any limitation to its use in peptic ulcer disease [70]. Since then, intensive study of the safety of cimetidine over 3 years of widespread clinical use has not changed this conclusion for the vast majority of patients. On current evidence the benefits still greatly outweigh the risks. The changes which have been made in the Prescribing Information affect mainly specific patient types and have been stimulated by the spontaneous voluntary reporting of adverse events by prescribers. The assessment of safety, therefore, still depends greatly on the continued vigilance of prescribing physicians and surgeons.

Acknowledgements

The authors would like to acknowledge the part played by the Medical Information Department of Smith Kline & French U.K., in particular John Amos, in compiling and maintaining the file of adverse events on which this paper was based. We also gratefully acknowledge the help of all the doctors who have reported adverse events, and discussed with us the clinical details of their patients.

References

1. Inman, W.H.W. and Evans, D.A. (1972): *Br. Med. J. 2*, 746.
2. 'Tagamet' Data Sheet, 1976.
3. 'Tagamet' Data Sheet, 1978.
4. Cross, S.A.M. (1977): *Acta Pharmacol. Toxicol. 41 (Suppl.)*, 116.
5. Robinson, T.J. and Mulligan, T.O. (1977): *Lancet 2*, 719.
6. Delaney, J.C. and Ravey, M. (1977): *Lancet 2*, 512.
7. Menzies-Gow, N. (1977): *Lancet 2*, 928.
8. Grimson, T.A. (1977): *Lancet 1*, 858.

9. Barbier, J.P. and Hirsch, J.F. (1978): *Nouv. Presse Méd. 7,* 1484.
10. Beraud, J.J., Monteil, A.L., Munoz, A. and Mirouze, J. (1978): *Nouv. Presse Méd. 7,* 2570.
11. Klotz, S.A. and Kay, B.F. (1978): *Ann. Intern. Med. 88,* 579.
12. McMillen, M.A., Ambis, D. and Siegel, J.H. (1978): *N. Engl. J. Med. 298,* 284.
13. Pomare, E.W. (1978): *Lancet 1,* 1202.
14. Quap, C.W. (1978): *Drug Intell. Clin. Pharm. 12,* 121.
15. Spears, J.B. (1978): *Am. J. Hosp. Pharm. 35,* 1035.
16. Vickery, T.R. (1978): *Drug Intell. Clin. Pharm. 12,* 242.
17. Wood, C.A., Isaacson, M.L. and Hibbs, M.S. (1978): *J. Am. Med. Assoc. 239,* 2550.
18. Deheneffe, Y., Reynaert, M. and Tremouroux, J. (1978): *Nouv. Presse Méd. 7,* 4303.
19. Edmonds, M.E., Ashford, R.F.U., Brenner, M.K. and Saunders, A. (1979): *J. R. Soc. Med. 72,* 172.
20. Schentag, J.J., Cerra, F.B., Calleri, G. et al. (1979): *Lancet 1,* 177.
21. Flind, A.C. (1978): *Br. Med. J. 2,* 1367.
22. Flind, A.C. (1978): *Lancet 2,* 1054.
23. Serlin, M.J., Sibeon, R.G., Mossman, S. et al. (1979): *Lancet 2,* 317.
24. Wallace, W.A., Orr, C.M.E. and Bearn, A.R. (1977): *Br. Med. J. 2,* 865.
25. Keighley, B.D. (1977): *Br. Med. J. 2,* 1022.
26. Gill, M.J. and Saunders, J.B. (1977): *Br. Med. J. 2,* 1149.
27. Ellis, D.J., Hamer, J.D. and Baker, S.E. (1977): *Br. Med. J. 2,* 1538.
28. Ball, J.R. (1978): *Br. Med. J. 1,* 235.
29. Spence, R.W., Celestin, L.R., McCormick, D.A. et al. (1978): In: *Proceedings of an International Symposium on Histamine H$_2$-Receptor Antagonists, Göttingen, 10th-11th November 1977,* p. 116. Editor: W. Creutzfeldt. Excerpta Medica, Amsterdam-Oxford-Princeton.
30. Baron, J.H., Alexander-Williams, J. and Bennett, J.R. (1979): *Br. Med. J. 1,* 169.
31. Gudmand-Hoyer, E., Birger Jensen, K., Krag, E. et al. (1978): *Br. Med. J. 1,* 1095.
32. Bulman, A.S. (1979): *Br. Med. J. 1,* 409.
33. Byron, J.W. (1977): *Agents Actions 7,* 209.
34. Craven, E.R. and Whittington, J.M. (1977): *Lancet 2,* 294.
35. Johnson, N.McI., Black, A.E., Hughes, A.S.B. and Clarke, S.W. (1977): *Lancet 1,* 1226.
36. Corbett, C.L. and Holdsworth, C.D. (1978): *Br. Med. J. 1,* 753.
37. James, C. and Prout, B.J. (1978): *Lancet 1,* 987.
38. Ufberg, M.H., Brooks, C.M., Bosanac, P.R. and Kintzel, J.E. (1977): *Gastroenterology 73,* 635.
39. Ufberg, M.H., Brooks, C.M., Bosanac, P.R. and Kintzel, J.E. (1978): *Gastroenterology 74,* 163.
40. Lopez-Luque, A., Rodriguez-Cuartero, A., Perez-Galvez, N. et al. (1978): *Lancet 1,* 444.
41. Gouffier, E., Schnurmann, D., Durepaire, H. and Vernant, J.B. (1978): *Nouv. Presse Méd. 7,* 2660.
42. Teichmann, R.K., Zumtobel, V. and Heberer, G. (1978): *Chirurg 49,* 397.
43. Littlejohn, G.O. and Urowitz, M.B. (1979): *Ann. Intern. Med. 91,* 317.
44. Al-Kawas, F.H., Lenes, B.A. and Sacher, R.A. (1979): *Ann. Intern. Med. 90,* 992.
45. Nouel, O., Pariente, E.-A., Slaoui, H. and Renoux, M. (1979): *Gastroenterol. Clin. Biol. 3,* 481.
46. De Galocsy, C. and van Ypersele de Strihou, C. (1979): *Ann. Intern. Med. 90,* 274.
47. Posnett, D.N., Stein, R.S., Graber, S.E. and Krantz, S.B. (1979): *Arch. Intern. Med. 139,* 584.
48. Selker, R.G., Moore, P. and LoDolce, D. (1978): *N. Engl. J. Med. 299,* 834.
49. Davis, T.G., Pickett, D.L. and Schlosser, J.H. (1980): *J. Am. Med. Assoc.* (In press.)
50. Reding, P., Devroede, C. and Barbier, P. (1977): *Lancet 2,* 1227.
51. Jeffreys, D.B. and Vale, J.A. (1978): *Lancet 1,* 828.
52. Bournerias, F., Ganeval, D. and Danan, G. (1978): *Nouv. Presse Méd. 7,* 2069.

53. Luciano, J.J., Theodorou-Touchais, A.M. and Souteyrand, P. (1978): *Nouv. Presse Méd. 7,* 4049.
54. Stimmesse, B., Daoudal, P., Neidhardt, A. and Ory, J.P. (1978): *Nouv. Presse Méd. 7,* 4233.
55. Ligumsky, M., Shochina, M. and Rachmilewitz, D. (1978): *Ann. Intern. Med. 89,* 1008.
56. Cohen, J., Weetman, A.P., Dargie, H.J. and Krikler, D.M. (1979): *Br. Med. J. 2,* 768.
57. Barber, S.G. and Hoare, A.M. (1979): *Horm. Metab. Res. 11,* 220.
58. Bohnet, H.G., Greiwe, M., Hanker, J.P. et al. (1978): *Acta Endocrinol. 88,* 428.
59. Peden, N.R., Cargill, J.M., Browning, M.C.K. et al. (1979): *Br. Med. J. 1,* 659.
60. Van Thiel, D.H., Gavaler, J.S., Smith, W.I. and Paul, G. (1979): *N. Engl. J. Med. 300,* 1012.
61. Elder, J.B., Ganguli, P.C. and Gillespie, I.E. (1979): *Lancet 1,* 1005.
62. Roe, F.J.C. (1979): *Lancet 1,* 1039.
63. Reed, P.I., Cassell, P.G. and Walters, C.L. (1979): *Lancet 1,* 1234.
64. Taylor, T.V., Lee, D., Howatson, A.G. et al. (1979): *Lancet 1,* 1235.
65. Buck, J.P., Murgatroyd, R.E., Boylston, A.W. and Baron, J.H. (1979): *Lancet 2,* 42.
66. Welsh, C.L., Craven, J.L. and Hopton, D. (1977): *Br. Med. J. 1,* 1413.
67. Taylor, R.H., Menzies-Gow, N., Lovell, D. et al. (1978): *Lancet 1,* 686.
68. Murray, C., Chapman, R., Isaacson, P. and Bamforth, J. (1978): *Lancet 1,* 1092.
69. Minoli, G., Terruzzi, V. and Rossini, A. (1978): *Lancet 1,* 1092.
70. Burland, W.L. (1978): In: *Proceedings of an International Symposium on Histamine H₂-Receptor Antagonists, Göttingen, 10th-11th November, 1977,* p. 238. Editor: W. Creutzfeldt. Excerpta Medica, Amsterdam-Oxford-Princeton.

Results of the Tagamet® Post Market Surveillance Program in the United States

L.M. Gifford, M.E. Aeugle, R.M. Myerson and P.J. Tannenbaum
Medical Affairs Department, Smith Kline & French Laboratories, Philadelphia, Pennsylvania, U.S.A.

Introduction

This paper presents the results of the initial phase (Phase 1) of the Tagamet® [cimetidine] Post Market Surveillance Program, which was conducted with the intention of gathering data on the effectiveness of cimetidine treatment in 10,000 outpatients. We believe that this survey, when complete, will be the first to include both initial and follow-up data on such a large number of patients.

Subjects and methods

Data collection followed a protocol designed in cooperation with the U.S. Food and Drug Administration late in 1977. Our professional service representatives contacted 1,232 physicians (60% family practitioners, 30% internists and 10% gastroenterologists) and asked each to provide data on at least 10 outpatients for whom they would prescribe cimetidine within the following 3 months. Patients already receiving cimetidine at the time the survey was initiated could be included, as long as they had not yet completed their course of therapy. Those who had completed their course of therapy prior to March 13, 1978, and those who were hospitalized during their entire course of cimetidine therapy, were not eligible for inclusion.

A 2-page case report form was used by the physicians to record the data requested (Figs. 1 and 2). Except for the routine demographic data, the information was requested in a relatively open-ended manner, allowing ample space for comments.

The question 'Is Tagamet® therapy continuing?' requires an explanation. Normally, the duration of therapy recorded on a case report form covers the entire course of therapy; in this case, however, patients could be enrolled in our surveillance program at any time during the specified 3-month period, and *all* case report forms were collected at the end of that time. Therefore, many patients had not yet completed their course of therapy when the case report forms were collected; the exact duration of therapy for such patients will be obtained during the follow-up phase.

The second page of the form requested data on any adverse effects noted, and also asked for information concerning changes in associated diagnostic conditions, changes in concomitant therapy, hospitalizations, and consultations.

Document
Number

'TAGAMET' SURVEILLANCE PROGRAM
TA-102

INSTRUCTIONS TO PHYSICIAN: Please use a check (√) in all cases, except where specific information is requested.

DEMOGRAPHY: PATIENT'S NAME: _____   DATE OF BIRTH: ___/___/___
                                                                              M   D   Y

HEIGHT: _____   WEIGHT: _____   SEX: _____   RACE: _____

                in.   lbs.

DATE OF
INITIAL VISIT: ___/___/___
            M   D   Y

Diagnosis: _____   Total Duration of Condition: <1 yr. ☐ >1 yr. ☐

Associated Conditions: _____

Concomitant Medication: _____

'TAGAMET' DOSE RECORD

	FROM (mo/day/yr)	TO (mo/day/yr)	TOTAL DAILY DOSE (mg)
Date 'Tagamet' Started	___/___/___	___/___/___	

COMPLETE THIS SECTION WHEN 'TAGAMET' IS DISCONTINUED OR WHEN CRF IS COLLECTED

RESULTS OF 'TAGAMET' THERAPY (Check Appropriate Blocks)

☐ 1. EXCELLENT – Symptom Free
☐ 2. GOOD   – Symptoms Substantially Relieved
☐ 3. FAIR   – Little Symptom Relief
☐ 4. POOR   – Poor Or No Relief
☐ 5. WORSE

Is 'Tagamet' therapy continuing?

YES ____   NO ____.   If "NO", give reason:

☐ Desired therapeutic effect obtained
☐ Other (Define): _____
_____
_____

If patient failed to return, describe follow-up efforts: _____

_____

_____

_____   _____
DATE   PHYSICIAN'S SIGNATURE

Fig. 1.   Page 1 of the case report form used in the Tagamet® Post Market Surveillance Program.

Document
Number

SINCE STARTING 'TAGAMET' THERAPY:

1) Did any adverse effects occur?   NO ___   YES ___.   If "YES", complete section below.

ADVERSE REACTIONS

ADVERSE REACTIONS (One per Line)	DATE OF ONSET (mo./day/yr.)	DATE CLEARED (mo./day/yr.)	SEVERITY			RELATION TO DRUG			ACTION		
			MILD	MOD.	SEVERE	NONE	QUEST.	RELATED	NONE	REDUCED	DISC.
	__/__/__	__/__/__									
	__/__/__	__/__/__									
	__/__/__	__/__/__									

2) Were there any changes in associated medical condition(s) or their treatment OR have any new medical conditions developed or any new therapies been initiated? NO ___ YES ___. If "YES", please describe:

CONDITION	TREATMENT

3) Has patient been hospitalized? NO ___ YES ___. If "YES", give reason and dates: _____

_____

_____

4) Has patient visited or have you consulted with another specialist? NO ___ YES ___ ; if "YES", give name of consultant, type of specialty, and describe condition:

_____

_____

_____

Did condition requiring hospitalization/consultation pre-date 'Tagamet' therapy?   NO   YES

_____   _____
DATE   PHYSICIAN'S INITIALS

Fig. 2. Page 2 of the case report form used in the Tagamet® Post Market Surveillance Program.

Results

Of the 1,232 physicians originally contacted by our professional service representatives, 1,049 submitted case report forms, a physician response rate of 85%. We received a total of 10,166 case report forms, an average of 9.7 forms per physician.

This paper is based on the analyses of 9,907 Phase 1 case report forms; we are still processing additional data from the remaining 259 forms. These 259 case report forms have already been individually reviewed by an information scientist and a clinical monitor, and there is no indication that they will have any significant effect on the overall safety data or any of the other data in the present report.

In order to include all adverse effects reported, we have used all 9,907 case report forms for that tabulation. However, 881 forms were excluded from other tabulations because the patients had failed to meet the inclusion criteria; that is, they had either completed their course of therapy prior to March 13, 1978, or had been hospitalized during their entire course of therapy. Therefore, all of the Tables presented in this paper (except Tables V and VI, which deal with adverse effects) are based on data from 9,026 outpatients undergoing cimetidine treatment during all or part of the designated data-collection period.

Table I shows the number and percentage of case report forms submitted, grouped by type of practice or specialty of the submitting physician. Over 50% of the reports came from general or family practitioners, about 25% from internists, and 15% from gastroenterologists.

Participating physicians used a number of different terminologies to indicate the same diagnoses; the primary gastroenterological diagnoses and the specific conditions treated in each of these categories are listed in Table II. The miscellaneous group includes a variety of gastrointestinal symptoms and nongastrointestinal primary diagnoses which accounted for the patient's visit to his or her physician. In the nongastrointestinal cases, an associated gastrointestinal condition was often listed as a secondary diagnosis, and, in such cases, was presumably the reason for cimetidine therapy.

The relief of symptoms during cimetidine therapy as evaluated by the physician is shown in Table III. There were no placebo controls in this study; however, the response reported corresponds very closely to the results previously observed in· rigorously-controlled clinical trials [1-8], and demonstrates that these benefits continue to be seen in routine clinical use.

Table I. Number and percentage of case report forms submitted, grouped by type of practice or specialty of the submitting physician.

Type of practice or specialty	Number (and %) of cases
General or family practitioners	4,951 (54.9)
Internists	2,405 (26.7)
Gastroenterologists	1,353 (15.0)
Internist/gastroenterologists	179 (2.0)
Not known	138 (1.6)
Total	9,026

Table II. Primary gastroenterological diagnoses and specific conditions treated in 9,026 patients.

Primary diagnosis Specific condition treated	Number of patients
Duodenal disease	4,208
Duodenal ulcer disease	3,875
Duodenitis	300
Duodenal deformity	33
Peptic disease	1,407
Peptic ulcer disease	1,174
Hyperacidity syndrome, gastric hyperacidity, gastric acidity	124
Acid peptic disease/syndrome, peptic gastrointestinal disease	76
Dyspepsia	33
Gastric disease	1,588
Gastritis	948
Gastric ulcer disease	635
Antritis	5
Esophageal disease	1,082
Hiatal hernia	559
Reflux esophagitis, gastroeso- phageal reflux, reflux	306
Esophagitis	184
Esophageal ulcer	33
Other frequently-reported GI	243
Marginal ulcer	70
Epigastric pain	42
Pyloric spasm	39
Gastroenteritis	32
Gastrointestinal bleeding	31
Pancreatitis	29
Zollinger-Ellison syndrome	18
Miscellaneous	480

Table III. Relief of symptoms during cimetidine therapy.

Quality of relief	Number (and %) of cases
Excellent	4,984 (55.3)
Good	2,845 (31.6)
Fair	404 (4.5)
Poor	252 (2.8)
Worse	35 (0.4)
Not known/deferred	506 (5.6)
Total	9,026

Table IV.   Duration of therapy.

Duration	Number (and %) of cases
< 1 week — 4 weeks	1,714 (19.0)
> 4 weeks — 8 weeks	2,690 (29.8)
> 8 weeks — 3 months	2,027 (22.5)
> 3 months — 4 months	954 (10.6)
> 4 months — 5 months	529 (5.9)
> 5 months — 6 months	320 (3.6)
> 6 months	792 (8.8)
Total	9,026

Table IV shows the duration of therapy as of the time the case report forms were collected. Most of the patients had received cimetidine for from 1-3 months; over 2,500 had received varying doses for more than 3 months. There are at least 2 opposing biases that influence this data: since inclusion criteria required some treatment during the specified 3-month period, the initial group of entrants would be biased toward a longer duration of treatment by including a disproportionate number of cases where prolonged treatment persisted into the collection period; however, on the other hand, patients who entered toward the close of the surveillance period will show only the duration of treatment up to the time the case report forms were collected. We expect that the total length of therapy per patient may be better reflected after we have completed the second phase of the surveillance program.

As mentioned earlier, our adverse effect data are based on all 9,907 case report forms evaluated; cases were not excluded from this tabulation even if hospitalized throughout their course of cimetidine therapy or if treatment was completed before the designated enrollment period, so all adverse effects reported to the participating

Table V.   Adverse effects in 9,907 patients, grouped by organ system affected.

System affected	Total number of effects reported	Number (and %) of patients reporting adverse effect
Gastrointestinal	254	208 (2.1)
Central nervous	136	108 (1.1)
Allergic/skin	55	46 (0.5)
Endocrine	25	24 (0.3)
Musculoskeletal	21	20 (0.2)
Urinary tract	19	19 (0.2)
Autonomic	14	14 (0.2)
Sensory organs	14	14 (0.2)
Cardiovascular	13	11 (0.2)
Blood	9	9 (0.1)
Miscellaneous	17	17 (0.2)
Total	577	

physicians are included. Table V shows the total number of adverse effects reported for each organ system, the number of patients reporting them, and the percentage of the total population surveyed that these patients represent. Adverse effects were reported by a total of 442 of the 9,907 patients, or 4.4%; since some patients reported more than 1 adverse effect, the total number of reporting patients is not additive.

The most frequently reported adverse effects in each organ system (10 or more reports) are shown in Table VI. Of the 254 events reported as possible gastrointestinal adverse effects, 30 occurred in circumstances strongly suggesting a relationship to cimetidine treatment. Of these, 27 involved nausea, vomiting and diarrhea. The other 3 reports were of epigastric pain or cramps. Of the 136 cases of central nervous system adverse effects, dizziness or dizzy feeling was reported most frequently (34 reports), followed by headache (23 reports). Three of the patients reporting dizziness were rechallenged with cimetidine; in all 3 cases, their dizziness was thought to be directly related to the drug.

Because of reports in the literature suggesting a possible relationship between cimetidine and mental confusion [9], blood dyscrasias [10] and endocrine effects [11], the adverse effects reported in these areas merit discussion. There were 5 reported cases of confusion in the surveillance program, none of which, as described, could be unequivocally related to cimetidine therapy. In addition, coma was reported in 1 patient, disorientation and unconsciousness in a second, and disorientation and hallucinations in a third; however, because of pre-existing underlying or associated conditions, the relationship between these reactions and cimetidine was considered questionable in these 3 patients as well.

Twenty-five adverse effects were reported in the endocrine system; 18 of these were gynecomastia and were considered to be related to cimetidine therapy. One of the patients who reported gynecomastia also reported sex inhibition. Sex inhibition

Table VI.   Most frequently-reported adverse effects.

Effect	Times reported
Diarrhea	98
Nausea and vomiting	81
Rash, hives, pruritus	41
Dizziness	34
Headache	23
Epigastric/stomach pain/cramps	23
Gynecomastia	18
Constipation	18
Gas	18
Sleepiness	17
Dry mouth	12
Muscular pain/pain	10
Miscellaneous	184
Total number of effects	577

was also reported by a female patient, loss of libido by a male, and poor sexual performance by another male.

Nine cases of hematological problems were reported. Only 1 of these was considered to be related to cimetidine: a patient on anticoagulants who had difficulty in regulation of prothrombin time because of excess anticoagulant effect. There were 2 cases of leukopenia reported, in both of which the relationship to cimetidine was considered questionable: 1 of these occurred in a female who was also receiving naproxen, whose white blood cell count dropped from 5,100 to 3,500 a month after starting cimetidine and returned to normal 3 weeks after stopping treatment; the other case occurred in a female with pre-existing breast cancer who had been receiving chemotherapy for years. Other hematological adverse effects reported were: 2 cases of petechiae and 1 each of 'irregular' prothrombin time, purpura, hemolysis, and anemia.

We were especially interested to know if there was any relationship between the occurrence of adverse effects and the duration of therapy. Our review showed that half of the patients reporting adverse effects were treated for more than 8 weeks; however, only 44 of the adverse effects reported had their *onset* after 8 weeks (Table VII). Gynecomastia stands out as the most common late adverse effect, although the total incidence was still quite low. Of the 11 cases where the time of appearance was noted, only 1 was reported with onset at less than 8 weeks, and that was seen in an 80-year-old male. New cases were still arising after 6 months on cimetidine, although there was no apparent increase in the rate of occurrence.

Table VIII shows the age and sex distribution of the patients under surveillance, and also of those who died during the surveillance period. Interestingly, 216 patients under the age of 16 received cimetidine treatment; the bulk of the patients, however, were in the 30-70 age group. There was an unexpectedly even division of males and females.

Sixty-five deaths were reported during the surveillance period; these cases have all been given special attention, and none appear to have been due to cimetidine therapy. Most of the deaths reported occurred in patients over the age of 60, and

Table VII. Onset of adverse effects which began after more than 56 days of cimetidine treatment.

Type of effect	Total reported	Days of treatment before onset				
		57-93	94-120	121-155	156-183	>184
Gynecomastia	10	3	2	1	1	3
Diarrhea	7	2	1	2	0	2
Nausea	5	3	1	1	0	0
Rash	4	3	1	0	0	0
Dizziness	2	1	0	1	0	0
Others	16*	8	0	4	0	4
Total	44	20	5	9	1	9

*This figure represents 1 case each of edema, purpura, vertigo, vomiting, cramps, muscle guarding, abdominal pain, angina pectoris, palpitation, constipation, joint aches, ulcer symptoms, tendinitis, bruises, increased prothrombin time, and gastrointestinal bleeding.

Table VIII.   Age and sex distribution of the patients under surveillance (total population), and of those who died during the surveillance period (deaths).

Age group	Total population				Deaths			
	Number	Male	Female	NL	Number	Male	Female	NL
Under 16	216	102	100	14	0	0	0	0
16-19	182	81	99	2	0	0	0	0
20-29	942	479	446	17	1	1	0	0
30-39	1,369	691	655	23	0	0	0	0
40-49	1,609	781	796	32	7	3	4	0
50-59	1,992	1,019	921	52	12	9	3	0
60-69	1,511	733	752	26	20	12	7	1
70 and over	1,205	518	667	20	24	16	8	0
NL	0	0	0	0	1	1	0	0
Totals	9,026	4,404	4,436	186	65	42	22	1

NL = not listed on the submitted case report form.

most of the patients who died were males; thus, the age and sex distribution of the patients who died is distinctly different from that of the total population of patients treated with cimetidine.

Nineteen of the deaths were tumor-related, and all of these occurred in patients whose tumors had been diagnosed prior to beginning cimetidine therapy. There were 17 deaths with cardiovascular diagnosis: 16 of these were related to pre-existing or recurring disease of the heart or the cerebral circulation, and 1 was a post-operative pulmonary embolus. Other deaths were due to chronic pulmonary disease, complications of gastrointestinal disease or automobile accident, or occurred after stopping treatment.

One of the purposes of the surveillance program was to search for important events that might not be attributed to cimetidine by the prescribing physician. Therefore, we asked physicians to provide a listing of any consultations, hospitalizations, changes in associated conditions, or new conditions which occurred during or following therapy..The absence of a control group limits our ability to evaluate the incidence of these events; however, we have examined them carefully. In none of these areas were there observations which were judged to be additional adverse reactions not previously observed.

Acknowledgments

Figures 1 and 2, and Tables I, III, V, VI and VIII have been reprinted from the April 18, 1980 issue of the *Journal of the American Medical Association,* with the permission of the American Medical Association.

References

1. Binder, H.J., Cocco, A., Crossley, R.J. et al. (1978): Cimetidine in the treatment of duodenal ulcer. *Gastroenterology 74,* 380-388.

2. Moshal, M.G., Spitaels, J.M. and Bhoola, R. (1977): Treatment of duodenal ulcers with cimetidine. *S. Afr. Med. J. 52*, 760-763.
3. Wulff, H.R. (1978): Cimetidine in the treatment of gastric ulcer. In: *Cimetidine: proceedings of the second International Symposium on histamine H_2-receptor antagonists*, pp. 217-221. Editors: W.L. Burland and M.A. Simkins. Excerpta Medica, Amsterdam-Oxford-Princeton.
4. Bader, J.-P., Morin, T., Mondor, H. et al. (1977): Treatment of gastric ulcer. In: *Cimetidine: proceedings of the second International Symposium on histamine H_2-receptor antagonists*, pp. 287-292. Editors: W.L. Burland and M.A. Simkins. Excerpta Medica, Amsterdam-Oxford-Princeton.
5. Bodemar, G., Norlander, B. and Walan, A. (1977): Cimetidine in the treatment of active peptic ulcer disease. In: *Cimetidine: proceedings of the second International Symposium on histamine H_2-receptor antagonists*, pp. 224-239. Editors: W.L. Burland and M.A. Simkins. Excerpta Medica, Amsterdam-Oxford-Princeton.
6. Lepsien, G., Weiser, H.F., Weber, K. et al. (1977): Treatment of reflux oesophagitis with cimetidine. In: *Cimetidine: proceedings of the second International Symposium on histamine H_2-receptor antagonists*, 259-270. Editors: W.L. Burland and M.A. Simkins. Excerpta Medica, Amsterdam-Oxford-Princeton.
7. Behar, J., Brand, D., Brown, F. et al. (1978): Cimetidine in the treatment of symptomatic gastroesophageal reflux. *Gastroenterology 74*, 441-448.
8. Petrokubi, R.J. and Jeffries, G.H. (1978): Cimetidine versus antacid in scleroderma with reflux esophagitis, a randomized double-blind controlled study. *Gastroenterology 74*, 5, Part 2. (Abstract.)
9. Schentag, J.J., Cerra, F.B., Calleri, G. et al. (1979): Pharmacokinetic and clinical studies in patients with cimetidine-associated mental confusion. *Lancet I*, 177-181.
10. Freston, J.W. (1979): Cimetidine and granulocytopenia. *Ann. Intern. Med. 90*, 264-265.
11. Van Thiel, D.H., Gavaler, J.S., Smith, W.I. Jr. and Paul, G. (1979): Hypothalamic-pituitary-gonadal dysfunction in men using cimetidine. *N. Engl. J. Med. 300*, 1012-1015.

Progress in histamine research

Chairmen: **R.W. Brimblecombe** *(Welwyn Garden City, United Kingdom)*
 G. Bertaccini *(Parma, Italy)*

Agonists and antagonists at histamine receptors

C.R. Ganellin
The Research Institute, Smith Kline & French Research Ltd., Welwyn Garden City, United Kingdom

Evidence for histamine receptors is based on the action of certain drugs which have been shown to specifically and competitively antagonise various pharmacological effects of histamine. These drugs have been used to classify the actions of histamine, and we now recognise 2 classes of histamine receptor [1, 2]. It seems worthwhile, therefore, to mention the most important chemical compounds used by pharmacologists as tools with which to analyse the actions of histamine.

Histamine H_1-receptor antagonists

The H_1-receptor antihistamines are too well-known to need much discussion. They are generally tertiary amines, which usually incorporate a short chain of atoms carrying 2 aryl substituents, as represented by the general formula in Figure 1. Like histamine, they possess the basic aminoalkyl chain, but their aromatic rings do not have much specific resemblance to histamine's imidazole ring. The H_1-receptor antihistamines also resemble histamine in that they are strongly basic and protonated at physiological pH; however, whereas histamine is a very hydrophilic molecule, the antihistamines are lipophilic. Indeed, there are structure-activity studies which show that, within a given structural type, there may be good correlations between some function of lipophilicity and antagonist potency [3].

There are some 30 antihistamines in therapeutic use, but only a few of these are in general use by pharmacologists (Fig. 2). The most popular agent appears to be mepyramine, probably because of its high potency and great specificity. Others are diphenhydramine, tripelennamine and triprolidine [4, 5]. Although histamine has no asymmetric centre and is therefore not capable of optical isomerism, the antagonist chlorpheniramine has a chiral centre and shows a good degree of stereo-

General formula for antihistamines showing protonated side chain:

Formula for histamine monocation:

Fig. 1. Comparison of H_1-receptor antihistamines and histamine. Both have a basic aminoalkyl chain.

Structure	R	Name	pA$_2$	Ref.
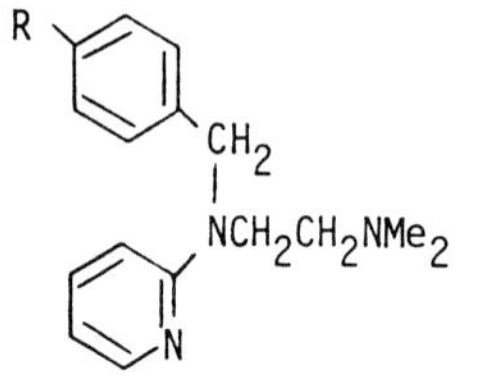	CH$_3$O	mepyramine	9.36	[4]*
			9.39	[5]**
	H	tripelennamine	9.00	[4]*
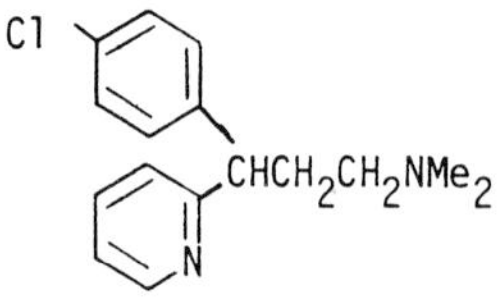		dl-chlorpheniramine	8.82	[4]*
			9.04	[5]**
		d-chlorpheniramine	9.30	[6]
		l-chlorpheniramine	7.84	[6]
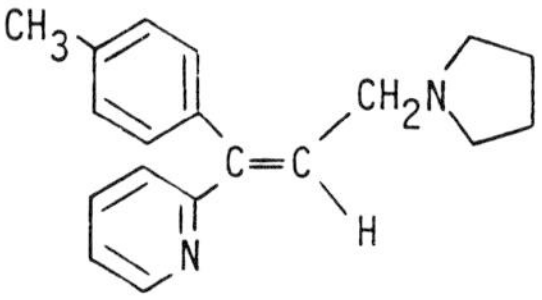		triprolidine	9.94	[5]**
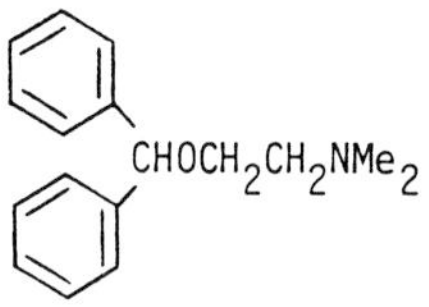		diphenhydramine	8.14	[4]*
			7.95	[5]**
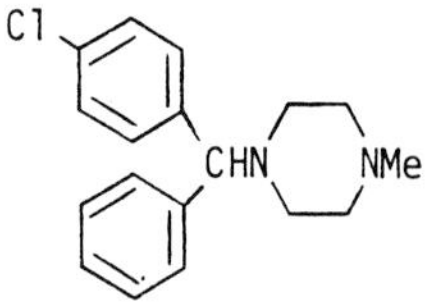		chlorcyclizine	8.63	[4]*

*Fig. 2.   Structures of some H$_1$-receptor antihistamines used in pharmacology, and reported pA$_2$ values for antagonism of histamine-stimulated contraction of guinea-pig ileum in vitro. The pA$_2$ value is the negative logarithm of the concentration of antagonist that necessitates a doubling of the histamine dose required to match the effect in the absence of antagonist. * = 10 minutes contact for equilibration; ** = 15-30 minutes contact for equilibration.*

specifity; thus d-chlorpheniramine is reported to be at least 35 times more potent than the l-isomer as an antagonist of histamine-stimulated contractions of the guinea-pig ileum in vitro [6], and the separation in vivo is reported to be even greater [7]. These stereoisomers are valuable tools for exploring possible H_1-receptor effects in other tissue systems; for example, a recent application has been their use in brain tissue binding studies [8, 9].

Name	Structure	ID_{50} (μmol/kg)	pA_2	Ref.
General formula	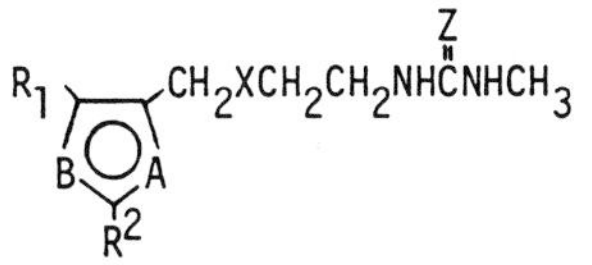 R_1 ⟨ring B—A, R^2⟩ $CH_2XCH_2CH_2NHCNHCH_3$ (Z above C)			
Burimamide	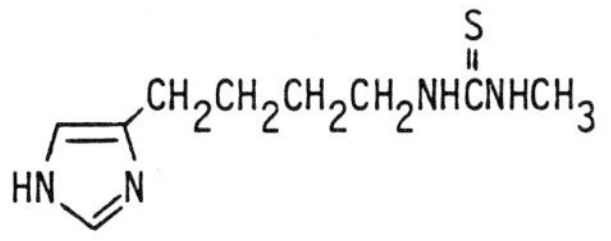 $CH_2CH_2CH_2CH_2NHCNHCH_3$ (S above C); imidazole (HN, N)	6.1	5.11	[2]
Metiamide	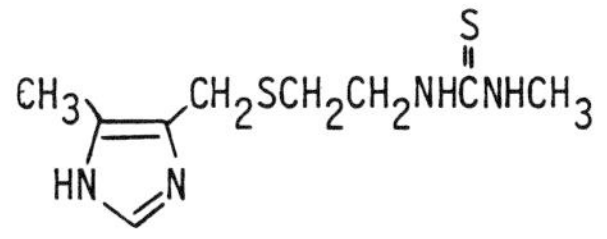 CH_3 —$CH_2SCH_2CH_2NHCNHCH_3$ (S above C); imidazole (HN, N)	1.6	6.04	[10]
Cimetidine	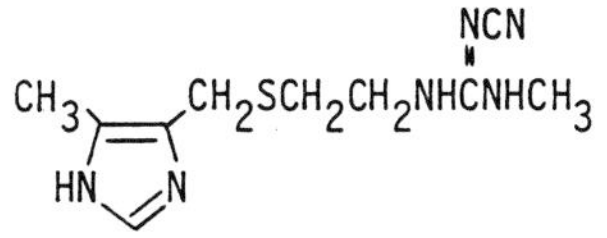 CH_3 —$CH_2SCH_2CH_2NHCNHCH_3$ (NCN above C); imidazole (HN, N)	1.4	6.10	[12]
Ranitidine	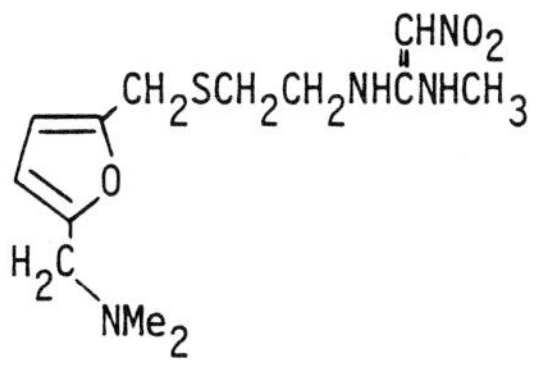 $CH_2SCH_2CH_2NHCNHCH_3$ (CHNO$_2$ above C); furan ring, H_2C—NMe_2	0.13	7.20	[14]
ICI-125211	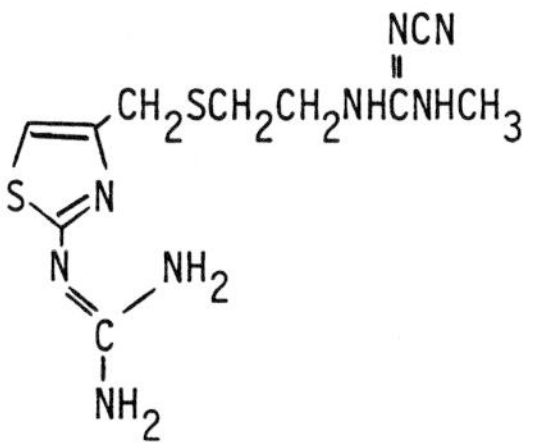 $CH_2SCH_2CH_2NHCNHCH_3$ (NCN above C); thiazole ring (S, N), N—C(NH$_2$)—NH$_2$		7.7	[15]

Fig. 3. *Structures of some histamine H_2-receptor antagonists, and activities determined both in vivo, as inhibitors of histamine-stimulated gastric acid secretion in the anaesthetised rat (see ID_{50} column), and in vitro, as inhibitors of histamine stimulation of the spontaneously-beating guinea-pig right atrium (see pA_2 column). ID_{50} = dose required to reduce acid secretion by 50%.*

Histamine H$_2$-receptor antagonists

Antagonists of histamine at its H$_2$-receptor first became available in 1972 as a result of work at our Institute. Those most widely used are burimamide, metiamide and, of course, cimetidine (Fig. 3). Like histamine, these compounds are imidazole derivatives with structurally-specific side chains, but they differ from histamine in 2 important respects: their side chains are longer and not basic (that is, the side chains are uncharged at physiological pH). The imidazole ring, however, is a base, and at pH 7 it exists as a mixture of charged and uncharged forms.

The H$_2$-receptor antagonists differ markedly in chemical structure from the H$_1$-receptor antihistamines. They are also much less basic and much less lipophilic; in fact they are quite polar molecules. Burimamide was used for the original definition and characterisation of H$_2$-receptors [2], but it was not considered to be sufficiently potent for therapeutic use. Metiamide was therefore developed as a more potent compound, which was also orally active [10]; a methyl group was substituted in the ring, and a sulphur atom introduced into the side chain in order to readjust the electronic characteristics of the imidazole ring [11]. Unfortunately, metiamide posed a potential toxicological problem and, for that reason, had to be replaced. Cimetidine was developed by replacing the sulphur atom of the thiourea group by cyanoimino, resulting in a cyanoguanidine [12]. So far as H$_2$-receptors are concerned, these groups appear to be isosteric [13].

Since the discovery of these drugs, other structural analogues have been mentioned in the patent literature, both from our own work and from work by others. Two new drugs, recently announced by other companies, are ranitidine [14] and ICI-125211 [15], both of which are claimed to be more potent than cimetidine (Fig. 3). They possess an obvious structural resemblance in the side chain, but it is of interest that they are not imidazole derivatives, although they do possess aromatic heterocyclic rings with basic substituents. Both compounds are stronger bases (higher pK$_a$) than is the imidazole ring of cimetidine. The above antagonists are summarised by the general formula in Figure 3. It should be appreciated, however, that this formula does not represent all the possibilities for defining the chemistry of an H$_2$-receptor histamine antagonist.

Selective agonists

The differentiation into 2 types of receptor is also supported by studies with agonists, which show relative selectivity. This is demonstrated very clearly by the effects of methyl substituents in the imidazole ring of histamine. Methyl substitution reduces potency relative to histamine [2], but in 4-methylhistamine (also known as 5-methylhistamine), H$_1$-receptor potency (measured in vitro as a stimulant of contractions of the guinea-pig ileum) is reduced by 500-fold, whereas H$_2$-receptor potency (determined in vitro as a stimulant of the rate of beating of the guinea-pig atrium, or in vivo as a stimulant of gastric acid secretion in the anaesthetised rat) is only reduced to 40% of histamine; thus, 4-methylhistamine is relatively specific as an H$_2$-receptor agonist. Conversely, 2-methylhistamine shows relative specificity for H$_1$-receptors. However, the degree of separation is less than for 4-methylhistamine; 2-methylhistamine has about 16% of the potency of histamine as an H$_1$-receptor agonist, and 2-4% at H$_2$-receptors.

These compounds have been very useful as tools for studying the pharmacology of histamine receptors. However, more specific compounds are available (Figs. 4 and 5).

Relatively selective H_1-agonists are heterocyclic analogues (Fig. 4). They retain the ring-nitrogen atom adjacent to the side chain, as in histamine, but do not possess the tautomeric NH, viz. 2-pyridylethylamine and 2-thiazolylethylamine [16]. The N-methyl derivative of 2-pyridylethylamine is available for human use and has the generic name betahistine (see, for example, [17]). There is a very good separation between H_1- and H_2-receptor activities of these compounds but there is still some residual H_2-receptor activity; this is especially evident on the guinea-pig atrium preparation. However, 2-pyridylethylamine and betahistine are only partial agonists on the guinea-pig atrium; compared with histamine, they do not achieve greater than 40-50% of the maximal response. Therefore, these compounds, although less active than 2-methylhistamine, are effectively more selective.

Name	Structure	H_1	H_2		
		G.P. ileum	G.P. atrium	Rat G.S.	Rat uterus
Histamine		100	100	100	100
2-methylhistamine	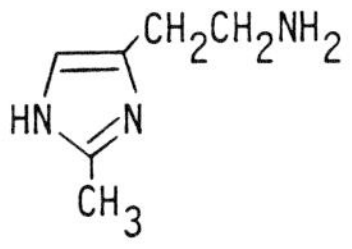	16.5 (15.1-18.1)	4.4 (4.1-4.8)	2.0	2.1
2-pyridylethylamine	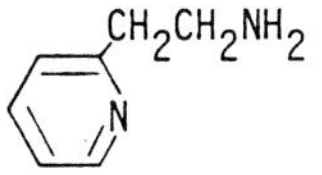	5.6 (5.0-6.3)	[2.5] 50% max.	∼ 0.2	< 0.05 20% max.
Betahistine	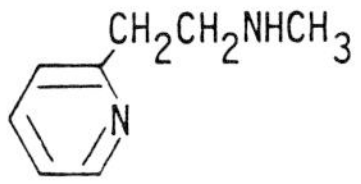	8.0 (7.2-8.8)	[1.5] 40% max.	∼ 0.2	
2-thiazolylethylamine	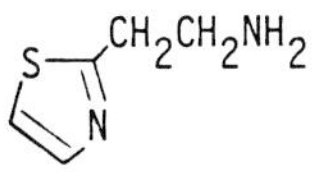	26 (20-32)	2.2 (2.0-2.5)	∼ 0.3	0.34 50% max.

Fig. 4. *Relatively selective H_1-receptor agonists (activities relative to histamine = 100, with 95% confidence limits given in parentheses). Activities determined by R.C. Blakemore and M.E. Parsons (Smith Kline & French Research Ltd.) on the following tissues: G.P. ileum (tested for stimulating contractions of the isolated guinea-pig ileum in the presence of atropine as described in [16]), G.P. atrium (tested for stimulation of rate in the spontaneously-beating isolated guinea-pig right atrium in the presence of propranolol as described in [19]), Rat G.S. (tested by rapid intravenous injection for stimulation of gastric acid secretion in the atropinised and vagotomised anaesthetised rat as described in [16]), and Rat uterus (tested for inhibition of electrically-evoked contractions of the isolated rat uterus in the presence of propranolol as described in [19]).*

Name	Structure	H$_1$	H$_2$			Ref.
		G.P. ileum	G.P. atrium	Rat G.S.	Rat uterus	
Histamine		100	100	100	100	
4(5)-methylhistamine	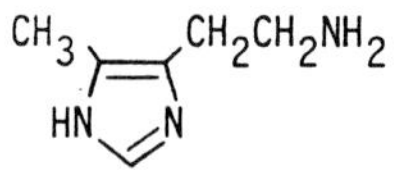 CH$_3$—CH$_2$CH$_2$NH$_2$ / HN—N	0.23	43	39	25	[2]
Betazole	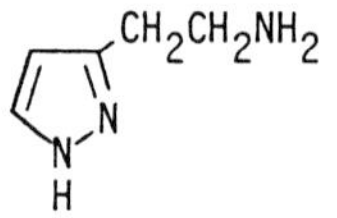 CH$_2$CH$_2$NH$_2$ / N–N / H	0.12	2.1	~0.5	0.11	
Dimaprit	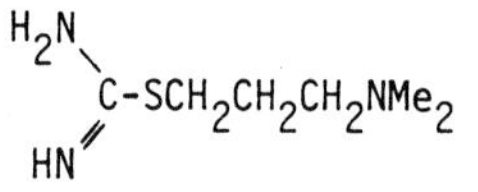 H$_2$N\C–SCH$_2$CH$_2$CH$_2$NMe$_2$ / HN⁄	< 10^{-4}	71	20	17	[19]
Impromidine	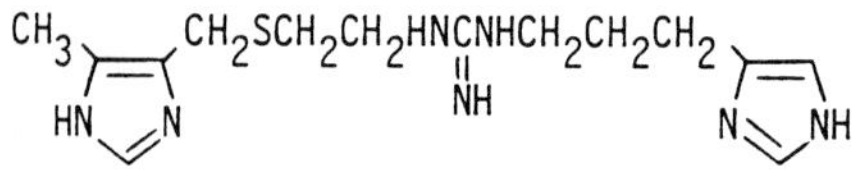 CH$_3$—CH$_2$SCH$_2$CH$_2$HNCNHCH$_2$CH$_2$CH$_2$ / HN—N ‖NH N—NH	< 10^{-3}	4,800	1,680	930 80% max.	[21]

Fig. 5.   *Relatively selective H$_2$-receptor agonists (activities relative to histamine = 100; see references for confidence limits). Activities determined by Blakemore and Parsons: see legend to Figure 4 for further details.*

Relatively selective H$_2$-agonists are shown in Figure 5. Betazole, which is the pyrazole analogue of histamine, is a very weak agonist, but it shows some selectivity towards H$_2$-receptors and has been widely-used clinically for over 20 years as a diagnostic agent for investigating gastric acid secretory capacity, expecially in North America (see, for example, [18]). Betazole is much less active than, and not as selective as, 4-methylhistamine. Of particular interest are the other 2 agonists shown in Figure 5, dimaprit and impromidine, which have a less obvious structural similarity to histamine.

Dimaprit, in which isothiourea replaces imidazole, is remarkably specific for H$_2$-receptors [19]. Its potency varies in comparison with histamine (71% on the guinea-pig isolated atrium, for example, and approximately 17-20% on the rat tissue systems). In vivo as a secretagogue in the anaesthetised cat, it is several times more potent than histamine. Dimaprit has no detectable activity at H$_1$-receptors. It is

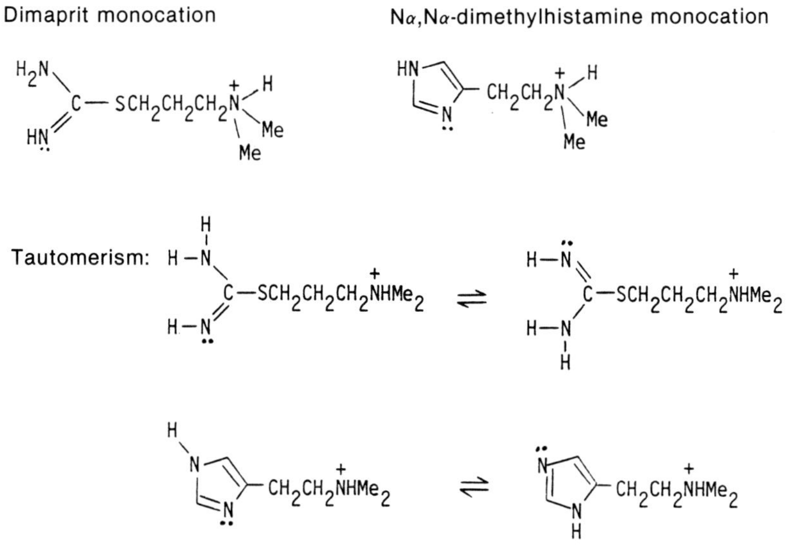

Dimaprit monocation | Nα,Nα-dimethylhistamine monocation

Tautomerism:

Fig. 6. Comparison of dimaprit and Nα,Nα-dimethylhistamine. The isothiourea group in dimaprit appears to function like imidazole in histamine. Both compounds can form monocations having side chain ⁺NH. Isothiourea and imidazole have N-H and N:, are planar, have 6π-electrons, and are tautomeric amidines.

named from the structure, di-methyl-amino-propyl-iso-thiourea. It forms a dihydrochloride salt and has 2 basic centres, the amino group and the isothiourea group. It may be compared with Nα,Nα-dimethylhistamine, the active form of which is considered to be the monocation as shown in Figure 6. Dimaprit can also form an analogous monocation, to the extent of about 5% at pH 7.4. Like dimethylhistamine, dimaprit possesses a side chain and terminal ⁺NH in this form, so that the isothiourea group appears to simulate imidazole. Like imidazole, isothiourea is a 6π-electron planar group which has the NH and N tautomeric amidine system [20]. One main difference from histamine is that the side chain of dimaprit has an extra CH_2 group.

The most remarkable of the selective agonists is impromidine; it is a complex structure, being a basic guanidine with 2 imidazole groups; half of the molecule has the same structural unit as in cimetidine. Impromidine does not stimulate H_1-receptors, and it is very much more potent than is histamine at H_2-receptors [21]. On the isolated guinea-pig atrium, impromidine is 48 times more potent than histamine. In the rat, impromidine is 17 times more potent as an inhibitor of evoked contractions of the uterus in vitro. However, on the uterus it only reaches 80% of the maximal effect of histamine, indicating that it is only a partial agonist, albeit a very potent one. This is the first compound that has been shown to be more potent than histamine on in vitro tissues.

Figure 7 shows structure activity comparisons between impromidine and some partial structures. SK&F-91486 (imidazolyl-propyl-guanidine) is a guanidine

Name	Structure	H$_2$-activity* Guinea-pig atrium
SK&F-91486	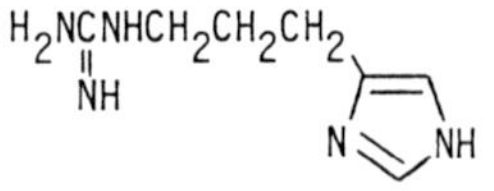 H$_2$NCNHCH$_2$CH$_2$CH$_2$ ‖ NH	Partial agonist 0.04 × histamine (31 ± 3% max.) pA$_2$ = 4.65
SK&F-92408	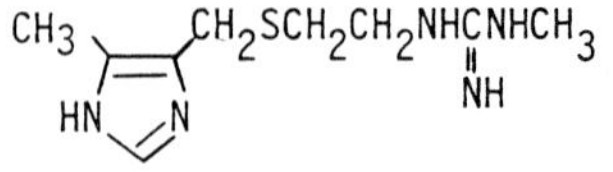 CH$_3$ ... CH$_2$SCH$_2$CH$_2$NHCNHCH$_3$ HN N ‖ NH	Weak antagonist pA$_2$ = 4.80
Impromidine	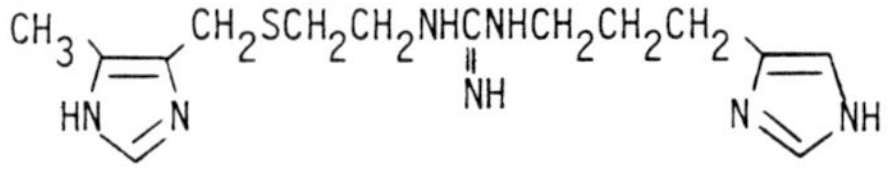 CH$_3$ ... CH$_2$SCH$_2$CH$_2$NHCNHCH$_2$CH$_2$CH$_2$ HN N ‖ NH	Potent agonist 48 × histamine

Fig. 7.   Impromidine and related guanidines. *In vitro in the presence of propranolol [21].

homologue of histamine, and was actually one of the important lead compounds in the development of the H$_2$-antagonists. It is a weak partial agonist [22], having about 4% of the potency of histamine as a stimulant of the isolated guinea-pig atrium but only reaching 30% of the maximal response. When tested as an antagonist of histamine it had a pA$_2$ of 4.65 (about 4% of the potency of cimetidine). Thus, SK&F-91486 has some affinity but low efficacy at H$_2$-receptors. SK&F-92408 is the guanidine analogue of cimetidine; it is not a partial agonist but a weak H$_2$-receptor antagonist of histamine [13], and on the isolated guinea-pig atrium it had a pA$_2$ of 4.8, which is about 5% of the activity of cimetidine. SK&F-92408 shows no stimulation and therefore has no efficacy at H$_2$-receptors, but it does have some affinity. Yet, for imidazolyl-propyl-guanidine, the addition of a group associated only with affinity (i.e. binding ability) in antagonist structures provides a remarkable 1,000-fold increase in stimulant activity. Not only has affinity increased, but so has efficacy, and this result must surely be telling us something about the way substances interact with receptors. The efficacy of impromidine must be less than that of histamine, however, since it is only a partial agonist on the isolated rat uterus. This means that the high potency is due to increased affinity for H$_2$-receptors. Thus it appears that the imidazolyl propyl guanidine group confers efficacy, and must resemble histamine at the receptor even though the side chain is longer, having 3 CH$_2$ groups whereas histamine has 2; the other side chain appears only to confer affinity.

Inactive substances as chemical controls

In addition to antagonists and agonists, a third category may be recognised: inactive compounds which, if they possess suitable chemistry, can be very useful to pharmacologists as controls. All drugs have properties in addition to their main pharmacological actions. Selective agonists and antagonists are valuable tools in the hands of pharmacologists for investigating the mechanism of histamine action in terms of histamine receptors, but sometimes it is not possible to construct adequate dose-

H_1/H_2	Active agent	Control	H_1	H_2	
			G.P. ileum	G.P. atrium	Rat G.S.
H_1 H_2	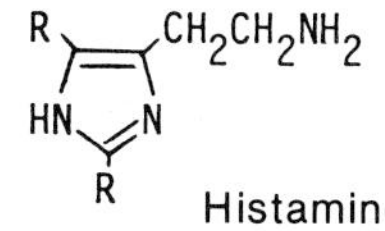 Histamine 2-MeH, 4-MeH	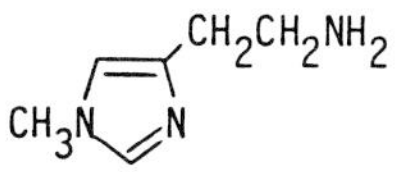 Tele-methyl-histamine	0.42	< 0.1	< 0.01
H_1	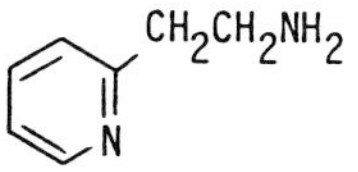 2-pyridyl-ethylamine	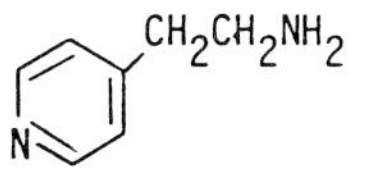 4-pyridyl-ethylamine	< 0.001	< 0.01	~ 0.4
H_2	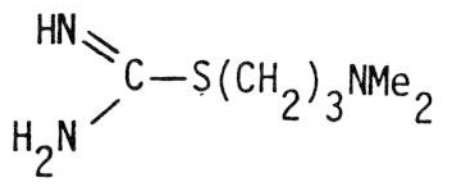 Dimaprit	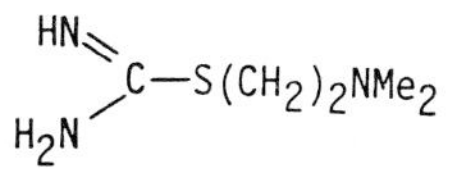 SK&F-91487 (nordimaprit)	< 0.01	<0.1	<0.1
H_2	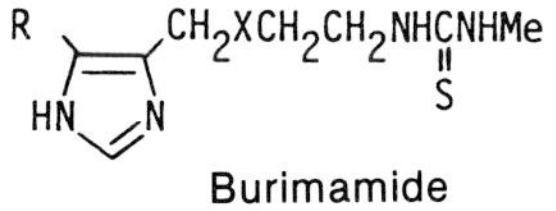 Burimamide Metiamide	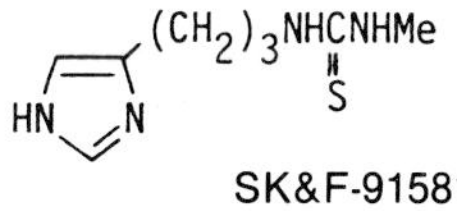 SK&F-91581 (norburimamide)	pA$_2$ < 4	pA$_2$ 3.9	-ve 250 μmol/kg

Fig. 8. Compounds for use as chemical controls (activities relative to histamine = 100). Activities determined by Blakemore and Parsons: see legend to Figure 4 for further details.

response relationships, and sometimes there may be apparent anomalies. Under these circumstances, a much less active compound which has many similar chemical properties but lacks the special chemistry needed for receptor interaction can be most valuable as a chemical control.

Convenient examples of chemical control substances are shown in Figure 8: tele-methylhistamine, which has some residual activity but is inactive at H_2-receptors and can be used for comparison with histamine itself or with 2- or 4-methyl-histamines; 4-pyridylethylamine, which has no H_1-receptor activity and may be used for comparison with 2-pyridylethylamine as an H_1-agonist; SK&F-91487 (nordima-prit), the lower homologue of dimaprit, which is inactive [20] and serves as a control for dimaprit when used as an H_2-receptor agonist; and SK&F-91581 (norburima-mide), which is the lower homologue of burimamide and is at least 100 times less potent than cimetidine or metiamide as a histamine antagonist at H_2-receptors.

References

1. Ash, A.S.F. and Schild, H.O. (1966): Receptors mediating some actions of histamine. *Br. J. Pharmacol. Chemother. 27*, 427-439.
2. Black, J.W., Duncan, W.A.M., Durant, G.J., Ganellin, C.R. and Parsons, M.E. (1972): Definition and antagonism of histamine H_2-receptors. *Nature (London) 236*, 385-390.
3. Rekker, R.F., Nauta, W.T., Bultsma, T. and Waringa, C.G. (1975): Integrated QSAR of H_1-receptor antagonists. *Eur. J. Med. Chem. 10*, 557-562.
4. Marshall, P.B. (1955): Some chemical and physical properties associated with histamine antagonism. *Br. J. Pharmacol. 10*, 270-278.
5. Ison, R.R., Franks, F.M. and Soh, K.S. (1973): The binding of conformationally re-stricted antihistamines to histamine receptors. *J. Pharm. Pharmacol. 25*, 887-894.
6. Van den Brink, F.G. and Lien, E.J. (1977): pD_2, pA_2 and pD_2' values of a series of compounds in a histaminic and a cholinergic system. *Eur. J. Pharmacol. 44*, 251-270.
7. Roth, F.E. and Govier, W.M. (1958): Comparative pharmacology of chlorpheniramine (chlortrimeton) and its optical isomers. *J. Pharm. Exp. Therap. 124*, 347-349.
8. Chang, R.S.L., Tran, V.T. and Snyder, S.H. (1979): Heterogeneity of histamine H_1-receptors: species variations in [^{3}H] mepyramine binding of brain membranes. *J. Neurochem. 32*, 1653-1663.
9. Hill, S.J., Emson, P.C. and Young, J.M. (1978): The binding of [^{3}H] mepyramine to his-tamine H_1-receptors in guinea-pig brain. *J. Neurochem. 31*, 997-1004.
10. Black, J.W., Duncan, W.A.M., Emmett, J.C., Ganellin, C.R., Hesselbo, T., Parsons, M.E. and Wyllie, J.H. (1973): Metiamide — an orally active histamine H_2-receptor an-tagonist. *Agents Actions 3*, 133-137.
11. Black, J.W., Durant, G.J., Emmett, J.C. and Ganellin, C.R. (1973): Sulphur-methylene isosterism in the development of metiamide, a new histamine H_2-receptor antagonist. *Na-ture (London) 248*, 65-67.
12. Brimblecombe, R.W., Duncan, W.A.M., Durant, G.J., Emmett, J.C., Ganellin, C.R. and Parsons, M.E. (1975): Cimetidine — a nonthiourea H_2-receptor antagonist. *J. Int. Med. Res. 3*, 86-92.
13. Durant, G.J., Emmett, J.D., Ganellin, C.R., Miles, P.D., Parsons, M.E., Prain, H.D. and White, G.R. (1977): Cyanoguanidine-thiourea equivalence in the development of the histamine H_2-receptor antagonist, cimetidine. *J. Med. Chem. 20*, 901-906.
14. Bradshaw, J., Brittain, R.T., Clitherow, J.W., Daly, M.J., Jack, D., Price, B.J. and Sta-bles, R. (1979): AH 19065: a new potent selective histamine H_2-receptor antagonist. *Br. J. Pharmacol. 66*, P464.
15. Yellin, T.O., Buck, S.H., Gilman, D.J., Jones, D.F. and Wardleworth, J.M. (1979): A potent new antisecretory drug on histamine H_2-receptors. *Pharmacologist 21*, A635.

16. Durant, G.J., Ganellin, C.R. and Parsons, M.E. (1975): Chemical differentiation of histamine H_1- and H_2-receptor agonists. *J. Med. Chem. 18*, 905-909.
17. Seipel, J.H. and Floam, J.E. (1975): Rheoencephalographic and other studies of betahistine in humans. I. The cerebral and peripheral circulatory effects of single doses in normal subjects. *J. Clin. Pharmacol. 15*, 144-154.
18. Breuer, R.I. and Kirsner, J.B. (1967): Present status of histalog gastric analysis in man. *Ann. N.Y. Acad. Sci. 140*, 882-895.
19. Parsons, M.E., Owen, D.A.A., Ganellin, C.R. and Durant, G.J. (1977): Dimaprit — [S-[3-(N,N-dimethylamino)propyl]isothiourea] — A highly specific histamine H_2-receptor agonist. Part 1. Pharmacology. *Agents Actions 7*, 31-37.
20. Durant, G.J., Ganellin, C.R. and Parsons, M.E. (1977): Dimaprit — [S-[3-(N,N-dimethylamino)propyl]isothiourea] — A highly specific histamine H_2-receptor agonist. Part 2. Structure-activity considerations. *Agents Actions 7*, 39-43.
21. Durant, G.J., Duncan, W.A.M., Ganellin, C.R., Parsons, M.E., Blakemore, R.C. and Rasmussen, A.C. (1978): Impromidine (SK&F 92676) is a very potent and specific agonist for histamine H_2-receptors. *Nature (London) 276*, 403-405.
22. Parsons, M.E., Blakemore, R.C., Durant, G.J., Ganellin, C.R. and Rasmussen, A.C. (1975): 3[4(5)-Imidazolyl]propylguanidine (SK&F 91486) — A partial agonist at histamine H_2 receptors. *Agents Actions 5*, 464.

Discussion

Bertaccini: As a pharmacologist, I greatly appreciated Dr. Ganellin's presentation of the relative potencies of the new compounds compared with the old ones, acting as agonists and antagonists of the H_2-receptors.

We have our own data to add to those of other workers, concerning different ratios of activity between histamine and various H_2-agonists in different preparations in which there are known to be classical H_2-receptors. What is Dr. Ganellin's opinion of the reason for these different ratios of activity? Is it possible that there are different H_2-receptor subtypes, or is it a question only of different experimental conditions and different test systems?

Ganellin: This is a very fundamental question — it is fundamental to consider the pharmacological classification of receptors. It is well-known in the adrenergic system, too, that there are differences in the ratios of agonist activity. There must be variations in affinity and efficacy, whatever those may mean (since they cannot easily be measured), and in the way in which the system responds. It has been suggested that activity may be affected by the density of receptors or the way in which the system responds to stimulation. Activity is measured relative to the natural transmitter substance, so the differences that occur have also to be explained relative to histamine, even if it is presumed that the receptors are equally sensitive to histamine. This is a fascinating question to which I have no real answer. On present evidence, however, I would say that it seems to be premature to invoke H_2-receptor subtypes.

Some speculations on the physiological control of gastric secretion

M.E. Parsons
The Research Institute, Smith Kline & French Laboratories, Welwyn Garden City, United Kingdom

Introduction

It is a well-known fact that, for many years, if one wanted to start a passionate argument among a group of gastroenterologists, all one needed to do was to state categorically that histamine has a key role in the normal physiological control of gastric acid secretion. The present paper briefly describes the background to this controversy and describes some recent results which throw light on the subject.

It was at the turn of this century when Edkins proposed his gastrin hypothesis [1]. He had found that extracts of the pyloric mucosa contained a gastric secretory stimulant and he concluded that this substance was released into the blood stream during digestion and activated the acid secretory cells of the fundic mucosa. Some 15 years later it was demonstrated that histamine was a potent stimulant of acid secretion [2] and, since histamine was found in the pyloric mucosa, the gastrin hypothesis fell into disrepute.

Observations such as those on the release of histamine into gastric juice during vagal stimulation [3] and histamine turnover studies [4] culminated in the common mediator hypothesis, championed by Code [5, 6]. Simply stated, the hypothesis says that secretagogues, other than histamine itself, do not act directly on the parietal cell, but via the release of endogenous histamine.

With the extraction, purification and then synthesis of gastrin [7], the pendulum swung in the other direction, so much so that an article was published in *Gastroenterology* entitled 'Control of gastric secretion: no room for histamine?' [8], suggesting that histamine was a pharmacological but not a physiological stimulant of gastric acid secretion.

The advent of the histamine H$_2$-receptor antagonists

What was hampering investigation of the relationship of histamine to the newly-identified hormone gastrin was the lack of a compound which antagonised the acid secretory stimulant effect of histamine. With the discovery that this effect was mediated via a second type of histamine receptor, the H$_2$-receptor, and the development of specific antagonists such as cimetidine [9], powerful new tools became available to gastroenterologists.

It has now been clearly demonstrated that H$_2$-antagonists can block histamine-stimulated gastric acid secretion in all species studied, including man [10]. Of perhaps greater significance is the fact that the secretory response to gastrin is equally

Table.   Inhibition of gastric acid secretion by cimetidine.

Preparation		Stimulant	Intravenous ED_{50} (μM/kg)
Rat:	lumen-perfused	Histamine	1.37
	stomach	Pentagastrin	1.40
Cat:	lumen-perfused	Histamine	0.85
	stomach	Pentagastrin	1.45
Dog:	Heidenhain	Histamine	1.70
	pouch	Pentagastrin	2.00

effectively blocked by histamine H_2-receptor antagonists. The Table shows the doses required to produce 50% inhibition of maximal acid secretion (ED_{50}) for cimetidine against histamine and pentagastrin in 3 different animal preparations. The figures are very similar for these 2 secretagogues, a result which closely links pentagastrin to histamine.

It has also been demonstrated that H_2-antagonists can inhibit the action of all other secretory stimulants, including stable choline esters, 2-deoxyglucose, insulin and food. Clearly, if it is accepted that cimetidine is a specific antagonist for histamine H_2-receptors (and a large volume of evidence both on gastric and non-gastric tissues has indicated that this is the case), then histamine certainly has a fundamental role to play in the normal physiological control of gastric acid secretion.

However, what exactly is the nature of this role? On the face of it, the ability of H_2-antagonists to inhibit the acid secretory stimulant effect of all types of secretagogues could be seen as providing convincing evidence in support of Code's common mediator hypothesis. Inherent in this hypothesis is the concept that histamine is an obligatory step between the interaction of gastrin and acetylcholine with their receptors and the production of acid.

In vitro studies

To gain a clearer view of the receptors involved, although not necessarily of the normal physiological control of secretion, necessitates moving away from in vivo studies, which are complicated by modulating influences such as vagal and local cholinergic tone and endogenous gastrin release.

An in vitro lumen-perfused whole rat stomach preparation which responds in a dose-related manner to a variety of gastric secretagogues has been developed at Smith Kline & French [11, 12]. Our studies have shown that the H_2-antagonist metiamide can inhibit histamine-stimulated acid secretion in vitro. By using a range of antagonist concentrations, a pA_2 value for metiamide was established which did not differ significantly from that obtained on non-gastric tissues containing H_2-receptors, such as the guinea-pig atrium and rat uterus. The ability of H_2-antagonists to inhibit histamine-stimulated acid secretion in vitro has also been reported by other workers using the isolated kitten mucosa [13] and the isolated whole mouse stomach [14].

In the isolated rat stomach, metiamide has also been shown to inhibit acid secretion stimulated by gastrin at the same concentrations as those effective against histamine [12]. However, as found in vivo, although the dose-response curves are shifted to the right the maximum response is depressed. An entirely satisfactory explanation for this result has yet to be found, but it is not incompatible with a 2-step model in which gastrin stimulates secretion via a release of histamine. The result certainly supports the hypothesis that gastrin acts, at least in part, via a histaminergic pathway.

The effect of the third of the triad of gastric secretory stimulants, acetylcholine, is resistant to blockade by H_2-antagonists [12]. Concentrations of metiamide some 1,000 times those effective against histamine and gastrin failed to inhibit acetylcholine-stimulated secretion. This result agrees well with studies carried out on the isolated kitten mucosa [13]. Rangachari, using the isolated primate gastric mucosa, has also confirmed that the secretory responses to histamine and pentagastrin are inhibited by metiamide, but that those to acetylcholine are resistant [15].

Taken overall, these results suggest that there exist both histamine H_2 and acetylcholine receptors on the gastric mucosa, but that gastrin acts indirectly via endogenous histamine.

As one simplifies the test preparation still further, the situation ironically becomes more complicated. For example, Berglindh and coworkers have developed a technique for isolating whole gastric glands from the rabbit mucosa [16]. Gastric acid secretion cannot be measured directly in this preparation, but the rate of oxygen consumption and the accumulation of the weak base aminophenazone (aminopyrine) are considered to reflect parietal cell function. This preparation responds to histamine and carbachol, and the response to the former is blocked by H_2-antagonists whereas that to carbachol is only inhibited by atropine. Of greater significance is the fact that the preparation fails to respond to pentagastrin. The authors suggested that this result could be interpreted as indicating that the gastrin receptors on the glands had been destroyed during the separation procedures. Alternatively, the receptors were intact but not located on the parietal cell membranes. The latter interpretation would be seen as favouring the concept that gastrin acts by liberating histamine but, in this preparation, in insufficient quantity to stimulate parietal cell function.

Isolated parietal cell studies

Recently a number of studies have been carried out using isolated parietal cell preparations of varying degrees of purity from a variety of mammalian species. Again oxygen uptake and aminophenazone (aminopyrine) accumulation are taken to reflect changes in H^+ secretion. Soll, using canine parietal cells, has shown that histamine, gastrin and carbachol stimulate oxygen uptake [17]. However, the responses to gastrin and to histamine alone are small. Responses to histamine are markedly potentiated by the addition of the phosphodiesterase inhibitor isobutyl methyl xanthine. The response to gastrin was not potentiated by isobutyl methyl xanthine. Stimulation of oxygen consumption by gastrin or pentagastrin has been confirmed by other workers using isolated rat parietal cells [18, 19] and parietal cells from the guinea-pig [20]. These results are difficult to reconcile with those of Berglindh who, as noted previously, failed to stimulate oxygen consumption in isolated gastric glands with pentagastrin. Interestingly, Albinus reported the failure of histamine and carbachol to increase oxygen uptake in guinea-pig parietal cell preparations [20]. These differences in results may relate to the species used, the techniques employed for the isolation of the cells and the purity of the cell preparations. Clearly, further work is necessary.

Comprehensive antagonist studies were also carried out by Soll, who found that metiamide could inhibit the response to histamine but not those to gastrin and carbachol, whereas atropine inhibited the carbachol-stimulated response but did not affect the responses to gastrin and histamine [17]. The response to gastrin was not inhibited by either an H_2-antagonist or an anticholinergic. From these results, he concluded that separate receptors exist on the parietal cell for the 3 major secretagogues and that gastrin does not act via a histaminergic pathway.

Binding studies

The existence of separate receptors would be given further confirmation by suitable specific binding studies. Two groups of workers, Lewin et al. in France [21] and Speir et al. in the United States [22], the former using tritiated gastrin and the latter using iodinated gastrin, have reported the presence of gastrin binding sites, presumed to be the gastrin receptor, in the rat gastric mucosa. Similarly, at a recent meeting in Montpellier, Lewin reported on the binding of C^{14}-histamine to H_2-receptors on guinea-pig gastric cells [23]. Finally, in 1978 Rosenfeld and coworkers described binding studies which provided evidence for the existence of specific muscarinic cholinergic receptors on the gastric mucosa [24]. These studies require confirmation and extension, but support the hypothesis of separate receptors for the 3 major secretagogues on the parietal cell.

Indirect studies

Mention must be made of other more indirect studies designed to increase our understanding of the control of gastric secretion.

Extra-cellular calcium appears to be an important factor in the control of secretagogue-induced acid secretion. It has been shown that removal of calcium from both the serosal and mucosal bathing fluids in the isolated perfused rat stomach preparation leads to a potentiation of the response to histamine [25]. If gastrin acts via release of endogenous histamine, then one might have expected the response to this secretagogue to be affected by calcium lack in the same way as histamine; in fact, however, removal of calcium ions from the bathing fluids had no significant effect on the response to gastrin [25]. In contrast, the response to acetylcholine is markedly inhibited by calcium lack, an effect which can be readily reversed by replacement of the calcium ions.

Therefore, although these results are interesting in terms of the light they throw on the underlying process of stimulus-secretion coupling, they do not support the hypothesis that the secretagogues act via a single pathway.

One of the cornerstones of Code's common mediator hypothesis was studies carried out on histamine turnover in the gastric mucosa. Kahlson's original observation that gastrin injection and feeding elevates mucosal histidine decarboxylase activity [4] has been confirmed many times. Cholinergic stimulants have also been reported to influence the activity of the enzyme, but whether this is a direct effect or an indirect one via release of endogenous gastrin has yet to be determined. In any case, nearly all the studies have been carried out in the rat and need extending to other species in which there is not even general agreement about the presence of a specific histidine decarboxylase in the gastric mucosa.

A large number of studies have been carried out to examine the relationship between gastric secretagogues and cyclic AMP in the gastric mucosa, and conflicting results have often been reported. However, most workers agree that histamine-stimulated acid secretion is accompanied by an increase in mucosal cyclic AMP content and in adenylate cyclase activity.

Studies carried out by Scholes and coworkers, using isolated gastric mucosal cells from canine gastric mucosa, showed that histamine caused a dose-dependent increase in cyclic AMP concentration, and that this effect of histamine was competitively antagonised by the H_2-antagonist metiamide [26]. The calculated pA_2 value for metiamide was very close to that reported on other non-gastric tissues, such as the guinea-pig atrium and rat uterus. Further studies with relatively specific H_1- and H_2-agonists, and the inactivity of typical H_1-antagonists such as mepyramine, led to the conclusion that the activation of adenylate cyclase by histamine is mediated via H_2-receptors.

If gastrin acts at least in part via release of endogenous histamine, then it might be expected to affect adenylate cyclase activity. Marked disagreement exists between various groups of workers regarding this question. In general, in vivo studies provide evidence supporting the concept of a gastrin-sensitive adenylate cyclase system in the gastric mucosa, but this is less certain in vitro. Recently, however, Becker and Ruoff, using human fundic mucosal tissue, identified such a system [27]. Histamine also activated adenylate cyclase in this preparation, an effect antagonised by cimetidine, but the H_2-antagonist was ineffective against pentagastrin-activated adenylate cyclase. This suggests that the 2 secretagogues acted via 2 distinct receptors.

Conclusions

If the balance of the in vitro evidence is in favour of 2 distinct receptors for histamine and acetylcholine and probably a third for gastrin, how can we account for the ability of a specific histamine H_2-receptor antagonist such as cimetidine to block all forms of secretagogue-induced secretion in vivo? Grossman and Konturek proposed a hypothesis involving receptor interaction [28]. In essence this meant that blockade of one receptor, say the H_2-receptor by metiamide, changed the properties of one or both of the other receptors, so that stimulation by gastrin or acetylcholine was less effective. However, Soll's studies on isolated parietal cell showed that the antagonists were specific for their appropriate receptors, and this argues against an interaction hypothesis. On the other hand, Soll has demonstrated potentiating interactions between the agonists [29]. Although there were some shortcomings in these studies, the fact that all of the potentiating interactions involve histamine (that is histamine plus gastrin, histamine plus carbachol and histamine plus gastrin plus carbachol) makes, perhaps, the ability of H_2-antagonists to inhibit all forms of acid secretion understandable, since these compounds would remove the potentiating effect of histamine. Many questions remain to be answered. For example, if gastrin has a direct action on acid secretion as well as being potentiated by histamine, why can its effect be totally abolished in vivo by an H_2-antagonist? Hopefully, questions of this type will be answered over the coming years.

References

1. Edkins, J.S. (1905): On the chemical mechanism of gastric secretion. *Proc. R. Soc. (London) Ser. B. Biol. Sci. 76,* 376.
2. Popielski, L. (1920): β-imidazolylathylamine und die Organextrakte; β-imidazolylathylamin als mächtiger Erreger der Magendrüsen. *Pflüg. Arch. Eur. J. Physiol. 178,* 214-226.
3. McIntosh, F.C. (1938): Histamine is a normal stimulant of gastric secretion. *Q. J. Exp. Physiol. 28,* 87-98.
4. Kahlson, G., Rosengren, E., Svahn, D. and Thunberg, R. (1964): Mobilization and formation of histamine in the gastric mucosa as related to acid secretion. *J. Physiol. (London) 174,* 400-416.
5. Code, C.F. (1956): Histamine and gastric secretion. In: *Histamine,* p. 189-219. Editors: G.E.W. Wolstenholme and C.M. O'Connor. Churchill, London.
6. Code, C.F. (1965): Histamine and gastric secretion: a later look, 1955-1965. *Fed. Proc. 24,* 1311-1333.
7. Gregory, R.A. and Tracy, H.J. (1961): The preparation and properties of gastrin. *J. Physiol. (London) 156,* 523-543.
8. Johnson, L.R. (1971): Control of gastric secretion: no room for histamine? *Gastroenterology 61,* 106-118.
9. Brimblecombe, R.W., Duncan, W.A.M., Durant, G.J., Emmett, J.C., Ganellin, C.R. and Parsons, M.E. (1975): Cimetidine — a non-thiourea H_2-receptor antagonist. *J. Int. Med. Res. 3,* 86-92.
10. Brimblecombe, R.W. and Parsons, M.E. (1977): Histamine H_2-receptor antagonists. In: *Pharmacological and biochemical properties of drug substances,* pp. 329-352. Editor: M.E. Goldberg. American Pharmaceutical Association, Washington.
11. Bunce, K.T. and Parsons, M.E. (1976): A quantitative study of metiamide, a histamine H_2-receptor antagonist, on the isolated whole rat stomach. *J. Physiol. (London) 258,* 453-465.
12. Bunce, K.T., Parsons, M.E. and Rollings, N.A. (1976): The effect of metiamide on acid secretion stimulated by gastrin, acetylcholine and dibutyryl cyclic adenosine $3',5'$ monophosphate in the isolated whole stomach of the rat. *Br. J. Pharmacol. 58,* 149-156.
13. Tepperman, B.L., Schofield, B. and Tepperman, F.S. (1975): Effect of metiamide on acid secretion from isolated kitten fundic mucosa. *Can. J. Physiol. Pharmacol. 53,* 1141-1146.
14. Angus, J.A., Black, J.W. and Stone, M. (1978): Comparative assay of histamine H_2-receptor antagonists using the isolated mouse stomach. *Br. J. Pharmacol. 62,* 445-446P.
15. Rangachari, P.K. (1979): Acid secretion by isolated primate gastric mucosa. *Am. J. Physiol. 236 (6),* E733-777.
16. Berglindh, T. and Obrink, K.T. (1979): Histamine as a physiological stimulant of gastric parietal cells. In: *Histamine receptors,* pp. 35-56. Editor: T.O. Yellin. SP Medical and Scientific Books, New York-London.
17. Soll, A. (1978): The action of secretagogues on oxygen uptake by isolated mammalian parietal cells. *J. Clin. Invest. 61,* 370-380.
18. Cheret, A.M., Girodet, J. and Lewin, M. (1977): Stimulation of isolated rat parietal cell by gastrin. In: *Hormonal receptors in digestive tract physiology,* p. 405. Editors: S. Bonfils, P. Fromageot and G. Rosselin. Elsevier North Holland, Amsterdam-New York-Oxford.
19. Jennewein, H.M., Herbst, M. and Waldeck, F. (1979): Functional oxygen consumption of isolated rat gastric mucosal cells in comparison to the in vivo function of the rat gastric mucosa. *N.S. Arch. Pharm. 307 Suppl.,* R52.
20. Albinus, M. (1979): Action of gastric secretagogues on the oxygen consumption in isolated gastric mucosal cells of the guinea-pig. *N.S. Arch. Pharm. 307 Suppl.,* R52.
21. Lewin, M., Soumaron, A. and Bonfils, S. (1977): Gastrin receptor sites in rat gastric mucosa. In: *Hormonal receptors in digestive tract physiology,* pp. 379-389. Editors: S.

Bonfils, P. Fromageot and G. Rosselin. Elsevier North Holland, Amsterdam-New York-Oxford.

22. Speir, G.R., Takeuchi, K. and Johnson, L.R. (1979): Binding characteristics and assay standardization of the gastrin receptor in rat gastric mucosa. *Gastroenterology 76,* 1253.

23. Lewin, M., Grelac, F., Cheret, A.M., Rene, E. and Bonfils, S. (1979): Direct evidence for histamine H_2-receptors on isolated guinea-pig gastric cells. In: *Hormonal receptors in digestion and nutrition.* (In press.)

24. Rosenfeld, G.C., Ecknauer, R., Johnson, L.R. and Thompson, W.J. (1978): Purified gastric mucosal parietal cells: demonstration of (^{3}H) QNB binding to cholinergic receptors. *7th International Congress of Pharmacology, Paris,* Abstract 319.

25. Bunce, K.T., Honey, A.C. and Parsons, M.E. (1979): Investigation of the role of extracellular calcium in the control of acid secretion in the isolated whole stomach of the rat. *Br. J. Pharmacol. 67,* 123-131.

26. Scholes, P., Cooper, A., Jones, D., Major, J., Walters, M. and Wilde, C. (1976): Characterization of an adenylate cyclase system sensitive to histamine H_2-receptor excitation in cells from dog gastric mucosa. *Agents Actions 6,* 677-682.

27. Becker, M. and Ruoff, H.J. (1979): Pentagastrin activation of adenylate cyclase in human gastric biopsy specimens. *Experientia 35 (b),* 781-782.

28. Grossman, M.I. and Konturek, S.J. (1974): Inhibition of acid secretion in dog by metiamide, a histamine antagonist acting on H_2-receptors. *Gastroenterology 66,* 517-521.

29. Soll, A. (1978): The interaction of histamine with gastrin and carbamylcholine on oxygen uptake by isolated mammalian parietal cells. *J. Clin. Invest. 61,* 381-389.

Discussion

Milton-Thompson (Gosport): It has been shown in both cat and dog that there is a higher acid response if histamine plus an H_1-antagonist are given than if histamine is given alone. Now, Dr. Parsons has shown that dimaprit also produces a higher response than histamine alone in both cat and dog. Would he care to speculate on the reason for this?

Parsons: Professor Bertaccini could probably also contribute to the answer to this question. Certainly both dimaprit and impromidine, referred to by Dr. Ganellin, produce a higher maximal acid secretory response both in the cat and the dog in in vivo situations. I believe I am correct in saying, Professor Bertaccini, that when you studied these compounds in in vitro systems, the maximum response was the same as that of histamine. That suggests that, in fact, it is probably an effect not on the gastric mucosa but, perhaps, on the vascular system, which then somehow limits — perhaps by limiting the access of histamine to the stomach — its maximal response. This is a phenomenon probably unrelated to the gastric mucosa.

Bertaccini: I completely agree with Dr. Parsons. I can add that, if histamine plus an H_1-antagonist are given in vivo, there is more or less the same response as with the H_2-agonists. Probably, therefore, these H_1-receptors are outside the stomach and can be modified by the action of H_1-antagonists. Thus, histamine can give its own response in the stomach.

Francavilla (Bari): Is cimetidine able to inhibit stimulation of acid secretion by theophylline or caffeine in isolated cells?

Parsons: I am sorry, but I do not know the answer to that question. With stimulation using, for example, dibutyryl cyclic AMP, it is certainly totally resistant to an H_2-antagonist. I have a feeling that the effects of theophylline have been shown to be inhibited by H_2-antagonists.

Bertaccini: How much does Dr. Parsons trust the kind of experiment performed by Soll, in terms of the technique? Is it possible to compare oxygen consumption with real acid secretion if there is more or less the same situation as far as interaction with receptors is concerned?

Parsons: I agree: I think that oxygen consumption is a very inadequate measure. Since Soll has added amidopyrine accumulation — although that also is subject to some criticism — this technique is now improved. I think we have to accept that he is probably measuring at least some part of hydrogen ion concentration, although I accept that even that is open to criticism.

Histamine receptors and gastrointestinal motility: an overview*

G. Bertaccini, C. Scarpignato and G. Coruzzi
Institute of Pharmacology, University of Parma, Parma, Italy

Introduction

There is a noticeable discrepancy between the enormous amount of papers in the recent literature on histamine and gastric secretion and the small number of papers on histamine and gastrointestinal motility.

The discovery of histamine H_2-receptors [1], and of their selective stimulants and inhibitors, represented an important step in the understanding of the physiology of gastric secretion; in some cases, though, this discovery actually contributed in a negative sense to explaining the effects of histamine on gut motility. In fact, several effects of the H_2-receptor blockers were immediately attributed to antagonism at the H_2-receptor level, without any consideration of the possible intrinsic non-specific actions which were found to be present, though in different degrees, with burimamide, metiamide and cimetidine. For this reason, it was suggested that the appropriate use of H_1- and H_2-receptor selective agonists *and* antagonists (at least 2 compounds of different structure for each group) which would respectively mimic or competitively inhibit the actions of histamine would be necessary to clearly establish that an effect of histamine was connected with an interaction amine-receptor [2].

Taking these premises into account, the effects of histamine on the motility of different segments of the gastrointestinal tract and the gallbladder, together with the different types of receptors involved, are shown in Tables I, III, V and VI. Some clinical effects of the commonly-used H_2-antagonists, as well as some nonspecific effects of these drugs on gastrointestinal motility, are shown in Tables II, IV and VII.

Histamine receptors in the lower esophageal sphincter

It is evident from Table I that receptors occurring in the lower esophageal sphincter (LES) are of different types in the various species examined. Moreover, the effect of histamine is rather erratic as we may observe both H_1- and H_2-receptor stimulation causing either LES contraction or relaxation. Species differences and different experimental conditions may explain the discrepancies, but we must also consider that several of the reported experiments were incomplete, with results obtained by using histamine plus only 1 kind of inhibitor, and arbitrarily extrapolated to the

*This work was supported by a grant from the Consiglio Nazionale delle Richerche, Rome, Italy.

Table I. Histamine receptors in the lower esophageal sphincter (LES).

Species	Receptors		Compound(s) used
	H_1	H_2	
Monkey [3]*	↓	↓	histamine
Australian opossum	↓	↓	histamine, H_1-agonists
(in vivo) [4]	(↑) ↓	0	histamine, H_1-agonists
American opossum	↑	↓	histamine, H_1- and H_2-agonists,
(in vitro and in vivo)			metiamide
[5, 6]			
Baboon	↑	0	histamine, H_1-antagonists,
(in vivo) [7]			cimetidine
Guinea-pig	↑	↓	histamine, H_1- and H_2-
(in vitro) [8]			antagonists
Rat	0	0	histamine
(in vitro) [8]			
Man	0	↑	histamine, H_1-antagonists,
(in vivo) [9]			cimetidine
Man		↑	betazole
(in vivo) [10]			
Man	↑ (↓) ?		histamine
(in vitro) [11]			
Man	↓?		histamine
(in vitro) [12]			

*In this and in the following Tables, only the most representative papers are reported.
↑ = contraction; ↓ = relaxation; 0 = no effect; ? = type of receptor not established.

other type of receptor. This was the case, for instance, with human LES, for which evidence of contraction induced by recent selective H_2-receptor agonists is still lacking. It has been reported that the inhibitory effect of histamine on the opossum LES was antagonized by tetrodotoxin [4]; this would suggest a neurally-mediated response independent from activation of H_1- or H_2-receptors. The data available suggest that the effects of histamine in vivo represent the net effect of stimulation of different receptors.

Results obtained with the H_2-inhibitors, which in most experiments have proved to be ineffective (Table II), support the hypothesis that endogenous histamine has no important effect on human LES, while exogenous histamine seems to stimulate human LES through activation of H_2-receptors, contrary to its effect in experimental animals (Table I).

Histamine receptors in the stomach

The effect of histamine on the stomach and its interaction with the different receptors is shown in Table III. It is evident that histamine usually produces contraction of the stomach muscle, an effect elicited predominantly through activation of H_1-receptors. Stimulation of H_2-receptors causes relaxation in the different species, with the exception of dog antrum, which appears to contract. Whereas the kind of receptor involved in relaxation of cat stomach and in contraction of kitten

Table II. Cimetidine and human LESP.

Dose and route of administration	Subjects	Effect
150 mg/hour intravenously [13]	H	(↑↓)
1.6 g/day for 6 weeks by mouth [14]	GER	↑
400 mg by mouth [15]	H	0
100 mg/hour intravenously [16]	H	0
400 mg by mouth [17]	H	↑
1.6 g/day for 8 weeks by mouth [18]	GER	0
4 mg/kg/hour intravenously [9]	H	↓
0.2 mg/kg/minute intravenously [19]	H and GER	0
1.2 g/day for 8 weeks by mouth [20]	GER	0

H = healthy subjects; GER = gastroesophageal reflux; ↑ = increase; ↓ = decrease; 0 = no effect.

Table III. Histamine receptors in the stomach.

Species and tissues	Receptors		Compound(s) used
	H_1	H_2	
Rat stomach (in vivo) [1]	↑	0	histamine, H_1-agonists
Rat stomach (in vitro) [21]	NT	↓	H_2-agonists
Rat pylorus (in vivo) [22]		↑*	histamine, H_1- and H_2- agonists and antagonists
Guinea-pig stomach (in vitro) [23]	↑	0	histamine, mepyramine, cimetidine
Dog antrum (in vitro) [24]	↑	↑	H_1- and H_2-agonists
Cat stomach (in vivo) [25]		↓?	histamine
Kitten and ferret fundus (in vitro) [26]		↑?	histamine
Cow forestomach (in vitro) [27]	↑	↓	histamine, mepyramine, metiamide

NT = not tested; ↑ = contraction; ↓ = relaxation; 0 = no effect; * = possible subtype of the classical receptors; ? = type of receptor not established.

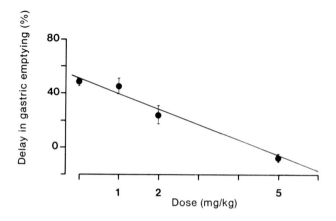

Fig. 1.   Dose-dependent inhibition of the effect of histamine (10 mg/kg) on gastric emptying by chlorpheniramine. The line is the calculated least regression line (r = -0.7646, n = 23, p < 0.001).

and ferret fundus was not established in the corresponding investigations [25, 26], those in the rat pylorus apparently did not belong to the classical histamine receptors, based on the equivocal results obtained with H_1- and H_2-receptor selective agonists and antagonists, and a subtype of histamine receptors has been hypothesized [22].

The problem of gastric emptying, which is strictly connected with histamine action on the stomach, has been thoroughly investigated in the rat [28]. Histamine delayed gastric emptying in a dose-dependent fashion, though high doses had to be used (1-10 mg/kg, administered intraperitoneally). This effect, which was mimicked by 2-aminoethylthiazole (an H_1-agonist), was inhibited, again in a dose-dependent fashion (Fig. 1), by chlorpheniramine (an H_1-antagonist), suggesting an action mediated through excitation of H_1-receptors. Apparently the situation in the monkey is exactly the opposite, since only H_2-receptors (whose stimulation causes an increased gastric emptying) seem to be involved [29]. In man, cimetidine is apparently devoid of any effect on gastric emptying (Table IV).

Table IV.   Histamine H_2-antagonists and human gastric emptying.

Compound	Dose and route of administration	Subjects	Effect
Metiamide [30]	400 mg, by mouth	DU	0
Cimetidine [31]	400 mg, by mouth	DU	0
Cimetidine [16]	100 mg/hour, intravenously	H	0
Cimetidine [32]	400 mg, by mouth	H	0
Cimetidine [33]	2 g/day for 8 weeks, by mouth	DU	0 (liquids)
Cimetidine [34]	2 g/day for 8 weeks, by mouth	DU	↑ (solids)

H = healthy subjects; DU = duodenal ulcer; 0 = no effect; ↑ = increase.

Histamine receptors in the intestine

Histamine contracts the bowel muscle in most species, though with consistent quantitative differences. A synopsis of the effects of histamine in different segments of the gut, together with the different receptors involved in the various experimental animals, is shown in Table V.

Because of the constancy and the reliability of its response to histamine and its complete lack of tachyphylaxis, guinea-pig ileum has been used for decades for the biological assay of the amine. Both an indirect and a more important direct action of histamine have been described: the first is represented by fast unsustained contractions, connected with stimulation of preganglionic sites in the intrinsic nervous system, and is inhibited by hexamethonium bromide, cooling and atropine; the second is represented by a sustained, more constant, atropine-resistant response, and is generally considered to be due to stimulation of histamine H_1-receptors. After 2 basic reports in which the competitive antagonism of mepyramine on the effect of histamine was demonstrated [46, 47], the guinea-pig ileum became the classical tool for the study of H_1-receptor agonists and antagonists.

In addition, there is evidence both for and against the occurrence of H_2-receptors (whose stimulation causes relaxation) in the intestinal muscle. Bareicha and Rocha e Silva were the first to claim that both duodenum and ileum of the guinea-pig contain a certain amount (12.4% and 15.7%, respectively) of true H_2-receptors with relaxant activity [35]. They based their assumption only on the potentiation caused by burimamide on the response of small doses of histamine. Other observations seemed to suggest the occurrence of H_2-receptors in guinea-pig ileum [37, 38, 41];

Table V.   Histamine receptors in the intestine.

Species and tissues	Receptors		Compound(s) used
	H_1	H_2	
Guinea-pig duodenum [35]	↑	↓	histamine, burimamide
Guinea-pig duodenum [36]	↓*		H_1- and H_2-agonists and antagonists
Guinea-pig ileum [37]	↓*		histamine, mepyramine, buri- mamide, 4-methyl histamine
Guinea-pig ileum [35]	↑	↓	histamine, burimamide
Guinea-pig ileum [38]	↑	↓	histamine, metiamide
Guinea-pig ileum [1]	↑	0	histamine
Guinea-pig ileum [39]	↑	0	histamine, tripelennamine
Guinea-pig ileum [40]	↑ ↓*	0	histamine, H_1- and H_2-agonists and antagonists
Guinea-pig ileum [41]	NT ↓*		clonidine, cimetidine
Chicken ileum [42]	↑	↓	histamine, metiamide
Rat ileum [43]	↑	NT	histamine
Guinea-pig tenia coli [43]	↑	NT	histamine, mepyramine
Rabbit ileum [44]	↑	NT	histamine, mepyramine
Rabbit colon [45]	↑	NT	histamine, mepyramine

NT = not tested; ↑ = contraction; ↓ = relaxation; 0 = no effect; * = possible subtype of the classical receptors.

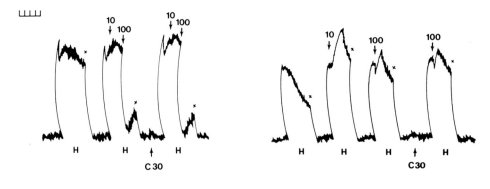

Fig. 2.   The relaxant activity of dimaprit, administered at arrows (↓), on the contraction induced by histamine (H) in whole ileum (left) and longitudinal muscle strip (right) of guinea-pig. C = cimetidine. Doses are given in µg/ml; time is in minutes. x = washing.

however, these reports were not sufficiently substantiated by the correct use of the available H_1- and H_2-receptor agonists and antagonists. Evidence indicating the absence of the classical H_2-receptors or the presence of subtypes of histamine receptors seems more conclusive [1, 39, 40, 48, 49]. Figure 2 shows a relaxant effect of dimaprit which is not abolished by cimetidine, indicating either a nonspecific effect of the H_2-agonist or a subtype of receptor which is apparently sensitive to dimaprit but insensitive to cimetidine.

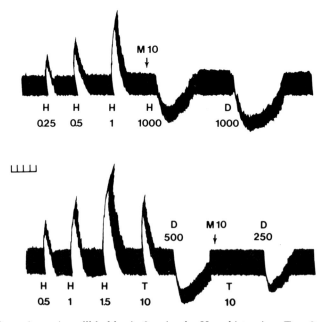

Fig. 3.   In situ guinea-pig gallbladder in 2 animals. H = histamine; T = 2-aminoethylthia-zole; M = mepyramine; D = dimaprit. All doses are given in µg/kg, and were administered intravenously; time is in minutes.

Table VI. Histamine receptors in the gallbladder.

Species	Receptors		Compounds used
	H_1	H_2	
Guinea-pig (in vitro) [50]	↑	↓	histamine, H_1- and H_2-antagonists, 4-methyl histamine
Guinea-pig (in vivo) [51]	↑	↓	histamine, H_1- and H_2- agonists and antagonists
Baboon (in vivo) [52]	↑	↓	histamine, diphenydramine, metiamide

↑ = contraction; ↓ = relaxation.

Histamine receptors in the gallbladder

Both types of histamine receptors were shown to occur in the gallbladders of the guinea-pig and the baboon. Stimulation of H_1-receptors induced by small doses of histamine or selective H_1-agonists caused a contraction, which was blocked by the classical antihistamine compounds. Stimulation of H_2-receptors induced by high doses of histamine after H_1-receptor blockade or by high doses of selective H_2-agonists caused relaxation of the gallbladder (Fig. 3). Moreover, a pretreatment with H_2-receptor antagonists significantly potentiated the stimulatory effect of histamine. The much higher doses of H_2-agonists required to induce relaxation of the

Table VII. Nonspecific actions of H_2-receptor blockers on the gastrointestinal tract.

Compound and dose	Species and tissue	Effect	Reference
Burimamide 50-200 mg/kg, intramuscularly	Rat stomach (in vivo)	Relaxation	[53]
Burimamide 10 mg/kg, intravenously	Rat pylorus (in vivo)	Contraction	[22]
Burimamide 'large doses'	Guinea-pig ileum (in vitro)	Inhibition	[1]
Metiamide 1 mg/kg/minute, intravenously	Rat stomach (in vivo)	Relaxation	[54]
Cimetidine 100 mg/kg, intraperitoneally	Gastric emptying rat (in vivo)	Delay	[55]
Cimetidine 25 μg/ml	Guinea-pig ileum (in vitro)	Naloxone-like action	[56]
Cimetidine 37.5 μg/ml	Rat antrum (in vitro)	Inhibition of TRH-induced contractions	[57]

gallbladder, in comparison with the small amounts required to induce contractions, are consistent with the hypothesis that H_1-receptors are predominant in the cholecystis, or at least that they are more susceptible to the action of their selective stimulants. The clear-cut situation concerning the presence of histamine receptors in the gallbladder, and the effect of their stimulation in the in vitro and in vivo guinea-pig and in the awake baboon, is shown in Table VI.

An interesting problem from a pharmacological point of view is that of the possible occurrence of a nonspecific effect of the classical H_2-blockers. Those concerning gastrointestinal motility are summarized in Table VII. It is evident from this Table that the nonspecific effects occurred with doses of the H_2-blockers decidedly higher than those required to inhibit histamine-stimulated gastric secretion (a classical effect of H_2-receptor stimulation). It is obvious that the use of such high doses cannot be employed for identification of a definite type of histamine receptor.

Conclusions

The distribution of histamine in the gastrointestinal tract is consistent with the idea that the amine has a function in secretion rather than in motility, but there are many important factors which cannot be disregarded, such as the turnover rate of histamine, the number and the susceptibility of receptors at the specific targets, and the interaction with other humoral and nervous mediators. We still do not know how many endogenous substances are involved in gut motility, or what the role of hormonal neural, vascular or metabolic influences on the effect of histamine could be. In vitro experiments have shown that histamine may affect intestinal muscle in particular experimental conditions, even in very small amounts, while in vivo studies have not been sufficiently reliable, because of a number of indirect systemic actions which can mask the effect of histamine on gut motility.

It is most probable that histamine does not have a primary role in peristalsis, as it does in gastric secretion; however, the possibility that the amine may play a physiological role in the regulation of gastrointestinal motility cannot be excluded, even if direct evidence for such a role is still lacking. Receptors involved in the motor response to histamine are predominantly of the H_1-type (mediating contraction) and to a lesser extent of the H_2-type (usually mediating relaxation but, in some cases, also contraction). A certain heterogeneity in the H_2-receptor population pointed out in several investigations [58-60], together with some contrasting findings obtained with H_1- and H_2-agonists and antagonists, suggests that subtypes of the classical histamine receptors may also occur in the gastrointestinal tract.

Of course it is fully possible that this situation represents only an artifact connected with the experimental conditions, and with the different measuring systems used in the various investigations.

References

1. Black, J.M., Duncan, W.A.M., Durant, C.J., Ganellin, C.R. and Parsons, E.M. (1972): Definition and antagonism of histamine H_2-receptors. *Nature (London) 236,* 385.
2. Bertaccini, G. (1978): Histamine H_2-receptors and gastric secretion. In: *Gastrointestinal hormones and pathology of the digestive system,* p. 69. Editors: M.I. Grossman, V. Speranza, N. Basso and E. Lezoche. Plenum Press, New York.
3. De Carle, D.J. and Glover, W.E. (1975): Independence of gastrin and histamine receptors in the lower oesophageal sphincter of the monkey and possum. *J. Physiol. (London) 245,* 78.

4. Goyal, R.Y. and Rattan, S. (1978): Neurohumoral, hormonal and drug receptors for the lower esophageal sphincter. *Gastroenterology 74*, 598.
5. Cohen, S. and Snape, W.J. (1975): Action of metiamide on the lower esophageal sphincter. *Gastroenterology 69*, 911.
6. De Carle, D.J., Brody, M.J. and Christensen, J. (1976): Histamine receptors in esophageal smooth muscle of the opossum. *Gastroenterology 70*, 1071.
7. Brown, F.C. and Castell, D.O. (1976): Histamine receptors on primate lower esophageal sphincter (LES) smooth muscle. *Clin. Res. 24*, A533.
8. Takayanagi, I. and Kasuya, Y. (1977): Effects of some drugs on the circular muscle of the isolated lower oesophagus. *J. Pharm. Pharmacol. 29*, 559.
9. Kravitz, J.J., Snape, W.J. Jr. and Cohen, S. (1978): Effect of histamine and histamine antagonists on human lower esophageal sphincter function. *Gastroenterology 74*, 435.
10. Castell, D.O. and Harris, L.D. (1970): Hormonal control of gastroesophageal sphincter strength. *N. Engl. J. Med. 282*, 886.
11. Misiewicz, J.J., Waller, S.L., Anthony, P.P. and Gummer, J.W.P. (1969): Achalasia of the cardia: Pharmacology and histopathology of isolated cardiac sphincteric muscle from patients with and without achalasia. *Q. J. Med. 38*, 17.
12. Burleigh, D.E. (1979): The effects of drugs and electrical field stimulation on the human lower oesophageal sphincter. *Arch. Int. Pharmacodyn. Ther. 240*, 169.
13. Bailey, R.J., Sullivan, S.N., MacDougall, B.R.D. and Williams, R. (1976): Effect of cimetidine on lower oesophageal sphincter. *Br. Med. J. 2*, 678.
14. Roesch, W., Lux, G., Schittenhelm, W. and Demling, L. (1976): Stimulation of lower esophageal sphincter pressure (LESP) by cimetidine. A double blind study. *Acta Hepato-Gastroenterol. 23*, 423.
15. Freeland, G.R., Higgs, R.H. and Castell, D.O. (1977): Lower esophageal sphincter response to oral administration of cimetidine in normal subjects. *Gastroenterology 72*, 28.
16. Osborne, D.H., Lennon, J., Henderson, M., Lidgard, G., Creel, R. and Carter, D.C. (1977): Effect of cimetidine on the human lower oesophageal sphincter. *Gut 18*, 99.
17. Siewert, R., Lepsien, G., Arnold, R. and Creutzfeldt, W. (1977): Effect of cimetidine on lower oesophageal sphincter pressure, intragastric pH and serum levels of immunoreactive gastrin in man. *Digestion 15*, 81.
18. Wesdorp, E. and Tytgat, G.N. (1978): A double-blind controlled trial of oral cimetidine in reflux oesophagitis. In: *Cimetidine*, p. 119. Editors: C. Harvengt, P.J. Deschepper, R. Bogaert, M. Cremer and P.C. Sharpe. Excerpta Medica, Amsterdam-Oxford-Princeton.
19. Blasi, A., Marletta, F., Monello, S., Mandalà, M.L. and Sala, L.O. (1978): Effects of cimetidine on LESP in normal subjects and patients with gastroesophageal reflux. In: *Proceedings of the VI World Congress of Gastroenterology*, p. 123. Editorial Garsi, Madrid.
20. Behar, J., Brand, D.L., Brown, F.C. et al. (1978): Cimetidine in the treatment of symptomatic gastroesophageal reflux. A double-blind controlled trial. *Gastroenterology 74*, 441.
21. Ercan, Z.S. and Turker, R.K. (1977): Histamine receptors in the isolated rat stomach fundus and rabbit aortic strips. *Pharmacology 15*, 118.
22. Bertaccini, G., Coruzzi, G., Molina, E. and Chiavarini, M. (1977): Action of histamine and related compounds on the pyloric sphincter of the rat. *Rend. Gastro-enterol. 9*, 163.
23. Gerner, T., Haffner, J.F.W. and Norstein, J. (1979): The effect of mepyramine and cimetidine on the motor responses to histamine, cholecystokinin and gastrin in the fundus and antrum of isolated guinea pig stomachs. *Scand. J. Gastroenterol. 14*, 65.
24. Fara, J.W. and Berkowitz, J.M. (1978): Effects of histamine and gastrointestinal hormones on dog antral smooth muscle in vitro. *Scand. J. Gastroenterol. 13*, 60.
25. Fasth, S., Hultén, L., Jahnberg, T. and Martinson, J. (1975): Comparative studies on the effects of bradykinin and vagal stimulation on motility in the stomach and colon. *Acta Physiol. Scand. 93*, 77.

26. Yates, J.C., Schofield, B. and Roth, S.H. (1978): Acid secretion and motility of isolated mammalian gastric mucosa and attached muscularis externa. *Am. J. Physiol. 234,* E319.

27. Ohga, A. and Taneike, T. (1978): H_1- and H_2-receptors in the smooth muscle of the ruminant stomach. *Br. J. Pharmacol. 62,* 333.

28. Scarpignato, C., Coruzzi, G. and Bertaccini, G. (1980): Effect of histamine and related compounds on gastric emptying of the rat. (Submitted.)

29. Dubois, A., Nompleggi, D., Myers, L. and Castell, D.O. (1978): Histamine H_2-receptor stimulation increases gastric emptying. *Gastroenterology 74,* A1028.

30. Richardson, C.T., Bailey, B.A., Walsh, J.H. and Fordtran, J.S. (1975): The effect of an H_2-receptor antagonist on food-stimulated acid secretion, serum gastrin, and gastric emptying in patients with duodenal ulcers. Comparison with an anticholinergic drug. *J. Clin. Invest. 55,* 536.

31. Richardson, C.T., Walsh, J.H. and Hicks, M.I. (1976): The effect of cimetidine, a new histamine H_2-receptor antagonist, on meal-stimulated acid secretion, serum gastrin, and gastric emptying in patients with duodenal ulcer. *Gastroenterology 71,* 19.

32. Heading, R.C., Logan, R.F.A., McLoughlin, G.P., Lidgard, G. and Forrest, J.A.H. (1977): Effect of cimetidine on gastric emptying. In: *Cimetidine,* p. 145. Editors: W.L. Burland and M.A. Simkins. Excerpta Medica, Amsterdam-Oxford-Princeton.

33. Forrest, J.A.H., Fettes, M., McLoughlin, G.P. and Heading, R.C. (1978): The effect of long-term cimetidine on gastric acid secretion, serum gastrin and gastric emptying. In: *Cimetidine: the Westminster Hospital Symposium,* p. 57. Editors: C. Wastell and P. Lance. Churchill Livingstone, Edinburgh.

34. Forrest, J.A.H., Fettes, M., McLoughlin, G.P. and Heading, R.C. (1979): Effect of long-term cimetidine on gastric acid secretion, serum gastrin and gastric emptying. *Gut 20,* 404.

35. Bareicha, I. and Rocha e Silva, M. (1975): Occurrence of H_2-receptors for histamine in the guinea-pig intestine. *Biochem. Pharmacol. 24,* 1215.

36. Bertaccini, G., Zappia, L. and Molina, E. (1979): 'In vitro' duodenal muscle in the pharmacological study of natural compounds. *Scand. J. Gastroenterol. 14,* Suppl. 54, 87.

37. Ambache, N., Killick, S.W. and Zar, A.M. (1973): Antagonism by burimamide of inhibitions induced by histamine in plexus-containing longitudinal muscle preparations from guinea pig ileum. *Br. J. Pharmacol. 48,* 362P.

38. Reinhardt, D., Ritter, E., Butzheinen, R. and Schümann, H.J. (1979): Relationship between histamine-induced changes of cyclic AMP and mechanical activity on smooth muscle preparations of the guinea pig ileum and the rabbit mesenteric artery. *Agents Actions 9,* 155.

39. Kenakin, T.P., Krueger, C.A. and Cook, D.A. (1974): Temperature-dependent interconversion of histamine H_1 and H_2 receptors in guinea pig ileum. *Nature (London) 252,* 54.

40. Bertaccini, G., Molina, E., Zappia, L. and Zséli, J. (1979): Histamine receptors in the guinea pig ileum. *Arch. Pharmacol. 309,* 65.

41. Fjalland, B. (1979): Evidence for the existence of another type of histamine H_2-receptor in guinea-pig ileum. *J. Pharm. Pharmacol. 31,* 50.

42. Chand, N. and De Roth, L. (1978): Occurrence of H_2-inhibitory histamine receptors in chicken ileum. *Eur. J. Pharmacol. 52,* 143.

43. Parrot, J.L. and Thouvenot, J. (1966): Action de l'histamine sur les muscles lisses. In: *Handbook of experimental pharmacology, 18/1,* p. 202. Editor: M. Rocha e Silva. Springer Verlag, Berlin.

44. Botting, J.H. (1975): Sensitivity of neonatal rabbit ileum to histamine. *Br. J. Pharmacol. 53,* 428.

45. Glover, W.E. (1979): Effect of dithiothreitol on histamine receptors in rabbit colon and guinea-pig ileum. *Clin. Exp. Pharmacol. Physiol. 6,* 151.

46. Arunlakshana, O. and Schild, H.O. (1959): Some quantitative uses of drug antagonists. *Br. J. Pharmacol. 14,* 48.

47. Ash, A.S.F. and Schild, H.O. (1966): Receptors mediating some actions of histamine. *Br. J. Pharmacol. 27,* 427.

48. Parsons, M.E. (1977): The antagonism of histamine H_2-receptors in vitro and in vivo with particular reference to the actions of cimetidine. In: *Cimetidine,* p. 13. Editors: W.L. Burland and M.A. Simkins. Excerpta Medica, Amsterdam-Oxford-Princeton.

49. Durant, G.J., Duncan, W.A.M., Ganellin, C.R., Parsons, M.E., Blakemore, R.C. and Rasmussen, A.C. (1978): Impromidine (SKF 92676) is a very potent and specific agonist for histamine H_2-receptors. *Nature (London) 276,* 403.

50. Waldman, D.B., Zfass, A.M. and Makhloef, G.M. (1977): Stimulatory (H_1) and inhibitory (H_2) histamine receptors in gallbladder muscle. *Gastroenterology 72,* 932.

51. Impicciatore, M. (1978): Occurrence of H_1- and H_2-histamine receptors in the guinea-pig gallbladder in situ. *Br. J. Pharmacol. 64,* 219.

52. Schoetz, D.J., Wise, W.E., LaMorte, W.W., Birkett, D.H. and Williams, L.F. (1978): Histamine receptors in the primate gallbladder. *Gastroenterology 74,* 1090.

53. Ridley, P.T., Groves, W.G., Schlosser, J.H. and Massenberg, J.S. (1973): H_2-antagonist action on interdigestive gastric acid secretion and motility in the rat. In: *International Symposium on histamine H_2-receptor antagonists,* p. 259. Editors: C.J. Wood and M.A. Simkins. Deltakos (UK) Ltd., London.

54. Black, J.W. and Spencer, K.E. (1973): Metiamide in systematic screening tests. In: *International Symposium on histamine H_2-receptor antagonists,* p. 23. Editors: C.J. Wood and M.A. Simkins. Deltakos (UK) Ltd., London.

55. Scarpignato, C. and Bertaccini, G. (1979): H_2-receptor antagonists and gastric emptying. (Unpublished.)

56. Takayanagi, I., Iwayama, Y. and Kasuya, Y. (1978): Narcotic antagonistic action of cimetidine on the guinea pig ileum. *J. Pharm. Pharmacol. 30,* 519.

57. Bruce, A.L., Behsudi, F.M. and Fawcett, C.P. (1979): Histaminergic involvement in thyrotropin-releasing hormone stimulation of antral tissue in the rat. *Gastroenterology 76,* 908.

58. Chand, N., Eyre, P. and DeRoth, L. (1979): Relaxant action of histamine on rabbit trachea: possible existence of third histamine receptor subtype. *Chem. Path. Pharmacol. 23,* 211.

59. Bertaccini, G., Molina, E., Vitali, T. and Zappia, L. (1979): Action of histamine receptor agonists and antagonists on the rat uterus. *Br. J. Pharmacol. 66,* 13.

60. Coruzzi, G., Bongrani, S. and Bertaccini, G. (1979): Histamine receptors in the heart and coronary vessels of rabbits. *Pharmacol. Res. Commun. 11,* 517.

Discussion

Milton-Thompson (Gosport): I was very interested in Professor Bertaccini's data on gastric emptying. Of course, this is a very difficult area methodologically. I would be interested in knowing how he measured gastric emptying in man, because we do not feel that we have found any completely satisfactory method of doing it.

Bertaccini: I have no data concerning man. The experiments from my laboratory were performed in the rat. However, I did cite data from the literature on cimetidine and gastric emptying in man in my paper. In the rat we used the phenol-red system, which is very simple and is a very reliable method.

Milton-Thompson: Yes, but of course it measures only liquid emptying.

Bertaccini: That is correct.

Mattila (Helsinki): There is an old belief among pharmacologists that the rat is not a suitable animal species for the investigation of histamine because, in many ways, it is resistant to histamine. Does Professor Bertaccini think that the data he presented concerning the action of histamine on the rat alimentary tract are relevant, bearing in mind that the rat is at least partially resistant to histamine?

Bertaccini: I agree to a certain extent with Dr. Mattila. However, both Dr. Ganellin and Dr. Parsons presented excellent data on histamine and rat gastric secretion, so it is probably not true that the rat is not a good species for histamine studies. Of course, it is not the best one; the guinea-pig is much better. I do not know whether the small standard errors were noticed, but what we observed in gastric emptying indicated that this is a good method. I would certainly not want to extrapolate any data obtained in the rat either to any other animal species or to man, but what we obtained in the rat is reliable for that species.

Harvey (Bristol): I am particularly interested in the gallbladder, and it is very puzzling to find 2 histamine receptors with opposite effects in the same organ, an organ which already has a powerful hormone which is believed to cause most of the contraction after food. Has Professor Bertaccini any observations on this, and has he studied the effects of cimetidine or interactions with cholecystokinin?

Bertaccini: We did not study interactions with cholecystokinin, but we studied guinea-pig gallbladder in situ with the usual system used for the biological assay of cholecystokinin. The tracing I presented was from my laboratory. We observed very good competitive antagonism between the relaxant effect of dimaprit, for instance, and the action of metiamide, and also between histamine or 2-thiazolyl ethylamine and mepyramine or chlorpheniramine.

Harvey: Which effect is dominant in real life? Is it the contraction or the relaxation that is the more important?

Bertaccini: Certainly it is the contraction. We did not observe the doses because they were very small, but only a few micrograms — or even a fraction of a microgram — of histamine is required to contract the gallbladder, whereas 100 μg is necessary to obtain relaxation. The population of H_1-receptors is predominant, so there is a predominant contraction effect. The relaxation can be obtained either by the use of very selective H_2-agonists, or after blockade of the action of the H_1-receptors.

Wingate (London): I wonder whether any of the things that Professor Bertaccini summarised have anything to do with physiology. One of the points that has become clear in recent years is that gastrointestinal smooth muscle deprived of its innervation — extrinsically denervated — so that it becomes a pharmacological preparation, behaves very differently from the same muscle in situ. There is, for instance, the peptide motilin, which was thought to have a dose-dependent contractile effect in vitro on smooth muscle. This effect is never seen in vivo, because it has a completely different effect on the innervation.

I add this comment because one might have the impression from Professor Bertaccini's talk that there are stimulatory or inhibitory effects of this nature. I am sure that there are effects of histamine, but I do not know whether this sort of system is one in which they can be displayed.

Bertaccini: Thank you for your comment. If I gave the impression that I was emphasising that the effects of histamine were physiological, I apologise. That was not my intention. Histamine is present in all the gastrointestinal tract, and now that there are so many substances known to be involved in gut motility I do not think that it is possible to say whether or not any one substance has a physiological effect. Probably the physiology concerns the interactions among all the substances present, and also between humoral agents and neural mediators. It is difficult to say whether an effect is physiological.

The effect of impromidine, a specific H_2-receptor agonist, on gastric secretion in man

Jane G. Mills, Richard H. Hunt*, U. Bangerter°, F. Halter°, W.L. Burland and G.J. Milton-Thompson*

*The Research Institute, Smith Kline & French Research Ltd., Welwyn Garden City; *Department of Gastroenterology, The Royal Naval Hospital, Haslar, Gosport, United Kingdom; and °Gastrointestinal Unit, University Hospital, Berne, Switzerland*

Introduction

Selective agonists for histamine at the H_2-receptor have been previously described [1-3], but these compounds are generally less potent than histamine. More recently, however, impromidine (Fig. 1) has been shown to be a very potent and specific agonist for H_2-receptors in animals and in man [4-6]. In vitro impromidine has been shown to have 10-50 times the potency of histamine at the H_2-receptor, and the H_2-receptor antagonist cimetidine has produced a dose-dependent parallel displacement of the impromidine dose response curve without depressing the maximum response; in vivo impromidine has been found to be a highly potent stimulant of gastric acid secretion in the rat, cat and dog.

In the present study, we evaluated the use of impromidine as a gastric secretagogue in healthy volunteers and in patients with peptic ulcer disease.

Subjects and methods

Forty patients (26 males and 14 females) with clinical signs and symptoms of peptic ulcer disease requiring further investigation of gastric secretory status were studied, along with 28 healthy male volunteers. In all cases, gastric secretory studies were carried out after an overnight fast, and gastric juice was collected in 10-minute aliquots by means of continuous aspiration. The volume and hydrogen ion concentration of each sample were determined. Correction for pyloric loss and reflux was made by means of a phenol red infusion technique in the healthy subjects

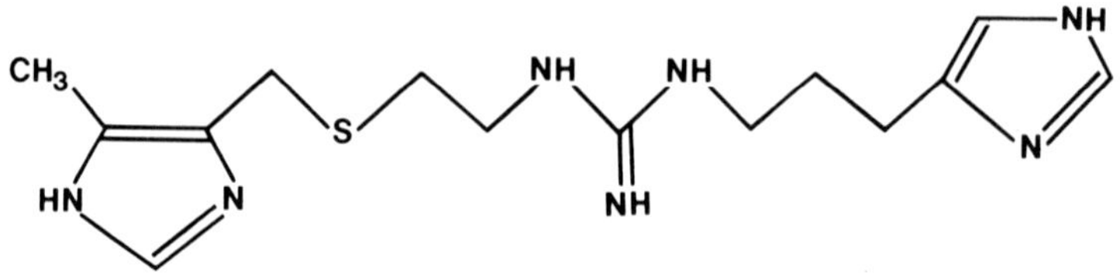

Fig. 1. *Structure of impromidine (SK&F-92676).*

[7, 8]. A dose response study was carried out in 4 of the healthy subjects. On the first study day, dose response curves to impromidine were constructed over the dose range 2.5-20 μg/kg/hour. On the second study day, cimetidine 0.5 mg/kg/hour was infused throughout the study period, and the dose response to impromidine was studied over the range 5.0-80 μg/kg/hour. Each dose of impromidine was infused for 60 minutes before increasing to the next dose, and dose-response curves were constructed using total gastric acid output over the last 30 minutes of each infusion period minus basal acid output as a measure of response.

The responses of patients and healthy subjects to an intravenous infusion of impromidine 10 μg/kg/hour were compared to responses obtained during the administration of pentagastrin 6 μg/kg/hour and histamine acid phosphate 40 μg/kg/hour. Similar comparative studies were made following the subcutaneous administration of impromidine and pentagastrin.

Pulse and blood pressure were monitored at 10-minute intervals during all studies involving the intravenous infusion of impromidine, including 1 group of 20 patients aged 55-78 years, 6 with histories of mild to moderate hypertension and 1 with coronary heart disease. Any other signs or symptoms either observed or reported were recorded. Venous blood samples were taken for routine haematological and biochemical analysis.

Data from the comparative studies were analysed by means of Wilcoxon's paired-rank sum test; data from the dose-response studies were subjected to analysis of variance for parallel-line assays.

Results

Following the intravenous infusion of impromidine alone, a significant linear

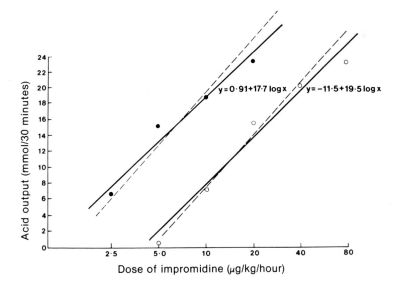

Fig. 2. Dose-response curves to impromidine with and without concomitant infusion of cimetidine 0.5 mg/kg/hour. Mean of 4 subjects. ●—● = impromidine; ○—○ = impromidine plus cimetidine; --- = best-fit parallel lines. (Reproduced from [5] with the permission of the authors and the editors of Gastroenterology.)

regression was seen over the dose range 2.5-20 µg/kg/hour ($p < 0.001$). Cimetidine 0.5 mg/kg/hour produced a marked inhibition of gastric acid output and a significant displacement of the log dose-response curve to the right ($p < 0.05$) (Fig. 2). In the presence of cimetidine, a significant linear regression was seen over the dose range 5.0-80 µg/kg/hour, and parallel-line assay showed that the best fit parallel lines were not significantly different from the natural regressions.

The results obtained during intravenous administration in healthy subjects and patients are shown in Figure 3. In healthy subjects, no difference was seen in peak or maximal acid output between the 3 secretagogues; the time course of the response was similar, although a higher acid output was seen after 20 minutes' infusion with pentagastrin. In patients, a clear difference was seen in the time course of the response to pentagastrin and impromidine, with significantly higher acid outputs seen over the first 40 minutes of infusion with pentagastrin; although mean peak acid output (PAO) and maximal acid output (MAO) were higher following the administration of pentagastrin, the differences did not reach statistical significance (for impromidine and pentagastrin, respectively: MAO = 17.4 ± 2.0 mmol/hour and 25.8 ± 4.1 mmol/hour; PAO = 28.9 ± 3.8 mmol/hour and 33.1 ± 4.8 mmol/hour).

Similar results were seen following the subcutaneous administration of impromidine and pentagastrin (Fig. 4). A more rapid secretory response was seen following the injection of pentagastrin, but no difference was seen in peak acid output (following impromidine and pentagastrin, respectively: mean of 9 healthy subjects = 40.3 ± 2.2 mmol/hour and 48.9 ± 4.2 mmol/hour; mean of 10 patients = 25.4 ± 6.3 mmol/hour and 29.7 ± 4.2 mmol/hour).

Facial flushing was seen in all of the healthy subjects and in 36 of the 40 patients, both during the infusion of impromidine 10 µg/kg/hour and following the injection of a single 10 µg/kg dose. The onset of flushing was gradual, and the flushing increased in intensity as the dose of impromidine was increased.

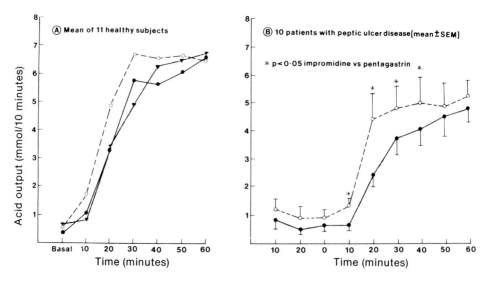

Fig. 3.   Gastric acid output during the intravenous infusion of impromidine, histamine and pentagastrin in 11 healthy subjects and 10 patients. ●—● = *impromidine 10 µg/kg/hour;* ▲—▲ = *histamine 40 µg/kg/hour;* ○---○ = *pentagastrin 6 µg/kg/hour.*

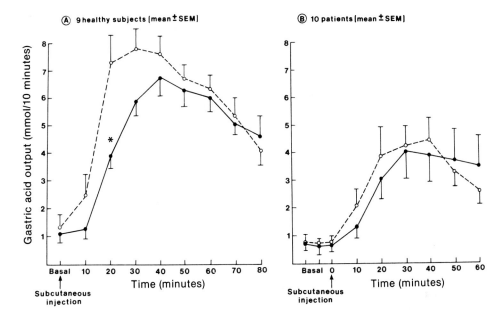

Fig. 4. *Gastric acid output following subcutaneous injection of impromidine 10 μg/kg/hour and pentagastrin 6 μg/kg/hour in 9 healthy subjects and 10 patients.* •——• = *impromidine;* ○---○ = *pentagastrin;* * p < 0.01.

During the comparative studies in healthy subjects, an increase in pulse rate was seen during the infusion of all 3 secretagogues. The increase in pulse rate following pentagastrin occurred early and was transient; during the infusion of impromidine and histamine, pulse rate increased after 10 minutes by 11 ± 2.5 and 16 ± 3.5 beats/minute (mean ± SEM), respectively; this increase in pulse rate was maintained throughout the infusion period, and was accompanied by a significant reduction in diastolic blood pressure of 16 ± 3.8 mm Hg for impromidine and 23 ± 4.8 mm Hg for histamine.

In the group of 10 patients aged 26-56 years, no change in pulse rate was seen during the infusion of pentagastrin. During the infusion of impromidine in these patients, a small but significant increase in pulse rate was seen 15 minutes after the start of the infusion, with a continued small increase during the rest of the infusion period: pulse rate before infusion was 72 ± 2.7 beats/minute (mean ± SEM), and 45 minutes after infusion began it was 80.4 ± 3.1 beats/minute (p < 0.02). On termination of the infusion, pulse rate returned to pre-infusion levels. No significant changes were seen in either diastolic or systolic blood pressure in patients in this age range.

In the group of 20 patients aged 55-78 years, 6 of whom had histories of mild to moderate hypertension, pulse rate increased during the infusion from 73 ± 2.7 beats/minute (mean ± SEM) to 81 ± 2.8 beats/minute, a significant difference (p < 0.01) (Fig. 5). Fifteen minutes after termination of the infusion, pulse rates had returned to resting values. Diastolic blood pressure fell by a mean of 9 mm Hg during the infusion period, but no changes were seen in systolic blood pressure (Fig. 5).

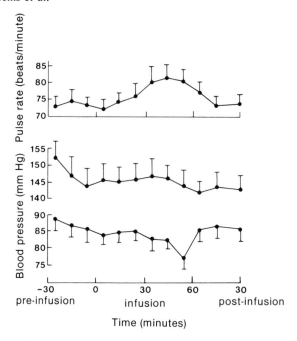

Fig. 5.   The effect of intravenous infusion of impromidine 10 μg/kg/hour on pulse rate and blood pressure in 20 patients aged 55-78 years. Mean ± SEM.

Mild to moderate frontal headache was reported by 8 of the 68 subjects following the administration of impromidine, and nausea or abdominal discomfort by 13 of the 40 subjects receiving pentagastrin. Following the intravenous infusion of histamine acid phosphate, 6 of 11 subjects reported headache. No clinically significant changes were seen during haematological and biochemical monitoring.

Discussion

These results confirm that impromidine is a potent gastric secretagogue in healthy man and in patients with peptic ulcer disease, with an effect comparable to that of either histamine or pentagastrin at the doses used in clinical practice. The gastric secretory response to pentagastrin appears to be more rapid in onset than the response to impromidine but, no significant differences were seen in peak acid output. Similar differences in the time course of the response have been reported between pentagastrin and histamine [9].

Stimulation of gastric acid output was dose-dependent, and cimetidine 0.5 mg/kg/hour caused a significant parallel displacement of the dose-response curve to the right, a finding consistent with direct competitive antagonism. In vitro studies have demonstrated the specificity of impromidine for the H_2-receptor; the results in man, while they are not conclusive, support the conclusion that impromidine is a potent and specific H_2-receptor agonist.

The cardiovascular effects of histamine in the cat and the dog are mediated via both H_1- and H_2-receptors [10-12] and the role of histamine-induced changes in heart rate and blood pressure in man has been studied in some detail [13]. In the present study, impromidine 10 μg/kg/hour produced only small changes in both pulse and diastolic blood pressure, but cardiovascular responses appeared to be dose-dependent and meant that the dose of impromidine was not increased above 20 μg/kg/hour. Consequently, no conclusions may be drawn with respect to the dose required to produce a maximal acid response.

Impromidine was well-tolerated in healthy subjects and in young peptic ulcer patients, as well as in older patients, some of whom had mild cardiovascular disease. This latter group of patients might have been expected to be more sensitive to the cardiovascular effects of impromidine but, in fact, only minor changes in pulse rate and diastolic blood pressure were seen.

Impromidine is a specific H_2-receptor agonist, and as such may have advantages over histamine and pentagastrin in routine tests of gastric secretory function; more particularly, it provides an important tool for the further investigation of the role of histamine at H_2-receptors in man.

References

1. Black, J.W., Duncan, W.A.M., Durant, G.J., Ganellin, C.R. and Parsons, M.E. (1972): Definition and antagonism of histamine H_2-receptors. *Nature (London) 236*, 385-390.
2. Durant, G.J., Emmett, J.C., Ganellin, C.R., Roe, A.M. and Slater, R.A. (1976): Potential histamine H_2-receptor antagonists. 3. Methylhistamines. *J. Med. Chem. 19*, 923-928.
3. Parsons, M.E., Owen, D.A.A., Ganellin, C.R. and Durant, G.J. (1977): Dimaprit — [5-[3-(N,N-dimethylamino)propyl]isothiourea] — A highly specific histamine H_2-receptor agonist. I. Pharmacology. *Agents Actions 7*, 31-37.
4. Durant, G.J., Duncan, W.A.M., Ganellin, C.R., Parsons, M.E., Blackmore, R.C. and Rasmussen, A.C. (1978): Impromidine (SK&F 92676) is a very potent and specific agonist for histamine H_2-receptors. *Nature (London) 276*, 403-404.
5. Hunt, R.H., Mills, J.G., Beresford, J., Billings, J.A., Burland, W.L. and Milton-Thompson, G.J. (1980): Gastric secretory studies in man with impromidine (SK&F 92676) — A specific histamine H_2 receptor agonist. *Gastroenterology 78*, 505-511.
6. Bangerter, U., Schlup, M., Liechti, N., Hacki, W.H. and Halter, F. (1979): Clinical experience with impromidine, a highly specific histamine H_2-receptor agonist. *Gut 20*, A938.
7. Hobsley, M. and Silen, W. (1969): Use of an inert marker (phenol red) to improve accuracy in gastric secretion studies. *Gut 10*, 787-795.
8. Hobsley, M. (1974): Pyloric reflux; a modification of the two-compartment hypotheses of gastric secretion. *Clin. Sci. Mol. Med. 47*, 131-141.
9. Halter, F., Buerki, V. and Richterich, R. (1968): Histamin und Pentagastrin Infusiontest. *Schweiz. Med. Wochenschr. 98*, 305-307.
10. Black, J.W., Owen, D.A.A. and Parsons, M.E. (1975): An analysis of the depressor responses to histamine in the cat and the dog: involvement of H_1- and H_2-receptors. *Br. J. Pharmacol. 54*, 319-324.
11. Owen, D.A.A. (1977): Histamine receptors in the cardiovascular system. *Gen. Pharmacol. 8*, 141-156.
12. Flynn, S.B. and Owen, D.A.A. (1975): Histamine receptors in peripheral vascular beds in the cat. *Br. J. Pharmacol. 55*, 181-188.
13. Boyce, M.J. and Wareham, K. (1980): Histamine H_1- and H_2-receptors in the cardiovascular system of man. *This volume*, p. 280.

Discussion

Venables (Newcastle-upon-Tyne): I am puzzled by, and would like to hear speculation on the possible explanation of, why impromidine has a slower effect than pentagastrin. That suggests a very different mechanistic effect.

Mills: In fact, a similar difference has been seen in patients when the effects of pentagastrin and histamine are compared. The rate of onset of the effect of histamine is slower than that of pentagastrin, as has been shown by Professor Halter, one of my colleagues.

Venables: It is not my personal experience. Is it possible that there is something different about the patients that makes them respond so differently?

Mills: I am not sure that they did respond differently. In some series of studies we see a more marked difference in the rate of onset in the healthy subjects, and in others in the patients, but it is a consistent feature. The statistics and the methodology used in the 2 sets of studies are slightly different, which probably accounts for the small changes in significance.

Lorenz (Marburg): We have been dealing mainly with subpopulations of ulcer patients. Has Ms. Mills any information about whether patients who show, say, a low pentagastrin response may have a high impromidine response? Are there such individuals, or is there no possibility of discriminating among individuals in this way?

Mills: To date, we have no such discrimination. There is one example of a patient in the group who failed to respond to impromidine who similarly failed to respond to pentagastrin.

Lorenz: When impromidine and pentagastrin were compared, was this done in a random sequence?

Mills: Yes, the order of drug administration was randomised.

The role of histamine in the cardiovascular system and in acute inflammatory responses: a review of current evidence

D.A.A. Owen, S.B. Flynn, R.W. Gristwood, C.A. Harvey and D.F. Woodward
Department of Pharmacology, Smith Kline & French Research Ltd., Welwyn Garden City, United Kingdom

Introduction

Despite numerous studies made since Dale and his colleagues first described the effects of histamine on cardiovascular function [1-4], no clear definition of the physiological or pathological role of histamine within the cardiovascular system has yet been achieved.

The hypothesis that histamine may contribute to or control aspects of cardiovascular function has been popular and is supported by much circumstantial evidence, but a *proven* role for histamine remains to be established. The difficulty of defining such a role for histamine can be traced to a number of causes, including: species variation in the cardiovascular response to histamine; the uncertainty of extrapolation of data from animal models, particularly models of pathologies, to physiological and clinical conditions; and, most decisively, the lack (until recently) of effective and selective antagonists of all the actions of histamine on cardiovascular function.

Several conclusions, however, *have* been drawn. For example: histamine can modify function throughout the cardiovascular system; histamine is stored within mast cells in the heart and immediately adjacent to blood vessels, and a variety of pathological conditions involving cardiovascular malfunction are associated with histamine release and mast cell degranulation; blood vessels, through the presence of the enzyme histidine decarboxylase, possess the capacity to synthesize histamine. Induction of this enzyme, and the resultant increased synthesis of histamine, has been measured under a wide variety of stressful conditions associated with altered cardiovascular function [5, 6].

Currently, the availability of histamine H_2-receptor antagonists used with H_1-receptor antagonists provides the means to inhibit histamine-induced changes in cardiovascular function, and the appropriate use of both histamine H_1- and H_2-receptor antagonists in experimental and clinical studies should allow clarification of the role of histamine in cardiovascular control. Such studies may also identify new and valuable therapeutic roles for these antagonists.

The present paper will describe some of the important effects of histamine in the cardiovascular system, identify the receptors involved in these responses, and illustrate how effective and selective antagonism of histamine can be achieved.

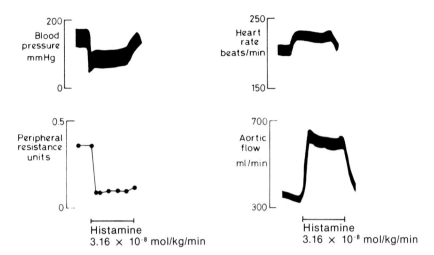

Fig. 1.   In anaesthetised cats, histamine infused intravenously for 5 minutes (as indicated by the bar) lowers arterial blood pressure, increases heart rate, decreases total peripheral resistance and increases aortic blood flow (measured by use of an electromagnetic flow probe around the aorta).

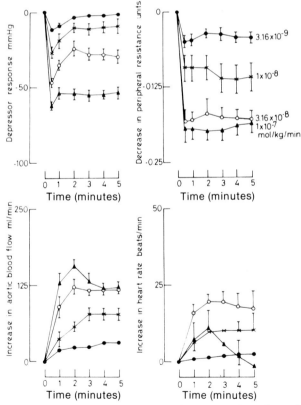

Fig. 2.   The haemodynamic effects of histamine infusions are dose-dependent over the dose range 3.16×10^{-9} to 1×10^{-7} mol/kg/minute. All results are means $\pm$ SEM of studies in 8 anaesthetised cats.

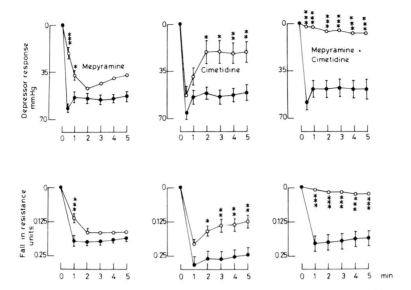

Fig. 3. *Dose-response curves (mean ± SEM) in 6 anaesthetised cats, before (●—●) and after (○—○) treatment. The fall in blood pressure (upper panels) and in total peripheral resistance (lower panels) during the infusion of histamine 1×10^{-7} mol/kg/minute is significantly modified by H_1-receptor blockade with mepyramine 12.5 µmol/kg (left-hand panels) and by H_2-receptor blockade with cimetidine 2 µmol/kg/minute (centre panels), although a substantial response persists. Abolition of the histamine responses can be achieved by combined treatment with both mepyramine and cimetidine (right-hand panels). Significant inhibition is indicated by asterisks.*

Effect of histamine on haemodynamics

Histamine is an effective depressor substance in all species except the rabbit, including man. The fall in blood pressure during administration of histamine is due to a decrease in total peripheral resistance which is adequate to reduce blood pressure despite the concomitant increase in cardiac output (Fig. 1). The haemo-dynamic response to histamine is dose-dependent (Fig. 2), and involves both hista-mine H_1- and H_2-receptors. The responses to histamine are significantly modified by either H_1- or H_2-receptor blockade, but can be abolished only by simultaneous use of both types of antagonist (Fig. 3). Thus, the haemodynamic response to circulat-ing histamine can be abolished by a combination of H_1- and H_2-receptor antagonists, whereas a substantial response to histamine persists if only 1 type of antagonist is administered.

Effect of histamine on cardiac function

Histamine is an effective cardiac stimulant in most species, although this parameter is subject to some species variation. Studies of the action of histamine on cardiac function have usually been made in guinea-pig hearts in vitro; the data currently available, although limited, suggest that responses of the guinea-pig heart to hista-

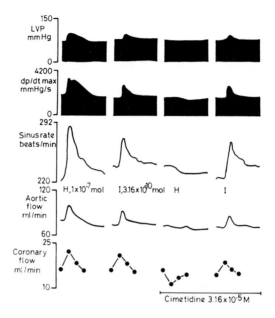

Fig. 4.   Both histamine (H) and isoprenaline (I) cause cardiac stimulation in the isolated working heart of the guinea-pig. The responses to histamine are abolished by cimetidine, which does not modify the responses to isoprenaline.

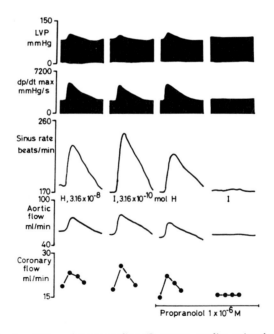

Fig. 5.   Both histamine (H) and isoprenaline (I) cause cardiac stimulation in the isolated working heart of the guinea-pig. The responses to isoprenaline are abolished by propranolol, which does not modify the responses to histamine.

mine are similar to those of primate hearts, including the human heart [7-9].

Studies of the isolated working heart of the guinea-pig have indicated that histamine, like isoprenaline, increases the rate of force of beating of the heart, and also increases cardiac output, coronary flow and external pressure-volume work. The response to histamine is dose-dependent and can be competitively inhibited by cimetidine, with pA_2 values between 6.25 and 6.59 on all parameters. Inhibition of responses to histamine, but not isoprenaline, by cimetidine is illustrated in Figure 4; propranolol, however, in concentrations adequate to abolish isoprenaline responses, does not inhibit histamine (Fig. 5).

Thus, the direct cardiac stimulant actions of histamine are associated with H_2-receptors, and can be abolished by cimetidine.

Effect of histamine on peripheral vascular beds

Histamine causes changes in function along the entire length of peripheral vascular beds. These actions of histamine may be studied in a variety of vascular beds, and reflect the acute inflammatory actions of histamine and include increases in local tissue blood flow, increases in local blood content, accumulation of macromolecules in tissues due to increases in vascular permeability, and tissue swelling. Typical responses to histamine on these parameters in skeletal muscle are illustrated in Figure 6.

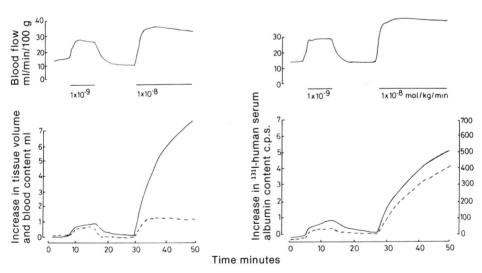

Fig. 6. *Traces from 2 similar experiments on skeletal muscle vasculature in anaesthetised cats. Left: histamine 1×10^{-9} and 1×10^{-8} mol/kg/minute, infused intra-arterially as indicated by the bars, causes dose-dependent increases in blood flow; the infusions also increase tissue volume (—) and tissue blood content (---); at the lower infusion rate, the increase in tissue volume is due mainly to the increase in blood content, while at the higher infusion rate substantial oedema occurs and the increase in tissue volume greatly exceeds the increase in blood content. Right: histamine is shown to cause similar increases in blood flow and tissue volume (—), but the large increase in tissue volume at the higher infusion rate is shown to be associated with substantial accumulation of ^{131}I-human serum albumin (---) due to the increase in vascular permeability to macromolecules.*

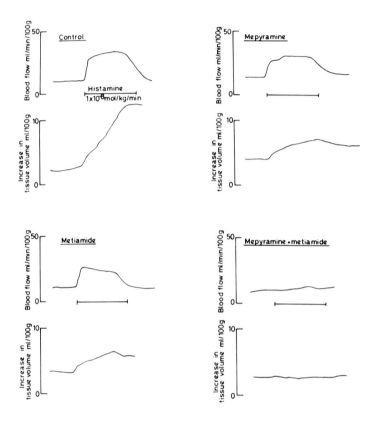

Fig. 7.   *Skeletal muscle vasculature in anaesthetised cats. Histamine 1 × 10⁻⁸ mol/kg/min-*
ute, infused intra-arterially for 3 minutes, causes a large increase in tissue blood
flow and tissue volume (oedema). A typical response to histamine in untreated cats is shown,
top left. In animals treated with mepyramine 1.25 × 10⁻⁵ mol/kg (top right) or metiamide 2 ×
10⁻⁶ mol/kg/minute (bottom left), histamine still increases blood flow, though the increase in
tissue volume is small. Mepyramine and metiamide together abolish the response to histamine
(bottom right).

The increase in blood flow during infusion of histamine persists in the presence of
either H_1- or H_2-receptor blockade, whereas the rate of oedema formation and
increase in vascular permeability are substantially reduced by either antagonist. The
response to histamine can be abolished only by combined H_1- and H_2-receptor
blockade (Fig. 7).

Histamine produces similar inflammatory effects on the blood vessels in skin, as
was first described by Sir Thomas Lewis in his studies on human skin [10]. The
vascular responses in skin can be determined precisely by measurement of surface
temperature, as an index of local blood flow, local accumulation of ^{125}I-human
serum albumin, as an index of vascular permeability, and oedema. Histamine elicits
each of these changes in a dose-dependent manner. After H_1-receptor blockade,
histamine still causes substantial vasodilatation, but does not increase vascular
permeability and causes very little oedema. After H_2-receptor blockade, some
vasodilatation also persists, and histamine still increases vascular permeability and

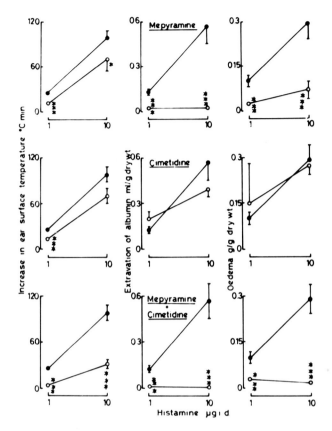

Fig. 8. *Cutaneous inflammation due to intradermal injections of histamine in guinea-pig ears, and the results of treatment with mepyramine and cimetidine. The left-hand panels show the effects of histamine (●—●) and modification by antagonists (○—○) on ear surface temperature (index of vasodilatation), the centre panels on vascular permeability, and the right-hand panels on oedema. Mepyramine 5 μmol/kg is shown to cause a small reduction in vasodilatation, to almost abolish the increase in vascular permeability, and to substantially reduce the oedema formation (top panels); cimetidine 500 μmol/kg also causes a small reduction in vasodilatation, but has no significant effect on vascular permeability or oedema formation (centre panels); a combination of mepyramine and cimetidine is shown to almost abolish vasodilatation, and to abolish increases in vascular permeability and oedema (bottom panels). All values are means ± SEM in 8-10 animals per group. Significant reductions are indicated by asterisks.*

causes oedema. Abolition of the vascular responses to histamine in skin, as elsewhere in the circulation, requires the simultaneous use of both H_1- and H_2-receptor antagonists (Fig. 8).

Acute cutaneous inflammatory responses can also be produced by mast cell degranulation, achieved by active anaphylaxis, with release of endogenous histamine and other vasoactive substances. The inflammation can be reduced by either H_1- or H_2-receptor blockade, and further reduced by the combination of antagonists (Fig. 9). Although the reduction in the inflammation by combined H_1- and H_2-

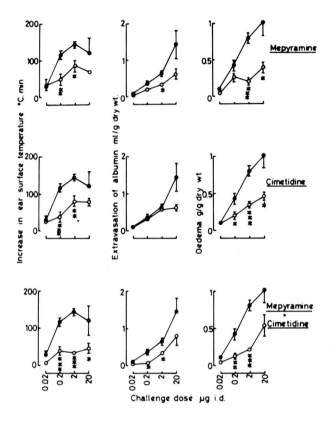

Fig. 9. Cutaneous anaphylaxis in guinea-pig ears. Antigen challenge (egg albumin) in sensitised animals causes increases in ear surface temperature (vasodilatation), as shown in the left-hand panels, increases vascular permeability (centre panels) and causes oedema (right-hand panels). Mepyramine 5 μmol/kg decreases the vasodilatation, the increase in vascular permeability and oedema (top panels). Cimetidine 500 μmol/kg is shown to decrease vasodilatation and oedema formation, but has no significant effect on the increase in vascular permeability (centre panels). A combination of mepyramine and cimetidine almost abolishes vasodilatation and significantly reduces the increase in vascular permeability and oedema (bottom panels). It is, however, clear that a substantial part of the permeability and oedema responses persist despite the use of a combination of mepyramine and cimetidine adequate to abolish vascular responses to histamine in this preparation. All control values (●—●) and treated values (○—○) are means ± SEM in a mean of 6 animals. Significant reductions are indicated by asterisks.

receptor blockade establishes a substantial role for histamine in cutaneous anaphylaxis, a refractory and therefore non-histamine component persists. This refractory component is due to the vascular effects of other mediators released in the anaphylactic response.

These studies in cutaneous anaphylaxis exemplify the value of using combined H_1- and H_2-receptor antagonists, in doses shown to effectively and selectively inhibit the vascular actions of histamine, to analyse the quantitative contribution of histamine in experimental and clinical cardiovascular pathology.

Conclusion

With the availability of both histamine H_1- and H_2-receptor antagonists adequate to provide effective and selective inhibition of the cardiovascular actions of histamine, progress towards an understanding of the role of histamine in the cardiovascular system, both in physiological and pathological control, should now be possible. The concept that histamine is important in cardiovascular control can be meaningfully tested, and important new therapeutic uses of these antagonists may be identified.

References

1. Dale, H.H. and Laidlaw, P.P. (1910): The physiological action of β-iminazolylethyla- mine. *J. Physiol. (London) 41,* 318-344.
2. Dale, H.H. and Laidlaw, P.P. (1911): Further observations on the action of β- iminazolylethylaminc. *J. Physiol. (London) 43,* 182-195.
3. Dale, H.H. and Laidlaw, P.P. (1919): Histamine shock. *J. Physiol. (London) 52,* 355- 390.
4. Dale, H.H. and Richards, A.N. (1918): The vasodilator actions of histamine and some other substances. *J. Physiol. (London) 52,* 110-165.
5. Schayer, R.W. (1960): Relationship of stress-induced histidine decarboxylase to circula- tory homeostasis and shock. *Science 131,* 226-227.
6. Schayer, R.W. (1965): Histamine and circulatory homeostasis. *Fed. Proc. 24,* 1295-1297.
7. Levi, R., Zavecz, J.H., Lee, C.H. and Allan, G. (1979): Histamine-drug-disease interac- tions and cardiac function. In: *Histamine receptors,* pp. 99-113. Editor: T.O. Yellin. Spectrum Press, New York.
8. Wolleman, M. and Papp, J.G. (1979): Blockade by cimetidine of the effects of histamine on adenylate cyclase activity, spontaneous rate and contractility in the developing prenatal heart. *Agents Actions 9,* 29.
9. Gristwood, R.W., Lincoln, J.C.R. and Owen, D.A.A. (1980): Effects of histamine on hu- man isolated heart muscle: comparison with effects of noradrenaline. *J. Pharm. Pharma- col. 32,* 145.
10. Lewis, T. (1927): *The blood vessels of the human skin and their responses.* Shaw and Sons Ltd., London.

Histamine H₁- and H₂-receptors in the cardiovascular system of man

M.J. Boyce and Kathleen Wareham
Clinical Research Department, The Research Institute, Smith Kline & French Research Ltd., Welwyn Garden City, United Kingdom

Introduction

The cardiovascular effects of histamine were first studied in man by Eppinger, who reported in 1913 that a single intravenous injection of histamine reduced blood pressure and caused flushing of the skin [1]; he gave no details of his results. In 1926, Harmer and Harris showed that single intravenous and subcutaneous injections of histamine reduced systolic and diastolic blood pressure and increased heart rate [2]. Weiss et al. could not confirm these blood pressure changes, despite using continuous infusions of histamine at doses which caused marked flushing and increases in heart rate [3, 4]. In 1945, Horton and co-workers reported a study in which continuous infusions of histamine caused dose-dependent falls in systolic and diastolic blood pressure and increases in heart rate [5]; in other studies, however, they failed to demonstrate any consistent changes in systolic blood pressure [6, 7].

In 1954, Duff and Whelan confirmed that histamine increased forearm blood flow and, in addition, showed that each of several compounds, now known to be H₁-antagonists, abolished the increase from a small dose of histamine but only attenuated the increase from larger doses [8]. Chipman and Glover subsequently demonstrated, in 1976, that the increase in forearm blood flow from a dose of histamine which was only attenuated by an H₁-receptor antagonist alone could be abolished by the addition of metiamide, a histamine H₂-receptor antagonist, indicating that the peripheral vasculature of man contains both histamine H₁- and H₂-receptors [9]. Dermatological studies also provided results consistent with the existence of both types of histamine receptor in human peripheral blood vessels [10].

Animal studies have shown species variation in the cardiovascular response to histamine [11]. The development of cimetidine, an H₂-receptor antagonist [12], and impromidine, a new, potent and highly specific H₂-receptor agonist [13], for use in man provides a unique opportunity for further pharmacological characterisation of histamine receptors in the human cardiovascular system. In this paper, we report preliminary findings from 3 studies in healthy volunteers. These studies are to be published in detail elsewhere.

Subjects and methods

STUDY 1

Doses of histamine acid phosphate 20, 40 and 80 μg/kg/hour were administered via an infusion pump at a constant rate for 5 minutes into a forearm vein of 6 subjects on 3 occasions, before and 10 minutes after intravenous chlorpheniramine 10 mg (an H_1-receptor antagonist), cimetidine 200 mg, or a combination of chlorpheniramine and cimetidine. Additional histamine doses of 160 and 320 μg/kg/hour were given after the combination of antagonists. The antagonists were randomised and the study was single-blind. One infusion of saline was included among each series of histamine infusions. The order of giving the saline infusion was unknown to the subject. Heart rate and blood pressure were recorded at 15- and 30-second intervals, respectively, for 1 minute before, during and 3 minutes after each infusion. Heart rate was measured with a heart rate meter and blood pressure with an automatic sphygmomanometer. The presence and distribution of flushing of the skin was noted, and at the end of each experiment the subject reported any symptoms. Heart rate was permitted to return to baseline and any flushing was allowed to resolve after an effective infusion of histamine.

STUDY 2

Rapid injections of impromidine were given into a forearm vein of 6 subjects via a 3-way tap connected to an intravenous cannula. Each injection of impromidine, diluted with saline to a constant volume, was flushed into the circulation with a fast-running saline drip connected to the remaining limb of the 3-way tap. Heart rate and blood pressure were recorded at 30-second intervals for 1 minute before and 8 minutes after injection of impromidine. Flushing and any symptoms were also recorded. Each subject was studied on 2 separate days, before and 10 minutes after intravenous cimetidine 200 mg or placebo. Treatment was randomised and the subject was unaware of the order of treatment. Doses of 0.05, 0.1, 0.2 and 0.3 mg of impromidine were given before and after placebo and before cimetidine; an additional dose of impromidine 0.4 mg was given after placebo; doses of 0.3, 0.6, 1.2, 1.8 and 2.4 mg of impromidine were given after cimetidine. One dose of saline was included among each series of impromidine doses, and the order of giving the saline infusion was unknown to the subject. Heart rate was permitted to return to baseline and any flushing was allowed to resolve after an effective dose of impromidine.

STUDY 3

Six subjects were given, on the same day and in a manner similar to the previous study, rapid intravenous injections of impromidine before (0.1, 0.2 and 0.3 mg) and 10 minutes after (0.6, 1.2 and 1.8 mg) intravenous cimetidine 200 mg. Blood pressure was recorded with an automatic sphygmomanometer before and at 1-minute intervals for 7 minutes after dosing with impromidine. In addition, heart rate, stroke volume, cardiac output and systolic time intervals were derived from the electrocardiogram and impedance cardiogram [14, 15] and continuously monitored on-line by a purpose-built minicomputer. Mean values for 25 heart beats were obtained for the time points when blood pressure was measured. Blood pressure and cardiac output values were used to calculate peripheral resistance.

Results

STUDY 1

Effects of histamine before treatment with the antagonists

Infusions of histamine caused dose-dependent flushing of the skin, falls in systolic and diastolic blood pressure and increases in heart rate. The time-response curves for systolic and diastolic blood pressure and heart rate for the 3 control experiments, 1 of which is shown in Figure 1, were similar in profile; the areas under the curves were not significantly different, indicating that the responses are reproducible. The changes in blood pressure were time- as well as dose-dependent. Systolic pressure fell maximally during the early phase of histamine infusion and thereafter tended to recover, despite continuing administration of histamine. Diastolic pressure fell concomitant with the early fall in systolic pressure, tended to recover slightly and then fell again in the late phase of the infusion. This secondary fall in diastolic pressure was best seen with the highest dose of histamine. The increases in heart rate were also time-dependent, heart rate tending to recover slightly during the mid-phase of histamine administration.

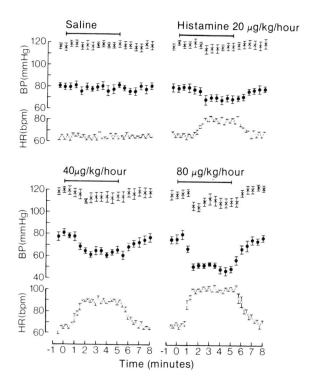

Fig. 1.   Histamine time-response curves before treatment with histamine antagonists. BP = systolic (x) and diastolic (•) blood pressure; HR = heart rate (○). (Mean ± SEM of 6 subjects.)

Table. Effect of chlorpheniramine and cimetidine, alone and in combination, on histamine-induced skin flushing.

| Antagonist | Subject | Saline | 5-minute infusion | | | | |
| | | | Histamine (µg/kg/hour) | | | | |
			20	40	80	160	320
Control*	1	—	+	+	+		
	2	—	+	+	+		
	3	—	+	+	+		
	4	—	+	+	+		
	5	—	+	+	+		
	6	—	+	+	+		
Chlorpheniramine	1	—	+	+	+		
	2	—	—	+	+		
	3	—	—	+	+		
	4	—	+	+	+		
	5	—	—	+	+		
	6	—	—	+	+		
Cimetidine	1	—	+	+	+		
	2	—	—	+	+		
	3	—	+	+	+		
	4	—	+	+	+		
	5	—	—	+	+		
	6	—	+	+	+		
Chlorpheniramine and cimetidine	1	—	—	+	+	+	+
	2	—	—	+	+	+	+
	3	—	—	—	+	+	+
	4	—	—	—	+	+	+
	5	—	—	—	—	+	+
	6	—	—	—	+	+	+

*Flushing occurred throughout the histamine dose range for all 3 control experiments. + = flushing present during infusion; — = flushing absent.

Flushing of the skin was observed in all subjects throughout the histamine dose range (Table). The distribution of flushing was dose-dependent: it first occurred on the face and then the neck, and tended to be confined to these areas with the lowest dose of histamine. As the dose of histamine was increased, flushing spread to involve the upper chest, upper limbs, lower chest, abdomen and lower limbs. Flushing of the lower legs and feet tended to occur only with the highest dose of histamine. Photographs of some subjects confirmed the impression that the *intensity* of the flush was also dose-dependent. All subjects experienced facial symptoms, usually described as a sensation of warmth, throughout the histamine dose-range. Some subjects reported more widely distributed skin symptoms and slight headache with the higher doses of histamine; overall, however, histamine was relatively well tolerated.

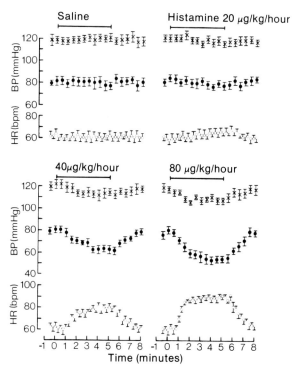

Fig. 2.   *Histamine time-response curves in the presence of chlorpheniramine. (Mean ± SEM of 6 subjects.)*

Effects of the antagonists

Chlorpheniramine alone. The H$_1$-antagonist attenuated the falls in systolic and diastolic blood pressure and the increase in heart rate, particularly during the early phase of histamine infusion and with the lowest dose of histamine (Fig. 2). Flushing and symptoms were abolished in 4 of the 6 subjects during the lowest dose of histamine (Table). Flushing was reduced in distribution during the higher doses of histamine, being confined to the upper part of the body.

Cimetidine alone. Cimetidine attenuated the fall in diastolic pressure and the increase in heart rate, particularly during the late phase of histamine infusion (Fig. 3). Systolic blood pressure was essentially unaffected. Flushing and symptoms were abolished in 2 subjects during the lowest dose of histamine (Table). Flushing was reduced in distribution during the higher doses, again being confined to the upper part of the body.

Chlorpheniramine and cimetidine in combination. The combination of antagonists abolished all effects of the 20 μg/kg/hour dose of histamine and caused greater attenuation of the flushing and diastolic blood pressure and heart rate changes induced by the 40 and 80 μg/kg/hour doses than was seen with either antagonist alone (Fig. 4 and Table). The combination was essentially no more effective than

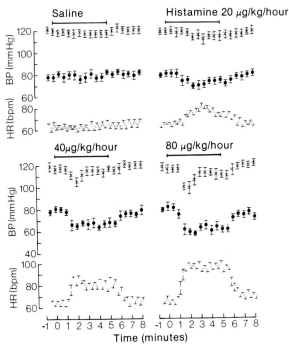

Fig. 3.   Histamine time-response curves in the presence of cimetidine. (Mean ± SEM of 6 subjects.)

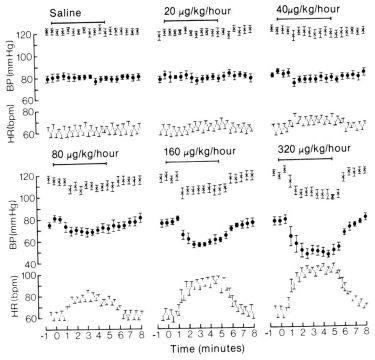

Fig. 4.   Histamine time-response curves in the presence of chlorpheniramine-cimetidine combination. (Mean ± SEM of 6 subjects.)

chlorpheniramine alone in modifying systolic blood pressure changes. Flushing was abolished in 4 subjects during the 40 µg/kg/hour dose, and in 1 subject during the 80 µg/kg/hour dose (Table). Even if flushing occurred with the 80 µg/kg/hour dose, it was usually confined to the face and neck. Two further doses of histamine 160 and 320 µg/kg/hour could be administered, thereby restoring the time-response curves for blood pressure and heart rate.

The time-dependent effects of the antagonists, alone and in combination, on the responses to the 80 µg/kg/hour histamine dose are seen more clearly in Figure 5.

Saline infusions

No subject experienced symptoms nor was flushing observed during any of the saline infusions (Table), and blood pressure and heart rate were essentially unchanged (Figs. 1-4).

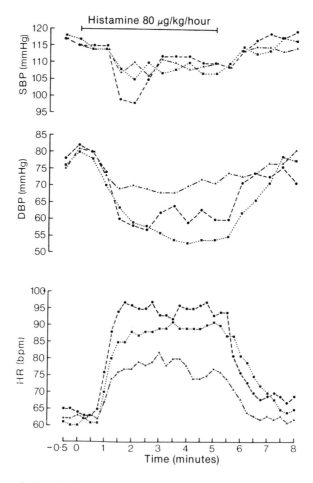

Fig. 5.   Effect of chlorpheniramine alone (■····■), cimetidine alone (●----●) and the combination (▲—▲) on systolic blood pressure (SBP), diastolic blood pressure (DBP) and heart rate changes induced by the infusion of histamine 80 µg/kg/hour for 5 minutes. (Mean of 6 subjects.)

STUDY 2

Control experiments with impromidine

Impromidine caused dose-dependent flushing (Fig. 6), falls in diastolic blood pressure and increases in heart rate (Fig. 7). Systolic blood pressure was essentially unchanged. There were no significant differences between the 3 control dose-response curves for changes in diastolic blood pressure and heart rate, indicating that the responses are reproducible. Flushing first appeared on the face and then neck and was confined to these areas with the smaller doses of impromidine. Larger doses of impromidine caused wider distribution of flushing in a manner similar to histamine. Again, photographs of some subjects confirmed the impression that the intensity of flushing was also dose-dependent. Flushing was usually accompanied by skin symptoms similar to those reported with histamine. None of the subjects experienced headache, and impromidine was well tolerated.

Effects of cimetidine

Compared with placebo, cimetidine caused significant displacement to the right of the dose-response curves for changes in diastolic blood pressure and heart rate ($p < 0.05$). Parallel-line assay showed that the dose-response curves were not significantly non-parallel. In the presence of cimetidine, no subject flushed after

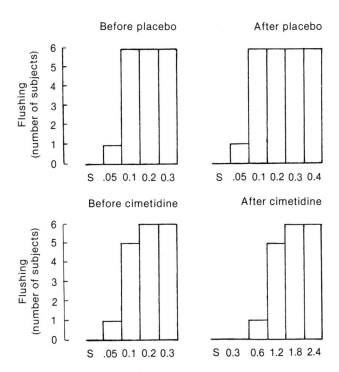

Fig. 6.   The effect of placebo and cimetidine on the presence of flushing induced by impromidine. Doses of impromidine are expressed in mg. S = saline.

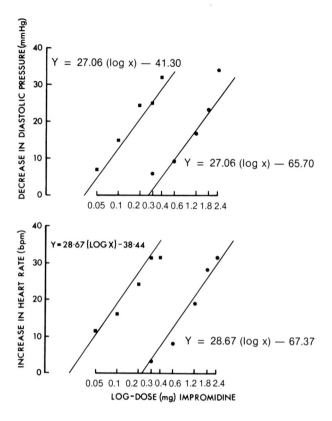

Fig. 7.   Effect of placebo (■) and cimetidine (●) on impromidine log dose-response curves for changes in diastolic pressure and heart rate. Values for impromidine 2.4 mg were omitted from the analysis. (Means of 6 subjects.)

impromidine 0.3 mg, whereas all subjects flushed extensively with this dose during control experiments. Flushing was restored as the dose of impromidine was increased (Fig. 6).

Saline injections

No subject experienced symptoms nor was flushing observed after any of the saline injections (Fig. 6), and blood pressure and heart rate were essentially unchanged.

STUDY 3

Control experiment

Impromidine 0.1-0.3 mg caused dose-dependent decreases in diastolic blood pressure, peripheral resistance (PR), pre-ejection period (PEP; onset of Q wave of electrocardiogram to onset of impedance cardiogram wave form, dZ/dt) and RZ interval (peak of R wave of electrocardiogram to peak of differentiated impedance cardiogram), and increases in heart rate, cardiac output (CO) and (dZ/dt)/RZ index

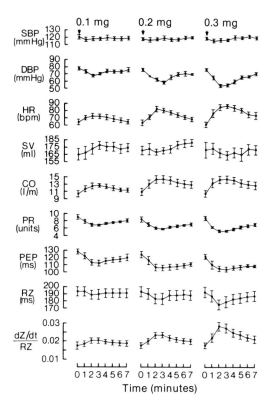

Fig. 8. Time-response curves for 3 doses of impromidine before treatment with cimetidine. (Mean ± SEM of 6 subjects.)

(Fig. 8). There were variable changes in stroke volume (SV), which tended to increase after the low dose of impromidine and to fall after the higher doses. Systolic blood pressure was again essentially unchanged.

Effects of cimetidine

Cimetidine antagonised the responses to impromidine. The larger doses of impromidine (0.6-1.8 mg) almost restored the time-response curves obtained during the control experiment (Fig. 9). Preliminary assessment of the data shows that the dose-response curves for changes in diastolic blood pressure, heart rate, peripheral resistance, cardiac output, pre-ejection period, RZ interval and (dZ/dt)/RZ ratio are displaced to the right in the presence of cimetidine.

Discussion

Infusions of histamine caused time- as well as dose-dependent changes in systolic and diastolic blood pressure. Rapid intravenous injections of histamine also cause falls in systolic and diastolic blood pressure; these falls are rapid in onset, transient and may be missed when blood pressure is recorded by the cuff method [Boyce and Wareham, unpublished observations]. The time of recording blood pressure and the

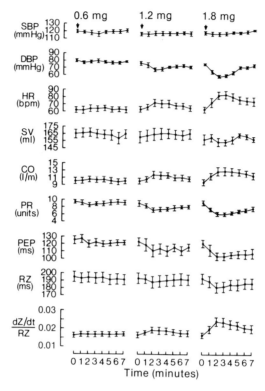

Fig. 9. Time-response curves for 3 doses of impromidine in the presence of cimetidine. (Mean ± SEM in 6 subjects.)

route of administration of histamine are therefore important factors in determining the blood pressure response to histamine, and may explain the variable results obtained in previous studies [1-7].

Chlorpheniramine and cimetidine each modified the blood pressure response to histamine in a time- and histamine dose-dependent manner. Chlorpheniramine alone attenuated the early falls in systolic blood pressure whereas cimetidine alone did not; the combination of antagonists was no more effective than chlorpheniramine alone in modifying systolic pressure changes. The combination was also no more effective than chlorpheniramine alone in reducing the overall changes in diastolic pressure induced by the smallest dose of histamine. When the dose of histamine was increased, however, the predominant effect of chlorpheniramine alone was to attenuate the early changes in diastolic pressure, giving a smoother profile to the time-response curves. The predominant effect of cimetidine alone on blood pressure was to attenuate late changes in diastolic pressure. These effects by histamine H_1- and H_2-receptor antagonists, alone and in combination, on the blood pressure responses to histamine are consistent with the existence of histamine H_1- and H_2-receptors in the peripheral blood vessels. That the dose-dependent flushing induced by histamine was also attenuated by chlorpheniramine or cimetidine alone, and to a greater extent by the combination, confirms that human skin blood vessels in particular contain both H_1- and H_2-receptors [10] which are widely distributed anatomically.

The antagonists modified heart rate responses in a manner similar to their modification of blood pressure. Chlorpheniramine alone tended to attenuate early increases in heart rate, whereas cimetidine tended to attenuate late increases. Again chlorpheniramine was as effective as the combination in modifying changes induced by the smallest dose of histamine, and the combination caused greater overall attenuation of the 40 and 80 μg/kg/hour histamine doses than either antagonist alone. These results are consistent with the existence of both histamine H_1- and H_2-receptors in the human heart. However, in vitro studies with human heart tissue indicate that the chronotropic response to histamine is mediated via H_2-receptors [16-18]. It seems likely, therefore, that secondary effects of histamine such as increased sympathetic tone, vagal withdrawal or catecholamine release from the adrenal medulla [19] contributed to the chronotropic response seen in our in vivo study.

In our second study impromidine, a specific H_2-receptor agonist, caused dose-dependent falls in diastolic pressure and increases in heart rate. In the presence of cimetidine, the log-dose response curves were displaced to the right, consistent with competitive antagonism at H_2-receptor sites in the peripheral blood vessels and heart. That impromidine flushing was also dose-dependent and antagonised by cimetidine provides further evidence for the existence of H_2-receptors in skin blood vessels [9].

The non-invasive method of impedance cardiography [14] was used in our third study to further explore the cardiovascular effects of impromidine. During the cardiac cycle a small impedance change occurs and a differentiator extracts the first time derivative of this impedance change, dZ/dt. In animals there is a linear relationship between dZ/dt and peak aortic flow, which forms the basis for calculating the stroke volume from thoracic impedance changes. PEP values derived from the impedance cardiogram show close correlation with those obtained from the carotid pulse [15], and PEP is a valid measure of left ventricular contractility in man [20]. The dZ/dt waveform can be used to obtain 2 additional measures of myocardial contractility, the RZ interval and the (dZ/dt)/RZ index [21, 22]. The results of our third study show that impromidine lowered diastolic pressure by reducing peripheral resistance. Although stroke volume increased with the lower dose of impromidine and fell with the higher dose, cardiac output increased throughout the impromidine dose-range. The dose-dependent reductions in PEP and RZ interval and increases in (dZ/dt)/RZ index are consistent with an inotropic effect of impromidine. All the responses to impromidine were antagonised by cimetidine. Preliminary assessment of the data shows that the dose-response curves for changes in diastolic blood pressure, heart rate, peripheral resistance, cardiac output and the contractility parameters are shifted to the right. These results are consistent with the interaction of impromidine at H_2-receptor sites on the peripheral blood vessels, causing vasodilatation, and the heart, causing positive chronotropic and inotropic responses. The cardiovascular effects of impromidine in man are therefore similar to those which have been obtained in experimental animals [23]. As with histamine, indirect cardiac effects mediated by reflexes associated with hypotension cannot be excluded. Catecholamine release from the adrenal medulla is unlikely, since this appears to be an H_1-receptor mediated phenomenon [19].

Chlorpheniramine slightly reduced baseline heart rate in the first study (see Fig. 5), perhaps related to the central sedative effect of this compound, as all subjects were drowsy. Otherwise, baseline cardiovascular parameters were essentially unchanged by the antagonists in any of the 3 studies. In normal subjects, oral cimetidine 1 g/day administered for 2 days did not affect the normal heart rate or blood pressure response to exercise, nor was the effect of β-blockade by propranolol exaggerated [24]. Resting heart rate, blood pressure and systolic time intervals of healthy subjects were essentially unchanged after oral cimetidine 1.6 g/day administered for 1 week [Warrington and Hamer, unpublished results].

Further studies with histamine agonists and antagonists should help establish whether cardiovascular histamine receptors play a role in health or disease in man.

Acknowledgements

D.D. Underwood of Smith Kline & French Maths Services analysed the data from the second study. The impedance study was carried out at the Clinical Research Centre, Northwick Park Hospital, in collaboration with Dr V. Balasubramanian.

References

1. Eppinger, H. (1913): Über eine eigentümliche Hautreaktion hervorgerufen durch Erga-min. *Wien. Klin. Wochenschr. 63,* 1414.
2. Harmer, I.M. and Harris, K.E. (1926): Observations on the vascular reactions in man in response to histamine. *Heart 13,* 381-394.
3. Weiss, S., Robb, G.P. and Blumgart, H.L. (1929): The velocity of blood flow in health and disease as measured by the effect of histamine on the minute vessels. *Am. Heart J. 4,* 664-691.
4. Weiss, S., Robb, G.P. and Ellis, L.B. (1932): The systemic effects of histamine in man. *Arch. Intern. Med. 49,* 360-396.
5. Peters, G.A., Horton, B.T. and Boothby, W.M. (1945): The effects of continuous intra-venous administration of histamine on basal metabolism in human beings. *J. Clin. Invest. 24,* 611-615.
6. Benson, A.J. and Horton, B.T. (1945): Effects of continuous intravenous administration of histamine on the blood pressure and pulse rates in cases of multiple sclerosis. *Mayo Clin. Proc. 20,* 113-119.
7. Wakim, K.G., Peters, G.A., Terrier, J.C. and Horton, B.T. (1949): The effects of intra-venously administered histamine on the peripheral circulation in man. *J. Lab. Clin. Med. 34,* 380-386.
8. Duff, F. and Welan, R.F. (1954): The effects of antihistamine substances on the response to histamine on the blood vessels of the human forearm. *Br. J. Pharmacol. 9,* 413-418.
9. Chipman, P. and Glover, W.E. (1976): Histamine H_2-receptors in the human peripheral circulation. *Br. J. Pharmacol. 56,* 494-496.
10. Greaves, M., Marks, R. and Robertson, I. (1977): Receptors for histamine in human skin blood vessels: a review. *Br. J. Dermatol. 97,* 225-228.
11. Owen, D.A.A. (1977): Histamine receptors in the cardiovascular system. *Gen. Pharma-col. 8,* 141-156.
12. Burland, W.L., Duncan, W.A.M., Hesselbo, T., Mills, J.G., Sharpe, P.C., Haggie, S.J. and Wyllie, J.H. (1975): Pharmacological evaluation of cimetidine, a new histamine H_2-receptor antagonist, in healthy man. *Br. J. Clin. Pharmacol. 2,* 481-486.
13. Durant, G.J., Duncan, W.A., Ganellin, C.R., Parsons, M.E., Blakemore, R.C. and Ras-mussen, A.C. (1978): Impromidine (SK&F-92676) is a very potent and specific agonist for histamine H_2-receptors. *Nature (London) 276,* 403-404.
14. Kubicek, W.G., Kottke, F.J., Ramos, M.U., Patterson, R.P., Witsoe, D.A., Labree, J.W., Remole, W., Layman, T.E., Schoening, H. and Garamela, J.T. (1974): The Minne-sota impedance cardiograph — theory and applications. *Biomed. Eng. (N.Y.) 9,* 410-416.
15. Balasubramanian, V., Mathew, O.P., Arun Behl, Tewari, S.C. and Hoon, R.S. (1978):

Electrical impedance cardiogram in derivation of systolic time intervals. *Br. Heart J. 40,* 268-275.

16. Wollemann, M. and Papp, J.Gy. (1979): Blockade by cimetidine of the effects of histamine on adenylate cyclase activity, spontaneous rate and contractility in the developing pre-natal heart. *Agents Actions 9,* 29-30.
17. Levi, R., Hordof, A., Edie, R. and Rosen, M. (1978): Histamine effects on human atria. *Circulation 58,* 105.
18. Gristwood, R.W., Lincoln, J.C.R. and Owen, D.A.A. (1980): Effects of histamine on human isolated heart muscle: comparison with effects of noradrenaline. *J. Pharm. Pharmacol.* (In press.)
19. Emmelin, N. and Muren, A. (1949): Effects of antihistamine compounds on adrenaline liberation from the suprarenals. *Acta Physiol. Scand. 17,* 345-355.
20. Sultan Ahmed, S., Levinson, G.E., Schwartz, C.J. and Ettinger, P.O. (1972): Systolic time intervals as measures of the contractile state of the left ventricular myocardium in man. *Circulation 46,* 559-571.
21. Siegel, J.H., Fabian, M., Lankav, C., Levine, M., Cole, A. and Nahmad, M. (1970): Clinical and experimental use of thoracic impedance plethysmography in quantifying myocardial contractility. *Surgery 67,* 907-917.
22. Hill, D.W. and Merrifield, A.J. (1976): Left ventricular ejection and the Heather index measured by non-invasive methods during postural changes in man. *Acta Anaesthesiol. Scand. 20,* 313-320.
23. Owen, D.A.A., Harvey, C.A. and Gristwood, R.W. (1979): Cardiovascular studies with impromidine (SK&F-92676), a new very potent and specific histamine H_2-receptor agonist. *J. Pharm. Pharmacol. 31,* 577-582.
24. Warburton, S., Opie, L.H., Kennelly, B.M. and Müller, F.O. (1979): Does cimetidine alter the cardiac response to exercise and propranolol? *S. Afr. Med. J. 55,* 1125-1127.

Discussion

Milton-Thompson (Gosport): Impromidine will be of interest to gastroenterologists because it has this specific H_2-agonist effect. When we were constructing our original dose-response curves, which Ms. Mills described earlier in this volume, the limiting factor about which we were concerned was the circulatory effects. For that reason, the dose was not increased beyond 20 μg/kg/hour by infusion; the main reason for that was that I was the subject involved, and did not want a higher dose to be given to me.

Would Dr. Boyce like to hazard a statement now, in the light of his experience, about what might be the maximum dose that can be safely used?

Boyce: My experience with impromidine is limited to the use of bolus injections. Dr. Burland is currently carrying out a study in normal subjects, using infusions of impromidine at doses of up to 50 μg/kg/hour. In the one subject so far studied there were falls in diastolic pressure and increases in heart rate. These cardiovascular responses were well-tolerated until reversed by intravenous cimetidine, when the subject became nauseated and vomited. Our work with bolus injections also suggests that the cardiovascular effects of impromidine should be permitted to resolve spontaneously.

Bertaccini: There seems to be some confusion about the type of histamine receptor involved in increases in vascular permeability. Could Dr. Owen please clarify this issue?

Owen: There are a number of points to be answered. The least clear aspect of the pharmacology of histamine-induced changes is the question of vascular permeability. Classically, from the time of the availability of H_1-receptor antagonists, researchers obtained the sort of data which I have shown on the guinea-pig ear, namely, that the H_1-receptor antagonists alone abolished the response to histamine.

There is, however, an increasing body of evidence that H_2-receptor antagonists can also inhibit this response. We have our own data in the cat skeletal muscle preparation, as I have shown. There are also some data in dog forelimb, recently reported from the United States, and also some studies on cat mesenteric vascular permeability in which the H_2-receptor antagonists were effective. In the case of the cat mesentery, the H_1-receptor antagonist was ineffective, a unique observation.

When it comes to the use of agonists, I am not sure whether the position has been clarified. I know of no instance where an H_1-receptor agonist failed to increase vascular permeability. In the 2 models that I have shown, H_1-receptor agonists are highly effective. Despite reports that H_2-receptor antagonists will inhibit the histamine response in some preparations, I know of no data that dimaprit, 4-methyl histamine or impromidine will increase vascular permeability.

Histamine receptors in human skin

M.W. Greaves and M.G. Davies
Institute of Dermatology, London, United Kingdom

There has recently been a renewal of interest in the basic and clinical pharmacology of histamine and antihistamines in the skin. A major factor has been the realisation that histamine is involved in a wider range of physiological and pathological events in the skin than was previously thought.

That histamine is involved in weal and flare reactions of the urticarial type was first proposed by Lewis in the 1920's [1]. Subsequent studies have given no grounds for major revision of this view, but studies of vascular and pharmacological changes occurring in the physical urticarias suggest that, at least in some forms of urticaria, other vasoactive mediators may be involved [2, 3]. It is now becoming increasingly clear that histamine is involved in the pathogenesis of skin lesions due to circulating immune complexes [4]. Histamine, released from basophils and platelets, permits sub-endothelial penetration of immune complexes in cutaneous venules, leading in turn to complement activation, vascular damage, granulocyte accumulation and leucocytoclasis. Histamine also plays an important regulatory role in delayed hyper-sensitivity reactions in the skin, including allergic contact dermatitis. Immigration of basophil leucocytes into affected skin is a feature of allergic contact reactions [5], and histamine released from these cells may regulate T-lymphocyte function through receptors on the T-lymphocyte cell membrane [6]. Histamine may also be important in non-immunological function of the skin. Epidermal cells bear histamine H_2-receptors [7], and the possibility should be entertained that histamine, derived from the dermis, may exert a regulatory role on epidermal cell growth and differentiation, possibly through a cyclic AMP-dependent mechanism.

It is widely recognised by clinicians that systemic antihistamine therapy is of variable and often rather poor effectiveness in the therapy of histamine-mediated skin diseases, including urticaria and eczema, and a number of explanations have been put forward to explain this fact. Clearly, mediators other than histamine could be responsible for the observed inflammatory changes. Because they combine with non-histamine receptors, these mediators would not be inhibited by antihistamines. Possible mediators include bradykinin, slow-reacting substance of anaphylaxis (SRS-A), prostaglandins and other hydroxy-acid metabolites of arachidonic acid. On the other hand, local concentrations of histamine in inflamed tissues may reach such high levels that systemically-administered antihistamines are ineffective, as suggested by Dale [8]. The discovery in 1966 of 2 subclasses of histamine receptor, subsequently termed H_1 and H_2, has provided an additional attractive explanation of the low effectiveness of classical (H_1) antihistamines [9].

Evidence for the representation of both classes of histamine receptor on human skin blood vessels has been obtained by study of the responses of human skin to synthetic histamine analogues in vitro. The synthetic histamine analogues 2-methyl histamine and 4-methyl histamine possess predominantly H_1- and H_2-agonist activity, respectively [10]. Intradermal injection of either of these agents causes local erythema and wealing; in addition, 2-methyl histamine (but not 4-methyl histamine) causes an axon reflex flare, since the flare due to 2-methyl histamine readily traverses an elastic band applied tightly adjacent to the site of injection [11]. In order to investigate the vascular responses to 2-methyl histamine and 4-methyl histamine further, dose-response curves were constructed for erythema and wealing due to intradermal injection of these agents in 17 healthy volunteer subjects [11]. These curves were repeated, after a 5-day interval, 2 hours after systemic administration of chlorpheniramine 4 mg and, after a further 5-day interval, 2 hours after cimetidine 200 mg given systemically. The results are illustrated in Figures 1 and 2. The dose-response curves for wealing for both 2-methyl histamine and 4-methyl histamine were flat, and no influence of the drug treatments on the magnitude of the weals could be discerned. In contrast, chlorpheniramine caused significant suppression of the area of erythema at the 2 highest doses ($p < 0.01$). Cimetidine had no detectable effect on erythema due to 2-methyl histamine. The erythema results with 4-methyl histamine were of particular interest: as expected, cimetidine caused significant suppression of erythema at all 3 doses ($p < 0.05$); however, chlorpheniramine unexpectedly also produced significant suppression of erythema for the 2 higher doses ($p < 0.025$). This could be due to lack of specificity of either 4-methyl histamine or chlorpheniramine; alternatively, 4-methyl histamine could have caused release of endogenous histamine in the injected skin. Taken as a whole, these studies provide persuasive evidence that human skin blood vessels bear both H_1- and H_2-receptors.

More recently, we investigated the role of histamine H_1- and H_2-receptors in the production of itching, using 4-methyl histamine and dimaprit as H_2-agonists, and 2-methyl histamine as an H_1-agonist [12]. The method used was that of Greaves and McDonald-Gibson [13]. Forearm skin was scarified until the stratum corneum was breached and the stratum Malpighii exposed. Overt bleeding, indicating dermal

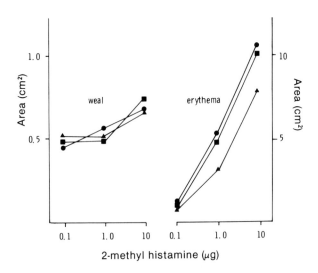

Fig. 1.   Weal and erythema responses to intradermal injection of 2-methyl histamine after placebo (•), chlorpheniramine 4 mg (▲), and cimetidine 200 mg (■). Each point represents the mean of observations in 17 subjects.

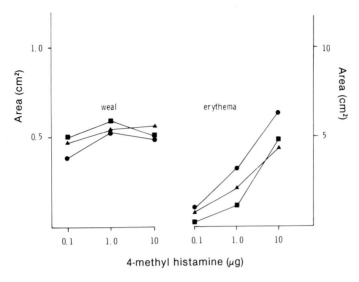

Fig. 2. Weal and erythema responses to intradermal injection of 4-methyl histamine after placebo (•), chlorpheniramine 4 mg (▲), and cimetidine 200 mg (■). Each point represents the mean of observations in 17 subjects.

damage, was avoided. The itch threshold for each agonist was determined by applying progressively increasing concentrations to the scarified site until the subject became conscious of itching (defined as a desire to scratch).

Twelve subjects were studied, and it was found that, over a wide range of concentrations, neither dimaprit nor 4-methyl histamine caused itching. However, 2-methyl histamine caused itching at a threshold concentration of 0.565 ± 0.15 mM/l (mean ± SEM). It is interesting to compare this value with the mean threshold concentration of histamine required to produce itching in the same subjects (Table). On a molar basis, the threshold concentration of histamine for itching was about half that of 2-methyl histamine. Administration of oral chlorpheniramine 4 mg 2 hours before determination of itch threshold caused the itch threshold for histamine to rise almost three times, but chlorpheniramine caused the itch threshold for 2-methyl histamine to rise by almost 5 times. Pre-treatment of scarified skin with either 4-methyl histamine or dimaprit did not lower the itch threshold for either histamine or 2-methyl histamine.

Tachyphylaxis for itching was studied using both histamine and 2-methyl histamine, and could be produced by both agents. While tachyphylaxis due to 2-methyl histamine could be overcome by the use of high concentrations of histamine, tachyphylaxis due to histamine persisted despite the application of high concentrations of 2-methyl histamine.

This data indicates that H_1-receptors, but not H_2-receptors, are involved in the production of histamine itching. However, the differences in response between histamine and 2-methyl histamine suggest that receptors other than histamine H_1- or H_2-receptors are also involved. Although there could be an additional subclass of histamine receptor, other non-histamine receptors may be affected, for example receptors for oligopeptides such as bradykinin, or short-chain fatty acid derivatives of arachidonic acid such as prostaglandins or non-prostaglandin hydroxy-acids. It is

Table.   Itch thresholds (mean ± SD) for histamine and 2-methyl histamine with and without prior administration of oral chlorpheniramine 4 mg.

Group	Number of subjects	Histamine (mM/l)	2-methyl histamine (mM/l)
Control	12	0.266 ± 0.028	0.565 ± 0.150
Chlorpheniramine	12	0.712 ± 0.221	2.813 ± 1.209

of interest that histamine is known to evoke prostaglandin formation in some tissues [14].

The presence of histamine H_1- and H_2-receptors on skin blood vessels has prompted exploration of the possibility that combined therapy with histamine H_1- or H_2-antagonists might be more effective in the suppression of histamine-mediated inflammatory reactions in the skin than therapy with either type of antihistamine by itself. This proposition was initially examined by studying the influence of H_1- and H_2-antihistamines alone and in combination on erythema and wealing due to several doses of intradermally-injected histamine and the histamine liberator compound 48/80. The trial was carried out in 12 healthy volunteer subjects on a randomised, double-blind basis [15]. It was found that both oral cimetidine 200 mg and oral chlorpheniramine 4 mg caused significant displacement of the dose-response curve for histamine erythema and wealing, when compared with placebo. Treatment with both cimetidine 200 mg and chlorpheniramine 4 mg caused a greater displacement of the histamine erythemal dose-response curve than either drug alone or placebo; the combination treatment was not, however, significantly more suppressive of wealing than either drug given singly. Broadly similar results were obtained on erythema and wealing due to compound 48/80. These findings were sufficiently encouraging to prompt exploration of the possible use of histamine H_2-receptor antagonists in therapy of inflammatory skin diseases due to histamine, some of which are reported elsewhere in this volume.

In conclusion, human skin blood vessels bear both H_1- and H_2-receptors, which mediate erythema and increased vascular permeability due to histamine. In addition, the histamine-induced axon reflex flare appears to involve H_1-receptors. Histamine-induced itching appears to be an H_1-receptor effect, but other receptors which are not H_2-receptors and which may be non-histamine in nature may also be involved. Experimentally-induced histamine erythema is more effectively suppressed by combined treatment with oral chlorpheniramine and cimetidine than by treatment with either drug alone. This has prompted exploration of the possible advantages of the combination in the clinical situation.

Acknowledgement

We thank the Sir Herbert Dunhill Trust for financial support for this study.

References

1. Lewis, T. (1927): *Blood vessels of the human skin and their responses,* p. 106. Shaw and Sons Ltd., London.

2. Bentley-Phillips, C.B., Eady, R.A.J. and Greaves, M.W. (1978): Cold urticaria: inhibition of cold-induced histamine release by doxantrazole. *J. Invest. Dermatol. 71,* 266.

3. Keahey, T.M. and Greaves, M.W. (1980): Cold urticaria: disassociation of cold-evoked histamine release and urticaria following cold challenge. *Arch. Dermatol. 116,* 174.

4. Kniker, W.T. and Cochrane, C.G. (1978): The localisation of circulating immune complexes in experimental serum sickness: the role of vasoactive amines and hydrodynamic forces. *J. Exp. Med. 127,* 119.

5. Wolf-Jurgensen, P. (1962): Cytological examination of experimental contact allergy using the skin window technique. *Acta Allergol. 17,* 547.

6. Rocklin, R.E. (1976): Modulation of cellular immune responses in vivo and in vitro by histamine receptor-bearing lymphocytes. *J. Clin. Invest. 57,* 1051.

7. Iizuka, H., Adachi, K., Halprin, K.M. and Levine, V. (1976): Histamine H_2-receptor adenylate cyclase system in pig skin (epidermis). *Biochim. Biophys. Acta 437,* 150.

8. Dale, H.H. (1948): Antihistamine substances. *Br. Med. J. 2,* 281.

9. Ash, A.S.F. and Schild, H.O. (1966): Receptors mediating some actions of histamine. *Br. J. Pharmacol. 27,* 427.

10. Black, J.W., Duncan, W.A.M., Durant, C.J., Ganellin, C.R. and Parsons, E.M. (1972): Definition and antagonism of histamine H_2-receptors. *Nature (London) 236,* 385.

11. Robertson, I. and Greaves, M.W. (1978): Responses of human skin blood vessels to synthetic histamine analogues. *Br. J. Clin. Pharmacol. 5,* 319.

12. Davies, M.G. and Greaves, M.W. (1980): Sensory responses of human skin to synthetic histamine analogues and histamine. *Br. J. Clin. Pharmacol.* (In press.)

13. Greaves, M.W. and McDonald-Gibson, W. (1973): Itch: the role of prostaglandins. *Br. Med. J. 2,* 608.

14. Blackwell, G.J., Flower, R.J., Nijkamp, F.P. and Vane, J.R. (1978): Phospholipase A2 activity of guinea-pig isolated and perfused lungs: stimulation and inhibition by anti-inflammatory steroids. *Br. J. Pharmacol. 62,* 79.

15. Marks, R. and Greaves, M.W. (1977): Vascular reactions to histamine and compound 48/80 in human skin: suppression by a histamine H_2-receptor blocking agent. *Br. J. Clin. Pharmacol. 4,* 367.

The results of clinical investigative studies with H_1- and H_2-antagonists in skin diseases

R. Marks and J. Horton*

*Department of Medicine, Welsh National School of Medicine, Heath Park, Cardiff; and *The Research Institute, Smith Kline & French Laboratories, Welwyn Garden City, United Kingdom*

Introduction

The debate as to whether it is serendipity or assiduous directed research which results in more useful drugs is enjoyable, persistent and not resolvable. It should be remembered, for example, that tetracyclines were first prescribed for acne and rosacea because it seemed that an antimicrobial effect was desirable, yet the observed success of the tetracyclines in the treatment of these diseases is probably due to their anti-inflammatory or anti-chemotactic effects, rather than to an 'antibiotic' action. Similarly, dapsone, which has been used with such good effect in the treatment of dermatitis herpetiformis, was originally prescribed because of its usefulness in treating leprosy; it was entirely serendipitous that the suppressive effect for dermatitis herpetiformis was found.

The commitment to finding an H_2-receptor antagonist which is effective in controlling gastric acid secretion and the ultimate success with cimetidine have quite accidentally provided dermatologists with the possibility of a new therapeutic tool. Is this serendipity or directed research?

In the present paper, we will present the results of some of our studies on the clinical use of cimetidine in dermatological conditions and, also, we will present a general review of this area. We hope that this will place the use of cimetidine in the treatment of skin disease in some perspective, and will perhaps provide some guidance for further clinical research.

Urticaria

We give a single simple name to this reaction, which is the final common pathway for a variety of transient or recurrent inflammatory disorders of the skin [1]. It has become customary to qualify the term urticaria with an identified aetiology such as solar urticaria, cold urticaria or penicillin urticaria; it may also be the manifestation of dermatitis herpetiformis, mastocytosis, Schönlein-Henoch purpura, a rare form of inherited amyloidosis, ascariasis or a paraproteinaemia. Clearly, every effort must be made to uncover any aetiological agency; unfortunately, the only qualification one can give to the great majority of urticarial disorders is 'annoying', since, despite exhaustive investigation, no aetiological agency can be discovered.

This 'idiopathic' group is the dermatologist's nightmare. Conventional H_1-antagonists are only marginally helpful, and then primarily in patients with urticaria of recent onset. Exclusion diets, psychotherapy and avoidance of acetylsalicylic acid are usually tried in turn, singly, in combination, and both with and without H_1-antagonists; patients so treated return to the clinic month after month with their urticarial symptoms intact.

Obviously, the advent of a more efficient means of histamine blockade raises the hopes of both physician and patient for a more efficient treatment of this disease, although it must be pointed out that new, more efficient treatments do not absolve the medical attendant from the responsibility of making a proper diagnosis. Antihistamines are suppressive agents, and should only be administered when the provoking cause of the urticaria cannot be identified and removed. In addition, it should be noted that histamine release may not be the only mechanism of urticaria: it has been suspected that the kinins are involved in some of the physical urticarias, and it is possible that the prostaglandins are responsible for at least the erythema in some urticarial diseases.

The rationale for the use of cimetidine in combination with an H_1-antagonist for the treatment of urticaria stems from the work of Marks and Greaves [2] and Robertson and Greaves [3], which is described by Greaves elsewhere in this volume. These workers found significant reduction in the flare response after the intracutaneous injection of histamine or H_1- and H_2-agonists when combined with cimetidine, as compared with the use of either the H_1- or the H_2-antagonist given alone. The weal response behaved less predictably, but was significantly better-suppressed with the combination than with either drug alone. Our own work, which is discussed in more detail below, has demonstrated that the threshold for pruritus induced by intracutaneous histamine or papain is significantly increased after administration of the cimetidine and H_1-antagonist combination, as compared with the use of the antagonists individually [4]; however, contradictory results obtained by Hagermark et al. [5] should also be mentioned: these authors blocked the 'axon reflex' with lidocaine, injected the antagonists with the histamine locally, and then found that 'H_2-receptors do not seem to be involved' in the skin response to histamine, other than in the 'direct vasodilatory response to histamine'. This appears to have been a very carefully-conducted experiment, but it is difficult to interpret because of the large number of materials injected at the same site, which may well have traumatised the area sufficiently to confuse the responses.

There have been 2 controlled trials of combined H_1- and H_2-antagonists in chronic idiopathic urticaria [6, 7], and 2 controlled studies with results which have not yet been fully analysed. In addition, there have been several open studies in which the effectiveness of the combination has been assessed [8, 9]. Unfortunately, although all of these studies employed a minimum dosage of cimetidine 1.6 g/day and chlorpheniramine 16 mg/day, a variety of criteria and protocols were used, making confident conclusions difficult. The study by Commens and Greaves used a 14-day double-blind cross-over design to compare the effects of chlorpheniramine, a combination of chlorpheniramine and cimetidine, and placebo [6]; both treatments were better than placebo and, although the combination seemed to give numerical superiority, the observed benefit was not statistically significant. The study by Shuster's group did not show any benefit from the combination of cimetidine and chlorpheniramine over chlorpheniramine alone, but there was no placebo treatment period in this study, and there were several dropouts [7]. The Phanuphak et al. study used a combination of cyproheptadine and cimetidine for a 10-day period and found that 50% of patients with resistant chronic urticaria (4 of 8!) responded with

Table I.   Effects of chlorpheniramine, cimetidine and the combination on dermographism, assessed by response to scratch by stylus in 16 patients allocated at random to 3 consecutive 2-week treatments. Data has been extracted from [10].

	Stylus setting	Chlorphen- iramine	Cimetidine	Combination
Mean weal	8	2.3	2.2	1.9
diameter (mm)	12	3.3	2.9	2.7
Mean flare	8	2.3	15.9	4.4
diameter (mm)	12	5.4	21.9	4.6
Overall assessment				
Improved		5	2	7
No change		2	3	7
Worse		8	10	1

90% or greater improvement [8]. Munro, at St. Bartholomew's Hospital in London, has completed a study of 25 patients with chronic urticaria treated with cimetidine 600 mg/day and either chlorpheniramine 16 mg/day or mebhydrolin 150 mg/day [9]; 18 of these patients showed either complete or marked improvement and 4 showed partial improvement. Treatment could be withdrawn completely from 5 individuals, while the others have remained well on maintenance treatment of up to 1 year.

Patients with severe dermographism were studied by Warin in Bristol [10] and Shuster in Newcastle [11]. These studies, which employed standardised stimuli and a double-blind design, demonstrated that the combination of cimetidine and chlorpheniramine was effective in suppressing weal formation. In the Bristol study, the 'overall assessment' certainly indicated that the combination was best (Table I); unfortunately, no placebo was used and it is difficult to draw quantitative and confident conclusions from the study because of this. There is an anecdotal observation which should be mentioned here, concerning the effect of therapy in patients with urticaria or dermographism. From an examination of patient records, it seems that the longer the urticaria or dermographism has been present prior to initiating treatment, the more effective combination therapy will be: patients who have had either of these complaints for more than 6 months are more likely to respond to treatment than those who have had urticaria or dermographism for a shorter time; if either complaint has been present for more than 1 year, two-thirds of the patients treated are likely to respond favourably, as assessed by patient preference and physician's overall assessment.

Pruritus

Easton and Galbraith reported the relief of intractable pruritus due to polycythaemia vera in a patient after treatment with 'combined antagonists' [12], and there have been a few other such anecdotal reports [13]. However, our own experience in such patients has not been very encouraging, although the doses we administered (no more than 1 g/day of cimetidine) may have been too low to be

Table II. Results of treatment of histamine- and papain-induced pruritus with H_1- and H_2-antagonists [4]. All values are mean thresholds to itch (means of the denominators of the highest dilutions causing itch) ± SD.

	Initial threshold	Placebo	Chlorphen-iramine	Cimetidine	Combination
Histamine dilution	144.9 ± 68.0	74.7 ± 58.8	55.6 ± 58.8	100.8 ± 83.1	22.8 ± 18.0*
Papain dilution	32.7 ± 25.4	29.0 ± 36.8	18.0 ± 17.8	19.7 ± 16.4	12.7 ± 17.9**

* = significantly less than placebo ($p < 0.005$) or cimetidine ($p < 0.01$); ** = significantly less than placebo ($p < 0.05$).

conclusive [14]. Harrison et al. did not find cimetidine of any help in relieving the pruritus of biliary cirrhosis [15].

We have examined the effect of chlorpheniramine 16 mg/day and cimetidine 1.6 g/day on itch induced by the technique of Greaves and McDonald-Gibson [16], in which histamine and papain solutions are applied 'intraepidermally' using light scarification [4]. Twelve healthy volunteers had their itch thresholds determined before and after 4 treatment periods of 3 days each, during which cimetidine, chlorpheniramine, a combination of these 2 drugs or placebo was administered. The results (Table II) indicate that the combination of H_1- and H_2-antagonists was more effective than either alone and, therefore, that H_2-receptors may well be involved in the mediation of the sensation of itch. This study also demonstrated the 'power of the placebo', which also significantly raised the threshold for itch!

Solar urticaria

Magnus studied the effect of monochromatic light on weal and flare production in 8 patients with solar urticaria after random double-blind allocation to 4 weeks' treatment with either chlorpheniramine, cimetidine, chlorpheniramine and cimetidine combination, or placebo [17]; both chlorpheniramine and the combination were significantly more effective than cimetidine alone or the placebo in reducing weal and

Table III. The results of treatment of solar urticaria with placebo, cimetidine, chlorpheniramine or the combination [17]. Weal and flare areas are given as the difference between pre- and post-treatment responses, and expressed in millimeters.

Treatment period (minutes)	Placebo		Cimetidine		Chlorpheniramine		Combination	
	Weal	Flare	Weal	Flare	Weal	Flare	Weal	Flare
5-15	4.0	17.4	3.1	86.9	10.5	225.0	13.5	206.4
20-30	2.6	17.8	11.7	28.3	16.0	224.1	15.7	144.7
35-50	1.4	−30.3	15.8	55.7	16.6	180.4	21.7	133.4
0-70	2.8	−52.7	7.4	17.0	15.0	164.6	15.2	107.6

flare. Compared with placebo, cimetidine alone significantly reduced the weal area at some time points (Table III).

Ultraviolet light-induced erythema

It appears from the studies of the Greaves group in London that a major part of the erythematous response to ultraviolet light is induced by the release of prostaglandins. However, not all the response at all times and to all wavelengths appears to be due to this class of mediators, and it seems more than possible that histamine may mediate part of the reaction. We devised 2 studies to examine this possibility: in both of them, 12 healthy volunteers were given twice the previously-determined minimal erythema dose on the back 4 times over a 4-week period; for the first study, either placebo, cimetidine, chlorpheniramine or a combination of cimetidine and chlorpheniramine was administered during the treatment periods while, in the second study, the alternative regimens were placebo, cimetidine, indometacin or a combination of cimetidine and indometacin. The erythema was assessed 6 and 8 hours after irradiation, on a 4 point arbitrary scale, and the results indicate that none of the treatment schedules significantly suppressed the erythema (Table IV). However, there was a definite suggestion of benefit in the period of treatment with chlorpheniramine and cimetidine, and it has to be admitted that the reason for the lack of significance in the results may well be the insensitive arbitrary scale used for assessment of erythema.

Table IV.   Results of H_1- and H_2-antagonists and indometacin in the suppression of ultraviolet light-induced erythema.

Assessment time after irradiation	Cimetidine	Chlorpheniramine	Combination	Placebo
6 hours	1.17	1.33	1.17	1.83
8 hours	2.00	2.08	1.67	2.00
Assessment time after irradiation	Cimetidine	Indometacin	Combination	Placebo
6 hours	0.95	0.77	0.77	0.95
8 hours	1.45	1.18	1.27	1.09

Psoriasis

This disorder affects some 2% of most populations examined and, as yet, treatment for it leaves much to be desired. Clearly, much interest surrounds the possible value of a 'combined attack' on histamine, as histamine may well play a role in the heightened epidermal cell production in a number of inflammatory dermatoses, including psoriasis. There certainly appear to be histamine receptors on keratinocytes [18].

Several anecdotal case reports have found their way into the literature suggesting that cimetidine may hasten resolution of psoriasis, such as that of Giacosa and others in a letter to the *Lancet* in December 1978 [19], but they are not very convincing. Wells, at Guy's Hospital in London, has used cimetidine treatment in several patients with psoriasis, and apparently some benefit has resulted. We have started a full double-blind study with a Latin Square design in which chlorphenira-mine, cimetidine, the combination or placebo is administered, and we hope to report on this shortly.

We have, in addition, just completed an investigation into the effect of histamine antagonists on epidermopoiesis, both stimulated and unstimulated. Sixteen normal volunteer subjects had an area on 1 forearm 'stripped' with adhesive tape to remove the stratum corneum and stimulate epidermal cell production over a 1-inch square site. Groups of 4 subjects were given either cimetidine, chlorpheniramine, the com-bination or placebo. The stripped site and the contralateral 'unstripped' skin were then biopsied. The biopsies were then sliced in half, 1 half being prepared histolo-gically and the other half being incubated for a 4-hour period in the presence of tri-tiated thymidine so as to label cells in the DNA synthesis phase of the mitotic cycle. Autoradiographs were then made. The histologically-prepared specimens were studied histometrically by methods we have previously established [20, 21], to ob-tain epidermal measurements. The autoradiographs were examined for labelled cells and the labelling indices determined. The results are shown in Tables V and VI; although they were not statistically significant, it appears that both H₁- and H₂-antagonists may decrease epidermal cell division in both stimulated and unstimula-

Table V. Effect of H₁- and H₂-antagonists on epidermal cell production and epidermal dimensions in unstimulated forearm skin (mean ± SD).

Treatment group	Labelling index (%)	MET (number of cells)	MET (μ)	MKh (μ)
Placebo	8.43 ± 2.8	3.98 ± 0.6	49.73 ± 4.1	12.60 ± 1.0
Chlorpheniramine	5.90 ± 1.2	3.42 ± 0.6	41.76 ± 2.5	12.34 ± 1.2
Cimetidine	5.88 ± 1.8	4.02 ± 0.3	49.18 ± 6.0	12.23 ± 1.0
Combination	5.53 ± 2.0	3.90 ± 0.6	50.97 ± 4.1	13.17 ± 0.9

MET = mean epidermal thickness; MKh = mean keratinocyte height (MET/μ).

Table VI. Effect of H₁- and H₂-antagonists on epidermal cell production and epidermal dimensions in 'stripped' forearm skin (mean ± SD).

Treatment group	Labelling index (%)	MET (number of cells)	MET (μ)	MKh (μ)
Placebo	28.55 ± 7.6	5.43 ± 1.0	72.97 ± 15.5	13.70 ± 1.8
Chlorpheniramine	21.02 ± 11.2	4.23 ± 0.5	52.96 ± 10.5	12.49 ± 1.6
Cimetidine	25.60 ± 14.1	4.58 ± 0.8	62.51 ± 13.4	13.59 ± 1.0
Combination	26.83 ± 8.4	4.57 ± 0.7	67.91 ± 10.5	15.02 ± 2.3

MET = mean epidermal thickness; MKh = mean keratinocyte height (MET/μ).

ted epidermis. Further studies, seeking to unravel the role of histamine in the epidermal component of the inflammatory dermatoses, are under way.

Other conditions

Atopic dermatitis is a common intractable and disabling dermatosis, and any possibility of helping patients with this condition should be pursued. In view of the persistent pruritus, the abnormal vascular responses, depressed delayed hypersensitivity and abnormal immediate hypersensitivity, it is reasonable to suggest that total histamine blockade with combined H_1- and H_2-antagonists may give some relief. Several controlled double-blind studies have been initiated, and we await the results with interest.

Histamine is released at an early stage in wounding and after thermal injury. It can reasonably be expected that H_1- and H_2-antagonists might reduce the inflammatory response consequent on such injury. Yoshioka et al. described beneficial effects on oedema formation in burns in rats [22], and we look forward to seeing the results of comparable clinical studies.

Lyons et al. found that cimetidine alone decreased sebum secretion rate in 10 patients with acne over a 6-week period [23]. Studies are under way to determine whether this is an H_2-receptor effect or an independent weak anti-androgenic effect [24]. This has fascinating implications and, if confirmed, will indicate that cimetidine could well play an important role in the treatment of acne.

In mastocytosis there are abnormal collections of mast cells which, after stimulation, release histamine, which is responsible for a variety of symptoms. Gerrard and Ko described a patient who was considerably helped by a combination of cimetidine and chlorpheniramine [25], and it is quite likely that similar patients will also be helped by such treatment.

It is clear that the role of histamine in modulating the immune response is both profound and complex. All aspects of the immune response seem affected by the elaboration of histamine and many of the cells involved appear to possess histamine receptors on their surfaces [26, 27]. It is possible that, in the future, such putative auto-immune disorders as alopecia areata and vitiligo, as well as some varieties of vasculitis and dermatitis herpetiformis, could be aided by treatment with H_1- and H_2-antagonists.

Conclusions

There is good evidence for the presence of H_2-receptors on skin blood vessels and some evidence to suggest their involvement in the mediation of itch. There is increasing evidence for the usefulness of a combination of cimetidine 1.6 g/day and chlorpheniramine 16 mg/day in the treatment of urticaria and dermographism. There is some slight evidence to suggest that cimetidine may be useful in the treatment of certain types of burn (including sunburn). In addition, cimetidine may have a place in the treatment of psoriasis and acne. However, many more studies are required to pinpoint the usefulness of the combination of H_1- and H_2-antagonists in these and other skin disorders.

References

1. Warin, R.P. and Champion, R.H. (1974): *Urticaria*. W.B. Saunders Company Limited, Eastbourne.
2. Marks, R. and Greaves, M.W. (1977) Vascular reactions to histamine and compound 48/80 in human skin: suppression by a histamine H₂-receptor blocking agent. *Br. J. Clin. Pharmacol. 4*, 367.
3. Robertson, I. and Greaves, M.W. (1978): Responses of human skin blood vessels to synthetic histamine analogues. *Br. J. Clin. Pharmacol. 5*, 319.
4. Davies, M.G. and Marks, R. (1979): The efficacy of histamine antagonists as antipruritics in experimentally-induced pruritus. *Arch. Dermatol. Res. 266*, 117.
5. Hagermark, O., Strandberg, K. and Gronneberg, R. (1979): Effects of histamine receptor antagonists on histamine-induced responses in human skin. *Acta Derm.-Venereol. 59*, 297.
6. Commens, C.A. and Greaves, M.W. (1978): Cimetidine in chronic idiopathic urticaria: a randomised double-blind study. *Br. J. Dermatol. 99*, 675.
7. Shuster, S. (1978): *The effect of cimetidine and chlorpheniramine in the treatment of idiopathic urticaria*. Smith Kline & French Report No. D 176, Welwyn Garden City.
8. Phanuphak, P., Schocket, A. and Kohler, P.F. (1978): Treatment of chronic idiopathic urticaria with combined H₁- and H₂-blockers. *Clin. Allergy 8*, 429.
9. Munro, D. (1978): *Cimetidine in the treatment of idiopathic and physical urticaria*. Smith Kline & French Report No. D 165, Welwyn Garden City.
10. Matthews, C.N.A., Boss, J.M., Warin, R.P. and Storari, F. (1979): The effect of H₁- and H₂-histamine antagonists on symptomatic dermographism. *Br. J. Dermatol. 101*, 57.
11. Shuster, S. and Cook, J. (1978): *The effect of cimetidine and chlorpheniramine in the treatment of dermographism*. Smith Kline & French Report No. D 186, Welwyn Garden City.
12. Easton, P. and Galbraith, P.R. (1978): Cimetidine treatment of pruritus in polycythemia vera. *N. Engl. J. Med. 299*, 1134.
13. Hess, C.E. (1979): Cimetidine for the treatment of pruritus. *N. Engl. J. Med. 300*, 370.
14. Scott, G.L. and Horton, R.J. (1979): Pruritus, cimetidine and polycythemia. *N. Engl. J. Med. 300*, 434.
15. Harrison, A.R., Littenberg, G., Goldstein, L. and Kaplowitz, N. (1979): Pruritus, cimetidine and polycythemia. *N. Engl. J. Med. 300*, 433.
16. Greaves, M.W. and McDonald-Gibson, W. (1973): Itch: role of prostaglandins. *Br. Med. J. 3*, 608.
17. Magnus, I.A. (1977): *Cimetidine dermatology studies: solar urticaria*. Smith Kline & French Report No. D 110, Welwyn Garden City.
18. Harper, R.A., Flaxman, B.A. and Chopra, D.P. (1974): Mitotic response of normal and psoriatic keratinocytes in vitro to compounds known to affect intracellular cyclic AMP. *J. Invest. Dermatol. 62*, 384.
19. Giacosa, A., Farris, A. and Cheli, R. (1978): Cimetidine and psoriasis. *Lancet 2*, 1121.
20. Holt, P.J.A. and Marks, R. (1976): Epidermal architecture, growth and metabolism in acromegaly. *Br. J. Med. 1*, 496.
21. Holt, P.J.A. and Marks, R. (1977): The epidermal response to change in thyroid status. *J. Invest. Dermatol. 68*, 299.
22. Yoshioka, T., Monafo, W.W., Ayvazian, V.H., Deitz, F. and Flynn, D. (1978): Cimetidine inhibits burn edema formation. *Am. J. Surg. 136*, 681.
23. Lyons, F., Cook, J. and Shuster, S. (1979): Inhibition of sebum excretion by an H₂-blocker. *Lancet 1*, 1376.
24. Funder, J.W. and Mercer, J.E. (1979): Cimetidine, a histamine H₂-receptor antagonist, occupies androgen receptors. *J. Clin. Endocrinol. Metab. 48*, 189.
25. Gerrard, J.W. and Ko, C. (1979): Urticaria pigmentosa: treatment with cimetidine and chlorpheniramine. *J. Pediatr. 94*, 843.

26. Avella, J., Madsen, J.E., Binder, H.J. and Askenase, P.W. (1978): Effect of histamine H_2-receptor antagonists on delayed hypersensitivity. *Lancet 1,* 624.
27. Plaut, M. (1979): Histamine, H_1- and H_2-antihistamines, and immediate hypersensitivity reactions. *J. Allergy Clin. Immunol. 63,* 371.

Discussion

Bertaccini: I would like to stress the importance of these studies, which have demonstrated the presence of both histamine H_1- and H_2-receptors in the skin, and to underline the rigour with which these studies were conducted, not only with histamine but also with selective stimulants of the H_1-receptors, with selective stimulants of H_2-receptors and with the respective antagonists. I believe that that is the best approach for this type of study.

Mosca (Naples): I would like a comment from Dr. Horton. Are the local immune changes, which have been studied by skin tests and which show an increased cellular response with greater erythema and induration, to be attributed to a vascular effect, as he has demonstrated, as well as to an inhibition of H-methyltransferase, or to stimulation of the cellular immune systems?

Horton: Most of the responses to histamine in the skin appear to be primarily vascular, rather than immunological. I do not think that the alterations in skin response to histamine are secondary to immunological changes, because they are too immediate in their occurrence.

Smolen (Vienna): Were the effects of the drugs or combinations of the drugs studied in pruritus senilis or in Hodgkin's disease, or just in volunteers?

Marks: These were normal, healthy volunteers in both studies.

Smolen: Is it clear that any pruritic condition arises from histamine, papain or similar substances?

Marks: As I said in my presentation, it has been tried in polycythaemia vera and some contradictory results have been obtained. It has also been used in the pruritus of uraemia. We are now involved in a study attempting to determine whether it is of any use in so-called idiopathic essential pruritus.

Mattila (Helsinki): Itch probably means a desire to scratch. This desire can be overcome by central sedatives. Many years ago, some papers were published on skin inflammation caused by poison ivy, which was relieved by those neuroleptics which have a central sedative action. Has Dr. Marks tried to use peripherally-acting histamine H_1-antagonists — because chlorpheniramine also acts on the central nervous system — in order to separate non-specific relief of desire to scratch from more specific effects?

Marks: That is a very good point. In fact, we have not done that; possibly we should. There is a famous experiment in which scratch was recorded and used as an index of itch by a well-known Northern British dermatologist. We have repeatedly tried to tell him that there are more components than scratching alone to the itch-scratch sequence. It may well be that agents which are effective in suppressing the central nervous system or, in fact, muscle-blocking agents or paralytic agents are picked up as anti-itch agents, when all they are really doing is stopping one point in the itch-scratch sequence.

Bertaccini: It is very difficult to find an H_1-antagonist which is completely devoid of central effects. The usual compounds which are available have more or less central effects, but it is very difficult to find a specific peripheral compound.

Bianchi (Milan): Dr. Marks mentioned mastocytosis. This is of considerable interest to gastroenterologists because of the intestinal problems. Has he had any personal experience with this?

Marks: No, none at all. There is one case report in which some supposed benefit from the use of cimetidine was described, as far as the skin symptoms are concerned.

The role of histamine in immune responses

M.R. Vickers, S.A. Arlington, C. Jones, D. Martin and M.A. Melvin
Smith Kline & French Research Ltd., Welwyn Garden City, United Kingdom

Introduction

In the first half of this century, a role for histamine as a mediator of immediate hypersensitivity and inflammation was established by the work of Dale and many others. Histamine, released from mast cells and basophils, can contract smooth muscle, increase vascular permeability, dilate arterioles and increase nasal and lacrimal secretion. These 'pro-inflammatory' actions of histamine are achieved largely via stimulation of a histamine H_1-receptor.

More recent studies have begun to uncover another important role for histamine in immunology: that of a regulator of cellular and humoral immune responses. Receptors for histamine have been identified on lymphocytes, mast cells, basophils, eosinophils and neutrophils. Stimulation of these receptors may be necessary for the development, maintenance and limitation of normal immunological reactivity. It is generally accepted that the regulatory actions of histamine are achieved via stimulation of a histamine H_2-receptor.

In this paper, the evidence for a histamine-mediated regulation of immune responses is reviewed, and some responses affected by histamine are discussed in more detail, in an attempt to clarify the nature of the histamine receptor involved. In addition, the question of a histamine H_2-receptor angatonist-mediated modulation of immunological reactivity is also considered.

In vitro immune responses altered by histamine

The in vitro immune responses known to be affected by histamine are listed in Table I.

Singh and Owen studied the maturation of murine fetal thymus stem cells in vitro, and found that the proportion of cells expressing T cell antigens is significantly increased by incubation with histamine [1]. The histamine stimulation is inhibited by the histamine H_2-receptor antagonist metiamide, but not by a histamine H_1-receptor antagonist. The relevance of this observation to in vivo events in unclear, but it may indicate that histamine has some regulatory role in T-cell differentiation in the thymus.

A number of studies have looked at the influence of histamine on T lymphocyte proliferation, induced by antigens and mitogens in man, in the mouse and in the guinea-pig [2-8]. Histamine inhibits T lymphocyte proliferation, apparently via histamine H_2-receptor activation. In the guinea-pig, passage of lymph node cells through a column of insolubilised histamine (i.e., histamine covalently bound to rabbit serum albumin and then attached to Sepharose® beads) removes a subpopula-

Table I. In vitro immune responses altered by histamine.

Response	Species	Effect	Receptor thought to be involved	Ref.
Maturation of thymocytes	mouse	stimulation	H₂	[1]
Antigen- and mitogen-induced T lymphocyte proliferation	man, mouse, guinea-pig	inhibition	H₂	[2-8]
Lymphokine production	guinea-pig, man	inhibition	H₂	[3, 10, 11]
T lymphocyte-mediated cytolysis	mouse	inhibition	H₂	[12, 13]
E-rosette formation of T lymphocytes	man (immune disorders)	inhibition	H₁ + H₂	[14, 15]
Haemolytic plaque formation	mouse	inhibition	ND	[18]
Antibody production	mouse	inhibition	ND	[19]
Lysosomal enzyme release	man	inhibiton	H₂	[20]
Cell movement	man, guinea-pig	inhibition, enhancement	H₁ H₂	[21, 22] [23, 24]
IgE-mediated histamine release	man	inhibition	H₂	[25, 26]

ND = not determined.

tion of histamine responsive cells, so that the proliferation of non-adherent cells is not inhibited by histamine [9]. It was suggested that the cells adherent to the histamine column were suppressor cells which could be activated by histamine. Recently, a soluble factor, histamine-induced suppressor factor (HSF), elaborated by histamine receptor-bearing T-lymphocytes of the guinea-pig, has been identified [10]. This factor reversibly inhibits the proliferation of lymphocytes in the absence of histamine. HSF is elaborated in small quantities by non-immune spleen and lymphnode cells but, following antigenic stimulation, much larger quantities are produced and activity is also detected in peripheral blood and thymus cells.

HSF also inhibits production of the lymphokine migration-inhibitory factor (MIF) by guinea-pig lymphocytes [10]. Studies with histamine H₁- and H₂-receptor antagonists indicate that HSF production is histamine H₂-receptor-mediated. In man, histamine suppresses production of the lymphokine which inhibits leucocyte migration (LIF), again by stimulating the elaboration of a soluble factor, LIF-production-inhibiting (LIF-PI) by T lymphocytes with receptors for histamine [11]. It is reasonable to assume that LIF-PI, produced by human lymphocytes, and HSF, produced by guinea-pig lymphocytes, are closely-related factors performing similar functions, and that by stimulating their production, histamine would act to limit cell-mediated hypersensitivity responses.

Lichtenstein et al. have shown that histamine inhibits the cytolytic activity of alloimmunised murine-effector T lymphocytes [12, 13]. This system has been studied extensively, and evidence has been presented that histamine interacts with histamine H₂-receptors to cause inhibition of cytolysis. The susceptibility to inhibition by histamine increases with time after immunisation to reach a peak on day 18; this may reflect an antigen-stimulated generation of a subpopulation of histamine-receptor-bearing, cytolytically-active T lymphocytes.

Histamine inhibits the E-rosette formation of T lymphocytes from patients with allergies, auto-immune diseases or recurrent infections [14, 15]. This action of histamine can be prevented by pre-incubation with the histamine H_2-receptor antagonist cimetidine and the histamine H_1-receptor antagonist mepyramine. E-rosette formation of T lymphocytes from healthy subjects is not altered by histamine. Thus, patients with increased immunological reactivity appear to develop a subpopulation of histamine-receptor-bearing T lymphocytes. The function of these cells remains unclear, but in view of a recent report of T-suppressor cells which bind to insolubilised histamine in the blood of patients with systemic lupus erythematosus or rheumatoid arthritis, but not in blood from normal subjects [16], it is tempting to speculate that they have some regulatory function. This observation in man is consistent with Lichtenstein's finding in the mouse, that histamine receptors develop, or are exposed, on a subpopulation of T lymphocytes, as they mature in immunological function [17].

Antibody-mediated responses are inhibited by histamine. Pre-incubation of spleen cells from mice that are immune to sheep erythrocytes with histamine inhibits haemolytic plaque formation [18]. Plaque formation involves secretion of antibody, antigen-antibody interaction, and fixation of complement, and it is not known which of these processes is affected by histamine. The type of histamine receptor involved has not been studied. Fallah et al. found that addition of histamine to in vitro primary cultures of spleen cells inhibited the IgM antibody plaque-forming cell response to sheep erythrocytes [19].

The cell type involved in a histamine-mediated inhibition of antibody production has been studied by Weinstein and Melmon [9]. They examined the ability of cells passed through histamine rabbit serum albumin-sepharose (HRS) columns to produce antibody in in vitro primary cultures. If murine spleen cells are separated in this way, the non-adherent cells are able to induce an enhanced antibody response to T cell dependent antigens such as sheep erythrocytes, but not to T cell independent antigens. Weinstein and Melmon suggested that the cells which adhere to the HRS columns are a subpopulation of cells which can be stimulated by histamine to cause a suppression of antibody formation. To support their suggestion, they studied the ability of fractionated spleen cells from mice made tolerant to sheep erythrocytes to transfer tolerance. Unfractionated spleen cells could transfer tolerance, but transfer of non-adherent cells resulted in a normal response to sheep erythrocytes. Cells which bind to HRS columns thus appear to be responsible for the state of tolerance. Furthermore, if these cells are freed from the column by gentle shaking and transferred to immune mice, then tolerance is induced. One interpretation of these data is that the HRS-adherent cells are suppressor cells, with receptors for histamine.

Histamine affects several functions of polymorphonuclear leucocytes. The release of the lysosomal enzyme β-glucuronidase from human neutrophils is inhibited by histamine [20], and the histamine inhibition can be reversed by the histamine H_2-receptor antagonist metiamide, but not by the histamine H_1-receptor antagonist chlorpheniramine. Histamine can influence the movement of eosinophils, neutrophils and basophils. In its own right, histamine is chemotactic for human and guinea-pig eosinophils, and this action appears to be independent of histamine H_1- or H_2-receptors [21, 22]. The chemotactic response of eosinophils to other agents may be either enhanced or inhibited by histamine. Enhancement of chemotaxis is seen with low concentrations of histamine and appears to be histamine H_1-receptor-mediated, whereas inhibition of eosinophil chemotaxis is seen with higher concentrations of histamine, and appears to be histamine H_2-receptor-mediated [21]. The inhibitory effect of histamine on eosinophil migration may be indirect, via a soluble factor released from mononuclear cells [22]. Histamine also inhibits the chemotactic response of human neutrophils to endotoxin [23] and of human basophils to C5a [24], both effects being mediated via histamine H_2-receptor stimulation. Histamine can also inhibit its own release from mast cells and basophils. Lichtenstein showed that exogenous histamine, added to actively sensitised human basophils incubated with specific antigen, suppressed the amount of endogenous histamine released [25, 26]. This inhibition of IgE-mediated histamine release was blocked by the histamine H_2-receptor antagonists metiamide and burimamide, but not by histamine H_1-receptor antagonists. Several groups then found that histamine H_2-receptor antagonists caused an increase in the level of extracellular histamine when added to an incubation of actively or passively sensitised mast cells from the guinea-pig [27], monkey [28] or dog [29], with specific antigen; these data were interpreted as a histamine H_2-receptor-mediated blockade of histamine release, although possible effects on histamine metabolism or a blockade of uptake of histamine into tissues were also considered.

In vivo immune responses altered by histamine

Histamine can be released by several different mechanisms. In immediate hypersensitivity, histamine is released following interaction between antigen and IgE antibody on the surface of mast cells and basophils. Many immunological reactions involve complement, and products of complement activation can also release histamine. In addition to these 2 well-known mechanisms of histamine release, it has recently been reported that antigens and mitogens induce the release of a histamine-releasing activity from mononuclear cells [30], and that phytohaemagglutinin (PHA) stimulates the generation of another factor from mononuclear cells of atopic patients, which enhances the IgE-dependent release of histamine from basophils [31]. Thus, mechanisms exist for the release of histamine in many immune responses.

Histamine-releasing cells participate in the whole range of immunological reactions. Mast cells and basophils are the source of the chemical mediators of immediate hypersensitivity. In response to lymphokine production and to chemotactic factors generated by complement activation, basophils accumulate at tissue sites of late and delayed hypersensitivity responses. Basophils are now thought to participate in allograft rejection [32, 33], and there appears to be a local tissue increase in histamine levels prior to clinical rejection of skin and kidney grafts in man [34]. There is also evidence that some failure to release or to respond normally to histamine may be instrumental in successful tumour growth and in parasitic evasion of host-immune defenses [35].

Histamine thus has the ability and the opportunity to regulate immunological responses, but there are few reports of histamine affecting immune responses in vivo (Table II).

The reported effects of histamine on the expression of delayed hypersensitivity are variable, but probably result from the use of different experimental conditions. We have found that histamine, administered subcutaneously at the same time as antigen challenge is made intradermally, fails to affect a delayed hypersensitivity

Table II.   In vivo immune responses altered by histamine.

Response	Species	Effect	Receptor thought to be involved	Ref.
Delayed hypersensitivity	guinea-pig, mouse	inhibition	?	[3, 36, 37]
Antibody production	mouse	inhibition	?	
Adjuvant arthritis	rat	inhibition	H_2	[38]
Recruitment of eosinophils	man (atopics)	enhancement	NS	[39]

NS = not studied; ? = not determined.

response in the guinea-pig, the reaction being assessed by measuring skin thickness and area of erythema. Rocklin injected histamine intradermally with the challenging dose of antigen, and in some cases observed a slight inhibition of an induration response in the guinea-pig [3, 36]. Schwartz studied cell-mediated footpad swelling in the mouse and found that histamine, given 3-6 hours after antigen challenge, inhibits the development of a delayed hypersensitivity response [37].

Histamine administration during the induction of delayed hypersensitivity causes a marked reduction of a subsequent delayed hypersensitivity response. The nature of the histamine receptor involved in this inhibition is not clear.

Histamine inhibits antibody production in in vitro primary cultures. We have studied antibody production to sheep erythrocytes in vivo in the mouse, measuring the response by a plaque-forming cell assay. Histamine, given prior to or around the time of immunisation, causes a marked reduction in the number of antibody-forming cells. The nature of the histamine receptor, and the cell with which histamine reacts, remain to be clarified.

The development of an adjuvant arthritis in the rat is inhibited by daily administration of histamine. Saeki reported that the histamine-mediated inhibition is reversed by the histamine H_2-receptor antagonist burimamide, but not by the histamine H_1-receptor antagonist mepyramine [38]. The mechanism of action of histamine in this model is not known, but from the inhibitory properties of histamine in vitro, effects on antibody production and lysosomal enzyme release are indicated.

In atopics, histamine can act as an eosinophil chemotactic factor in vivo [39]. Weinstein and Melmon assessed chemotactic activity using skin windows containing filters soaked in histamine or saline. Histamine failed to recruit eosinophils in normal subjects, but in atopic patients a 3-fold increase in eosinophil recruitment was seen with histamine [39]. This report associates histamine activity with immunological reactivity, and is consistent with several in vitro observations in which histamine-mediated inhibitory effects occurred after antigen challenge or were seen only with cells from patients with immune disorders [14-17].

Nature of the receptor involved in histamine-mediated modulation of immune responses

Histamine clearly has an important role as a modulator of immune responses, but it is *not* clear whether the regulatory actions of histamine are mediated via histamine H_2-receptor activation. There are many reports of a histamine H_2-receptor antagonist blocking a histamine response, but few experimenters have used more than 1 concentration of antagonist and, with the exception of Lichtenstein's work on histamine release and cell-mediated cytolysis [13, 26], there have been no attempts to obtain evidence of competitive inhibition.

Studies in our laboratories, using specific histamine H_2-receptor agonists and chemically-related compounds lacking histamine H_2-receptor agonist activity, indicate that the receptor at which histamine acts to regulate immunological responses is not identical to the histamine H_2-receptor as defined by Black et al. [40].

We have compared the ability of histamine and various histamine H_1- and H_2-receptor agonists to inhibit a phytohaemagglutinin-induced proliferation of human lymphocytes (Fig. 1). Histamine caused a dose-related suppression of the response to PHA, giving a maximum inhibition of 35% at 10^{-4} M. Of the 2 histamine H_1-receptor agonists studied, 2-thiazole-ethylamine was as active as histamine, while 2-pyridyl-ethylamine showed approximately 10% of the activity of histamine. The histamine H_2-receptor agonist 4-methyl-histamine, which at histamine H_2-receptors has 25-43% of the activity of histamine, was marginally more active than histamine as an inhibitor of lymphocyte proliferation. Further, the histamine H_2-receptor agonist dimaprit, with 19-70% of the activity of histamine at histamine H_2-receptors, produced a dramatic decrease in the response to PHA, causing complete inhibition at high concentrations. The order of activity of the histamine-receptor agonists tested is, therefore, not consistent with stimulation of a histamine H_2-receptor.

As a chemical control we tested nor-dimaprit, the lower homologue of dimaprit, which has no activity on classical histamine H_2-receptor systems such as gastric secretion, contraction of rat uterus and beating of guinea-pig atria. Nor-dimaprit,

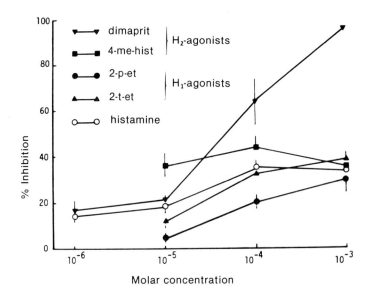

Fig. 1.   *Inhibition of phytohaemagglutinin-induced proliferation of human lymphocytes by histamine and histamine-receptor agonists. Mean ± SEM. 4-me-hist = 4-methyl-histamine; 2-p-et = 2-pyridyl-ethylamine; 2-t-et = 2-thiazole-ethylamine.*

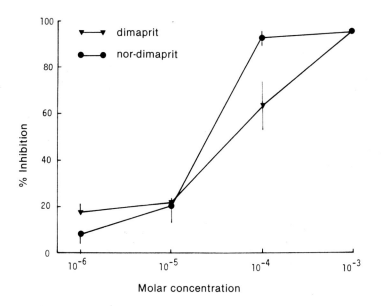

Fig. 2. Inhibition of phytohaemagglutinin-induced proliferation of human lymphocytes by dimaprit and nor-dimaprit. Mean ± SEM.

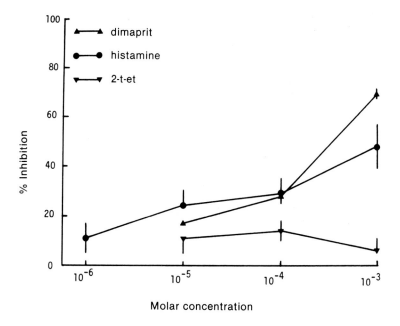

Fig. 3. Inhibition of the release of the lysosomal enzyme β-glucuronidase from human polymorphonuclear leucocytes by histamine, dimaprit and 2-thiazole-ethylamine. Mean ± SEM.

however, proved to be a more active inhibitor of lymphocyte proliferation than dimaprit (Fig. 2). It is possible that dimaprit and nor-dimaprit inhibit the PHA response by a different mechanism than does histamine, and this could be studied by attempting to block the response of these compounds with histamine H_2-receptor antagonists. However, the histamine H_2-receptor antagonists alone influence the PHA response and so, although we have seen a reversal of the effects of histamine, dimaprit and nor-dimaprit with cimetidine and metiamide, we have been unable to obtain evidence of competitive antagonism. Nevertheless, it is important to note that the histamine H_2-receptor antagonists affect the responses to histamine and to nor-dimaprit, a compound which lacks classical histamine H_2-receptor agonist activity, in a similar manner.

Lysosomal enzyme release from human neutrophils is inhibited by histamine, and the histamine inhibition is reversed by the histamine H_2-receptor antagonist metiamide. We have examined the ability of various histamine-receptor agonists to inhibit lysosomal enzyme release, and our results are similar to our findings with lymphocyte proliferation. Histamine produces a dose-related inhibition of lysosomal enzyme release (Fig. 3). The histamine H_1-receptor agonist 2-thiazole-ethylamine has very little effect, but the histamine H_2-receptor agonist dimaprit, which is less active than histamine at a classical histamine H_2-receptor, produces an inhibition indistinguishable from that of histamine at lower concentrations, but shows a greater maximum effect. Nor-dimaprit also inhibits lysosomal enzyme release, although in this system it is not more active than dimaprit (Fig. 4). Again, these data indicate that histamine does not act at a classical histamine H_2-receptor.

Studies in vivo are also consistent with histamine stimulation of a receptor other than a classical histamine H_2-receptor. Histamine inhibits antibody production to sheep erythrocytes in the mouse in a dose-related manner, giving a maximum reduc-

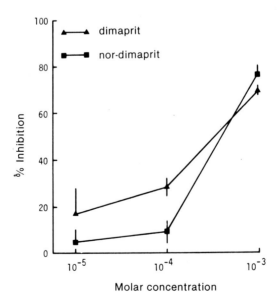

Fig. 4.   Inhibition of the release of the lysosomal enzyme β-glucuronidase from human polymorphonuclear leucocytes by dimaprit and nor-dimaprit. Mean ± SEM.

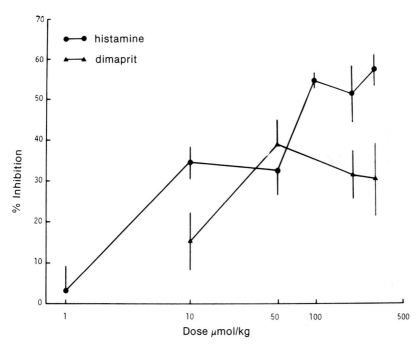

Fig. 5. Inhibition of antibody production to sheep erythrocytes in CBA mice by histamine and dimaprit. IgM plaque-forming cell numbers per spleen are determined. Mean ± SEM.

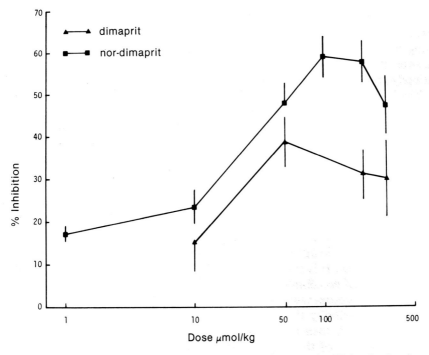

Fig. 6. Inhibition of antibody production to sheep erythrocytes in CBA mice by dimaprit and nor-dimaprit. IgM plaque-forming cell numbers per spleen are determined. Mean ± SEM.

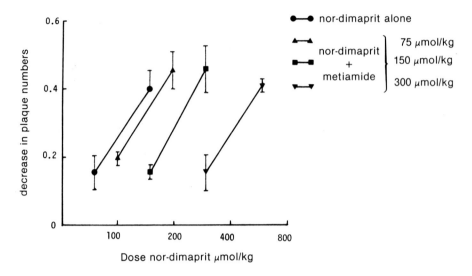

Fig. 7. Antagonism of nor-dimaprit by metiamide on antibody production to sheep erythrocytes in Swiss mice. IgM plaque-forming cell numbers per million spleen cells are determined. Mean ± SEM.

tion of 55% in IgM plaque-forming cell numbers; in contrast to our observations in vitro, dimaprit is less active than histamine as an inhibitor of antibody production, giving a maximum inhibition of 35% (Fig. 5). Consistent with the concept of a receptor distinct from a classical histamine H_2-receptor, nor-dimaprit inhibits antibody production, producing a maximum effect similar to that of histamine (Fig. 6). The histamine H_2-receptor antagonists do not affect antibody production in the mouse, and we were thus able to test whether the response to nor-dimaprit was subject to histamine H_2-receptor antagonism. Metiamide displaces the response to nor-dimaprit in a parallel dose-related fashion (Fig. 7). Similar results were found with other histamine H_2-receptor antagonists, but not with a chemically-related control compound lacking histamine H_2-receptor antagonist activity.

We have thus shown that the histamine H_2-receptor antagonists are effective surmountable inhibitors of the suppression induced by a compound which is not a classical histamine H_2-receptor agonist. The responses to histamine and to dimaprit are influenced by metiamide in a similar manner, suggesting that histamine, dimaprit and nor-dimaprit all act at the same receptor to cause an inhibition of immune responses. It is possible that this receptor is a histamine H_2-receptor, and that the failure of nor-dimaprit to stimulate histamine H_2-receptors in other systems reflects some heterogeneity in the receptors in different tissues. We should also consider the possibility that nor-dimaprit and dimaprit act indirectly, generating some factor which then acts at a histamine receptor. More data are required to identify the nature of the receptor stimulated by histamine in immunological systems, but our initial observations indicate that in some systems, contrary to published claims, the receptor involved is not a classical histamine H_2-receptor.

Modulation of immune responses by histamine H_2-receptor antagonists

Regardless of the precise nature of the receptor involved, histamine appears to act as a regulator of immunological responses, and the histamine H_2-receptor antagonists can block some of these regulatory actions. This has led to speculation that cimetidine may augment immunological reactivity in man, and cause potentially harmful exacerbations of immune disorders such as atopy and cell-mediated hypersensitivity. However, several million people have now taken cimetidine and there have been few reports suggesting any change in the ability of patients to respond immunologically. Animal studies with histamine H_2-receptor antagonists have also largely failed to uncover potentially harmful effects, although the short-term experiments which have been performed may not be relevant to long-term cimetidine therapy in man.

Histamine in vitro inhibits the release of endogenous histamine from basophils [25] and histamine H_2-receptors, which generally mediate relaxation, have been identified on respiratory smooth muscle [41]. In animal experiments in vivo, however, bronchoconstriction is not exacerbated by doses of cimetidine equivalent to the therapeutic dose [27-29], and in man, far from exacerbating bronchospasm, cimetidine may augment the beneficial effects of histamine H_1-receptor antagonists [42, 43]. Furthermore, immediate cutaneous hypersensitivity in man is not affected by cimetidine therapy [44, 45].

The effects of the histamine H_2-receptor antagonists on cell-mediated responses are not clear at present. Cimetidine, added to in vitro cultures of lymphocytes, can cause an augmentation of an antigen- or mitogen-induced proliferation of T lymphocytes [5, 6, 8, 46]. Using human lymphocytes, the response is extremely variable, both from subject to subject and in the same subject on different occasions. Most methods of lymphocyte separation do not remove all the basophils, and so histamine could be released from basophils following mitogen-stimulated generation of the histamine-releasing activity described by Thueson et al. [30]. Since histamine inhibits T lymphocyte proliferation, the apparent augmentation seen with cimetidine could result from a blockade of the histamine-mediated inhibition. There is one report of the responsiveness of lymphocytes to PHA before and after a course of cimetidine [47]. PHA-induced lymphocyte proliferation was measured in 9 patients with duodenal ulcers before and after a 2-week course of cimetidine 800 mg daily: in 8 of the 9 patients, there was some indication of an increased responsiveness to PHA after cimetidine therapy. No control patients were studied, and the authors do not state when the blood was taken relative to the last dose of cimetidine. If autologous serum which still contained appreciable quantities of cimetidine was used, then a blockade of histamine-mediated inhibition would explain the enhancement observed.

In animal studies, most groups have failed to show any effect with histamine H_2-receptor antagonists on either the induction or the expression of cell-mediated responses [3, 48, 49]. Askenase et al. did find that metiamide could reduce the expression of delayed hypersensitivity in the mouse, but only when very mild responses were induced with challenge doses of antigen just sufficient to produce a macroscopic end-point [50]. There are no reports of an exacerbation of cell-mediated hypersensitivity by histamine H_2-receptor antagonists in animals.

In man, there are several studies in which immune responsiveness has been assessed after cimetidine therapy. McGregor et al. measured leucocyte migration inhibition and serum immunoglobulin levels and looked for various auto-antibodies in 12 patients with acid-related dyspepsia, before and after a 28-day course of cimetidine [51]: any changes were compared with those observed in 5 healthy controls who did not receive cimetidine, and no alterations in immune responsiveness which could be attributed to cimetidine were observed. De Pauw et al. described results from 2 patients with Zollinger-Ellison syndrome, treated with histamine H_2-receptor antagonists for 16 months in 1 case and over 2 years in the other [52]: a large number of tests of immune function were made, and no immunological abnormalities were detected. André et al. measured serum immunoglobulin levels in 10 patients with duodenal ulcers before, during and after a 4-week course of cimetidine, and found a small decrease in the levels of IgA, IgM and IgG in some patients [53]; the reductions were less than 15%, and would probably not be statistically significant.

Two more recent papers describe apparently conflicting results. Avella et al. looked at delayed cutaneous reactions to PPD, Candida, Tricophyton and streptokinase-streptodornase (SK/SD) in 16 duodenal ulcer patients before and after a 6-week course of treatment during which half of them received cimetidine and half received placebo. A significant increase in both erythema and induration responses, measured at 24 and 48 hours, was observed after cimetidine, while after placebo there was an overall tendency for skin responses to decrease. This apparent augmentation of delayed hypersensitivity was most obvious for SK/SD, and at 48 hours increased induration was observed *only* after SK/SD challenge. Avella et al. explained their observations in terms of a cimetidine blockade of histamine action on regulatory T cells, although clearly vascular events and effects on histamine metabolism should also be considered. Their paper generated much discussion, the major criticism being directed towards the poor design of the study: the protocol was such that the 'before-treatment' skin test was read on day 1 and day 2 of cimetidine therapy, and the effects of cimetidine were assessed by skin tests performed after therapy had ended and therefore read 2 and 3 days after the last dose of cimetidine. It is therefore possible to interpret the data from this study in a completely opposite way.

Wolfe et al. examined both immediate and delayed hypersensitivity skin responses in 12 patients with allergic rhinitis, 6 of whom received cimetidine and 6 received placebo for 5 days [44]. No alteration in immediate cutaneous responses was observed, but the 48-hour induration reaction to SK/SD was increased in both cimetidine and control groups. SK/SD is the antigen to which an increased induration response was observed by Avella et al. after cimetidine therapy. The Wolfe et al. finding that both cimetidine-treated *and* control patients showed an increased response to SK/SD suggests that the first application of SK/SD primed all patients, resulting in increased sensitivity and therefore a greater response to a second application of antigen.

The main differences between the Avella and Wolfe studies were patient populations and duration of cimetidine therapy. As with the studies on lymphocyte proliferation, more data from controlled studies are required before any definite conclusions concerning the effects of histamine H_2-receptor antagonist therapy on cell-mediated hypersensitivity in man can be reached.

Evidence for a lack of effect of histamine H_2-receptor antagonists on immune responses in man has come from the use of cimetidine to prevent upper gastrointestinal haemorrhage in renal transplant patients. With the exception of Primack, who reported observations from only 2 patients [55], clinicians have found that the prophylactic use of cimetidine in renal transplant patients has no influence on the function of the graft, and does not cause an increase in either the number or the severity of rejection episodes [56-59].

The most interesting clinical reports have been descriptions of reversal of tolerance to 1-chloro-2,4-dinitrobenzene (DNCB) by cimetidine. Topical application of DNCB is used in the treatment of alopecia. Daman and Rosenberg gave cimetidine to a patient who had become tolerant to DNCB in an attempt to stimulate his cell-mediated immune responses [60]: after 2 days of treatment, tolerance was broken and the patient reacted again to DNCB. Breuillard and Szapiro later reported that of 30 patients treated topically with DNCB, 15 became tolerant [61]: cimetidine treatment was started, 5 patients dropped out of the study, in 4 patients there was no effect after 2 weeks' treatment with cimetidine, but in 7 patients tolerance was broken within 1 week. A histamine-mediated activation of suppressor cells would induce tolerance to DNCB in these patients, and the cimetidine effects could then be explained as a blockade of this histamine activation. There is much indirect evidence to support this speculation, and further studies in this area promise exciting results.

Conclusions

Histamine has an important regulatory role in normal immunological responses, and the development of some disease states may be due to a failure of histamine to regulate some part of the immune system. However, histamine H_2-receptor antagonists do not appear to cause any harmful exacerbation of either humoral or cell-mediated immune responses in normal individuals.

Acknowledgements

The skilled technical assistance of Mr K. Milliner and Mrs M. Turner is gratefully acknowledged.

References

1. Singh, U. and Owen, J.J.T. (1976): Studies on the maturation of thymus stem cells. The effects of catecholamines, histamine and peptide hormones on the expression of T-cell alloantigens. *Eur. J. Immunol. 6,* 59.
2. Artis, W.M. and Jones, H.E. (1975): Histamine inhibition of human lymphocyte transformation. *Fed. Proc. 34,* No. 1002.
3. Rocklin, R.E. (1976): Modulation of cellular-immune responses in vivo and in vitro by histamine receptor-bearing lymphocytes. *J. Clin. Invest. 57,* 1051.
4. Wang, S.R. and Zweiman, B. (1978): Histamine suppression of human lymphocyte responses to mitogens. *Cell. Immunol. 36,* 28.
5. Ogden, B.D. and Hill, H.R. (1979): Immune regulation by lymphocytes bearing H_1- and H_2-histamine receptors. *Clin. Res. 27,* 39A.
6. Helms, R.A. and Bull, D.M. (1979): The effect of cimetidine on histamine-modulated transformation of human lymphocytes. *Clin. Res. 27,* 267A.
7. Roszkowski, W., Plaut, M. and Lichtenstein, L.M. (1977): Histamine display on lymphocyte subpopulations. *Fed. Proc. 36,* No. 5146.
8. Beets, J.L. and Dale, M.M. (1979): Inhibition of guinea-pig lymphocyte activation by histamine and histamine analogues. *Br. J. Pharmacol. 66,* 365.
9. Weinstein, Y. and Melmon, K.L. (1976): Control of immune responses by cyclic AMP

and lymphocytes that adhere to histamine columns. *Immunol. Commun. 5,* 401.

10. Rocklin, R.E., Greineder, D.K. and Melmon, K.L. (1979): Histamine-induced suppressor factor (HSF): Further studies on the nature of the stimulus and the cell which produces it. *Cell. Immunol. 44,* 404.

11. Rigal, D., Monier, J.C. and Souweine, G. (1979): The effect of histamine on leucocyte migration test in Man. 1. Demonstration of a LIF-production inhibitor (LIF-PI). *Cell. Immunol. 46,* 360.

12. Plaut, M., Henney, C.S. and Lichtenstein, L.M. (1973): The effect of histamine on the cell-mediated immune response. *J. Clin. Invest. 52,* 64A.

13. Plaut, M., Lichtenstein, L.M. and Henney, C.S. (1975): Properties of a subpopulation of T cells bearing histamine receptors. *J. Clin. Invest. 55,* 856.

14. De Cock, W., De Cree, J. and Verhaegen, H. (1977): Restoration by levamisole of hista-mine-inhibited E rosette formation of T lymphocytes of patients with allergies. *Int. Arch. Allergy Appl. Immunol. 54,* 176.

15. De Cock, W., De Cree, J. and Verhaegen, H. (1978): Histamine-receptor bearing T lymphocytes in patients with allergy, autoimmune disease, or recurrent infection. *Clin. Immunol. Immunopathol. 11,* 1.

16. Tartakovsky, B., Segal, S., Shani, A., Karniely, Y. and Bentwich, Z. (1979): Suppressor role of histamine-receptor-bearing lymphocytes in patients with systemic lupus erythema-tosus and rheumatoid arthritis. *Isr. J. Med. Sci. 515,* 194.

17. Roszkowski, W., Plaut, M. and Lichtenstein, L.M. (1977): Selective display of histamine receptors on lymphocytes. *Science 195,* 683.

18. Melmon, K.L., Bourne, H.R., Weinstein, Y., Shearer, G.M., Kram, J. and Bauminger, S. (1974): Hemolytic plaque formation by leukocytes in vitro. Control by vasoactive hormones. *J. Clin. Invest. 53,* 13.

19. Fallah, H.A., Maillard, J.L. and Voison, G.A. (1975): Regulatory mast cells. 1. Suppres-sive action of their products on an in vitro primary immune reaction. *Ann. Immunol. (Pa-ris) 126C,* 669.

20. Busse, W.W. and Sosman, J. (1976): Histamine inhibition of neutrophil lysosomal enzyme release: an H_2-histamine receptor response. *Science 194,* 737.

21. Clark, R.A.F., Sandler, J.A., Gallin, J.I. and Kaplan, A.P. (1977): Histamine modula-tion of eosinophil migration. *J. Immunol. 118,* 137.

22. Kownatzki, E., Till, G., Gagelmann, M., Terwort, G. and Gemsa, D. (1977): Histamine induces release of an eosinophil-immobilising factor from mononuclear cells. *Nature (London) 270,* 67.

23. Anderson, R., Glover, A. and Rabson, A.R. (1977): The in vitro effects of histamine and metiamide on neutrophil motility and their relationship to intracellular cyclic nucleotide levels. *J. Immunol. 118,* 1690.

24. Lett-Brown, M.A. and Leonard, E.J. (1977): Histamine-induced inhibition of normal hu-man basophil chemotaxis to C5a. *J. Immunol. 118,* 815.

25. Lichtenstein, L.M. and Gillespie, E. (1973): Inhibition of histamine release by histamine controlled by H_2-receptor. *Nature (London) 244,* 287.

26. Lichtenstein, L.M. and Gillespie, E. (1975): The effects of the H_1 and H_2 antihistamines on 'allergic' histamine release and its inhibition by histamine. *J. Pharmacol. Exp. Ther. 192,* 441.

27. Dulabh, R. and Vickers, M.R. (1978): The effects of H_2-receptor antagonists on anaphylaxis in the guinea-pig. *Agents Actions 8,* 559.

28. Chakrin, L.W., Krell, R.D., Mengel, J., Young, D., Zaher, C. and Wardell, J.R. (1974): Effect of a histamine H_2-receptor antagonist on immunologically-induced mediator release in vitro. *Agents Actions 4,* 297.

29. Krell, R.D. and Chakrin, L.W. (1976): Histamine H_2-receptor antagonism in in vitro and in vivo canine models of allergic asthma. *Pharmacologist 18,* 204.

30. Thueson, D.O., Speek, L.S., Lett-Brown, M.A. and Grant, J.A. (1979): Histamine-

releasing activity (HRA). I. Production by mitogen- or antigen-stimulated human mononuclear cells. *J. Immunol. 123,* 626.

31. Bamzai, A.K. and Kretschmer, R.R. (1978): Enhancement of antigen-induced leukocyte histamine release by a mononuclear cell-derived factor. *J. Allergy Clin. Immunol. 62,* 137.

32. Dvorak, H.F. (1971): Role of the basophilic leukocyte in allograft rejection. *J. Immunol. 106,* 279.

33. Dvorak, H.F., Mihm, M.C. Jr., Dvorak, A.M., Barnes, B.A., Manseau, E.J. and Galli, S.J. (1979): Rejection of first-set skin allografts in man. The microvasculature is the critical target of the immune response. *J. Exp. Med. 150,* 322.

34. Moore, T.C., Thompson, D.P. and Glassock, R.J. (1971): Elevation in urinary and blood histamine following clinical renal transplantation. *Ann. Surg. 173,* 381.

35. Askenase, D.W. (1977): Role of basophils, mast cells and vasoamines in hypersensitivity reactions with a delayed time course. *Prog. Allergy 23,* 199.

36. Rocklin, R.E., Greineder, D., Littman, B.H. and Melmon, K.L. (1978): Modulation of cellular immune function in vitro by histamine receptor-bearing lymphocytes: mechanism of action. *Cell. Immunol. 37,* 162.

37. Schwartz, A. and Gershon, R.K. (1978): Activation of regulatory T cells by histamine. *Fed. Proc. 27,* 1353.

38. Saeki, K., Wake, K. and Yamasaki, H. (1976): Inhibition of adjuvant arthritis by histamine. *Arch. Int. Pharmacodyn. Ther. 222,* 132.

39. Weinstein, A.M., Gallin, J.I. and Kaplan, A.P. (1979): Eosinophil chemotactic activity of histamine in vivo. *J. Allergy Clin. Immunol. 63,* 207.

40. Black, J.W., Duncan, W.A.M., Durant, G.J., Ganellin, C.R. and Parsons, M.E. (1972): Definition and antagonism of histamine H_2-receptors. *Nature (London) 236,* 385.

41. Eyre, P. and Chand, N. (1979): Preliminary evidence for two subclasses of histamine H_2-receptors. *Agents Actions 9,* 2.

42. Schachter, E.N., Gerstenhaber, B. and Brown, S. (1978): Histamine receptors in the airways of healthy subjects. *Clin. Res. 26,* 635A.

43. Eiser, N.M., Guz, A., Mills, J. and Snashall, P.D. (1978): Effect of H_1- and H_2-receptor antagonists on antigen bronchial challenge. *Thorax 33,* 534.

44. Wolfe, J.D., Plaut, M., Norman, P.S. and Lichtenstein, L.M. (1979): The effect of an H_2-receptor antagonist on immediate and delayed skin test reactivity in man. *J. Allergy Clin. Immunol. 63,* 208.

45. Smith, J.A., Mansfield, L.E. and Nelson, H.S. (1979): The effect of cimetidine on the immediate cutaneous response to allergens. *Ann. Allergy 42,* 353.

46. Gifford, R.R.M., Hatfield, S.M. and Schmidtke, J.R. (1979): Cimetidine-induced modulation of human lymphocyte blastogenesis. *Proc. Am. Assoc. Cancer Res., 7th Annual Meeting 20,* 164.

47. Robertson, A.J., Peden, N.R., Saunders, J.H.B., Gibbs, J.H., Potts, R.C., Brown, R.A., Wormsley, K.G. and Swanson-Beck, J. (1979): Cimetidine and the immune response. *Lancet 2,* 420.

48. Sutton, T.J. (Personal communication.)

49. Dale, M.M. (1977): The effect of metiamide on cell-mediated immune reactions in the guinea-pig. *Br. J. Pharmacol. 60,* 441.

50. Schwartz, A., Askenase, P.W. and Gershon, R.K. (1977): The effect of locally-injected vasoamines on the elicitation of delayed type hypersensitivity. *J. Immunol. 118,* 159.

51. McGregor, C.G.A., Ogg, L.J., Smith, I.S., Cochran, A.J., Gray, G.R., Gillespie, G. and Forrester, J. (1977): Immunological and other laboratory studies of patients receiving short-term cimetidine therapy. *Lancet 1,* 122.

52. De Pauw, B.E., Lamers, C.B.H.N., Wagener, D.J.Th. and Festen, H.P.M. (1977): Immunological studies after long-term H_2-receptor antagonist therapy. *Lancet 2,* 616.

53. André, F., Druguet, M. and André, C. (1978): Traitement par la cimétidine et immunité humorale. *Gastroenterol. Clin. Biol. 2,* 8.

54. Avella, J., Binder, H.J., Madsen, J.E. and Askenase, P.W. (1978): Effect of histamine H_2-receptor antagonists on delayed hypersensitivity. *Lancet 1,* 624.

55. Primack, W.A. (1978): Cimetidine and renal-allograft rejection. *Lancet 1,* 284.

56. Doherty, C.C. and McGeown, M.G. (1978): Cimetidine and renal-allograft rejection. *Lancet 1,* 1048.

57. Rudge, C.J., Jones, R.H., Bewick, M., Weston, M.J. and Parsons, V. (1978): Cimetidine and renal-allograft rejection. *Lancet 1,* 1154.

58. Charpentier, B. and Fries, D. (1978): Cimetidine and renal-allograft rejection. *Lancet 1,* 1264.

59. Jones, R.H., Rudge, C.J., Bewick, M., Parsons, V. and Weston, M.J. (1978): Cimetidine: prophylaxis against upper gastrointestinal haemorrhage after renal transplantation. *Br. Med. J. 1,* 398.

60. Daman, L.A. and Rosenberg, E.W. (1977): Acquired tolerance to dinitrochlorobenzene reversed by cimetidine. *Lancet 2,* 1087.

61. Breuillard, F. and Szapiro, E. (1978): Cimetidine in acquired tolerance to dinitrochlorobenzene. *Lancet 1,* 726.

Immunological studies in patients treated with cimetidine, and the influence of cimetidine on skin-graft survival in mice

H.P.M. Festen, J.H.M. Berden* and B.E. de Pauw°
Divisions of Gastroenterology, *Nephrology and °Hematology, Department of Medicine, St. Radboud Hospital, Nijmegen, The Netherlands

Introduction

Studies by Plaut and his colleagues [1, 2] and by Rocklin [3] have demonstrated histamine H_2-receptors on T lymphocytes. Therefore, concern has been expressed about the possibility of immunological side-effects in patients undergoing treatment with H_2-receptor antagonists. The inhibition of histamine H_2-receptor bearing T cells by cimetidine may enhance the delayed type hypersensitivity reaction, and some observations in vivo [4] and in vitro [5] support this hypothesis. If it is true, an increase in the rejection of renal allografts might occur in patients on cimetidine, and this has also been previously reported [6, 7]. Other studies, however, are in contrast with these findings [8, 9]. We studied the influence of cimetidine on the immune response in 2 models: on several immunological parameters in man, and on skin-graft survival in mice.

Materials and methods

Nine patients (6 males and 3 females) with peptic ulcer but otherwise healthy were studied before, during and after treatment with cimetidine. Parameters studied included: lymphocyte counts, stimulation of lymphocyte cultures with various mitogens, assessment of immunoglobulin levels and skin testing for delayed type hypersensitivity with a battery of antigens. Treatment with cimetidine 1.6 g/day was started on day 3 after the results of skin tests were read, and stopped on day 40; the last tests were performed 2 days later. Blood cimetidine levels were assessed at the same time as the during and after treatment tests.

Lymphocytes were cultured following the procedure described by du Bois et al. [10]. Aliquots of a 1 ml suspension containing 300,000 lymphocytes/ml were cultured at 37°C. Cultures were stimulated by adding 25 μg of phytohemagglutinin (PHA), 25 μg of pokeweed mitogen (PWM) or a cocktail of the 5 different antigens used for skin tests. Mixed lymphocyte cultures were made by mixing 0.5 ml of a patient's lymphocyte suspension with 0.5 ml of the suspension of a healthy control. Unilateral stimulation in the mixed lymphocyte cultures was measured by blocking lymphocyte suspensions one-way by preincubation with mitomycin. All cultures were carried out in triplicate. PHA cultures were harvested on day 3, and all other cultures on day 6. To determine DNA synthesis, ^{14}C-thymidine was added 24 hours

Table I.   Antigenic differences of strain combinations used.

Donor → recipient combination	H-2 complex			Non H-2 loci
	Haplotype	Specificities		
		Private	Public	
$C_{57}Bl_{10}$ → $B_{10}LP$	b → b	—	—	H-3, H-13 and probably 2 others [12]
$B_{10}Br$ → $B_{10}A$	k → a × b	H-2D.32	H-2.7	—
$B_{10}D_2$ → $B_{10}A$	d → a × b	H-2K.31	H-2.34	—
$B_{10}D_2$ → $C_{57}Bl_{10}$	d → b	H-2K.31 H-2D.4	H-2.3, 8, 10, 13, 34, 40, 41, 42, 43, 44, 47, 49	—
PVG/c → $C_{57}Bl_{10}$	Xenogeneic graft			

before termination of the cultures. The lymphocytes were harvested on millipore microfiber glass filters and ^{14}C-thymidine uptake was measured in counts/minute with a liquid scintillation counter. A healthy volunteer, the same for each patient, served as a control in all tests. Skin tests were performed by intradermal injection of 0.1 ml of *Candida albicans* extract, intermediate-strength purified protein derivative, mumps skin-test antigen, streptodornase with streptokinase, and trichophyton allergenic extract in the forearm. Erythema and weal size were measured (in mm^2) and recorded after 24, 48 and 72 hours.

Maximum responses to each antigen before, during and after treatment were compared. Skin tests, which were also performed in 11 healthy controls at similar intervals, were regarded as increased when augmented by 100% or more, and as decreased when reduced by 50% or more. A reaction of less than 20 mm^2 was considered a negative test, and was discarded.

In our study in inbred mice, donor tail skin was grafted onto the flank of the recipient by a modified 'fitted graft' technique [11]. Five different combinations were used, with increasing antigenic disparity. Histo-incompatibility increases from a number of weak non-H-2 differences, an H-2D difference, an H-2K difference to a complete H-2 complex disparity and a xenogeneic difference (Table I).

The recipients received cimetidine 0.5 mg in 0.1 ml of saline (25 mg/kg of body weight) by intraperitoneal injection until rejection occurred, with 8-hour intervals between doses. Control animals were treated similarly, with saline 0.1 ml alone.

Results

In patients, blood cimetidine levels during treatment were 1.30 ± 0.29 μg/ml (mean ± SEM); after treatment these levels were nil in all patients. The total number of lymphocytes (mean ± SEM) did not change during the course of the study: it was 2.0 ± 0.2 × 10^9/l before and during treatment, and 2.1 ± 0.1 × 10^9/l after treatment. Results of lymphocyte transformation tests were expressed as a patient to

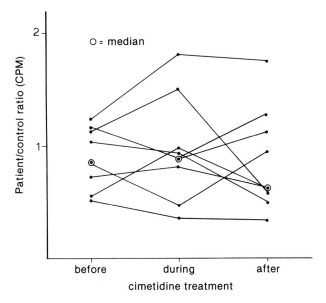

Fig. 1.   The effect of treatment with cimetidine on PHA-induced lymphocyte transformation in 9 patients.

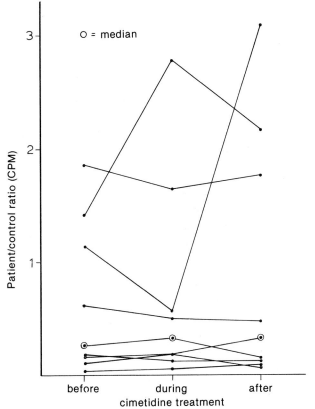

Fig. 2.   The effect of treatment with cimetidine on lymphocyte transformation induced by a cocktail of 5 antigens in 9 patients.

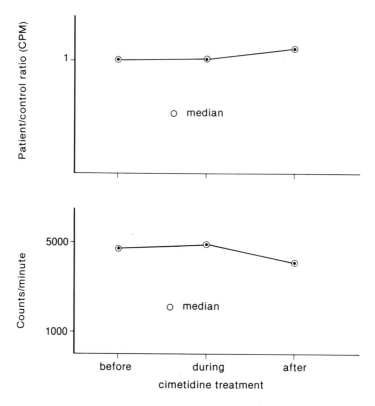

*Fig. 3.   The effect of treatment with cimetidine on PWM-induced lymphocyte transforma-
tion (top), and in mixed lymphocyte cultures (bottom). Data presented are the median of
observations in 9 patients.*

control ratio of counts/minute (CPM), except in mixed lymphocyte cultures where
they were expressed as counts/minute.

The results of cultures stimulated by PHA and by the cocktail of antigens are
shown in Figures 1 and 2, respectively. Although a few patients showed changes in
response, reactions in most patients were unchanged and the differences that were
seen were not significant.

A similar pattern was seen in the cultures stimulated by PWM and in the mixed
lymphocyte cultures, and this similarity can be seen in Figure 3; for the sake of
simplicity, only median values are shown. Stimulating and responding capacity of
patient lymphocytes in one-way mixed lymphocyte cultures did not alter.

No changes were observed in IgG, IgA or IgM levels, and all of these remained
within normal ranges (Fig. 4).

The number of skin tests which increased and decreased was not significantly
different between the cimetidine and control groups (Table II); as changes in
erythema did not differ significantly from those in induration, only the latter are
shown in this Table. When the results for each antigen were evaluated separately, no
significant differences were seen either.

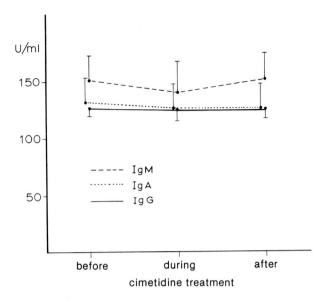

Fig. 4. The effect of treatment with cimetidine on immunoglobulin levels in 9 patients (mean ± SEM).

Table II. The effect of cimetidine treatment on response to skin test.

	before vs. during		before vs. after		during vs. after	
	cimetidine	control	cimetidine	control	cimetidine	control
total number of skin tests	37	41	41	44	41	45
induration increased	19	21	22	31	15	21
induration decreased	2	6	8	5	14	4

In mice, no difference in graft survival time was seen between the cimetidine and saline groups (Fig. 5). Results in donor-recipient combinations with low antigenic disparity were not different from those in combinations with higher antigenic disparity.

Discussion

In the present study, we did not find any change in immunological parameters in man during cimetidine treatment. Neither was any change observed after the drug was discontinued, and blood cimetidine concentrations were nil.

We did not find the pronounced increase in reactions to skin tests for delayed type hypersensitivity which was reported by Avella et al. [4]. The results of lymphocyte transformation tests stimulated by a cocktail of skin-test antigens, which correlate well with skin tests [13], confirmed this observation. Two other T-cell tests (PHA

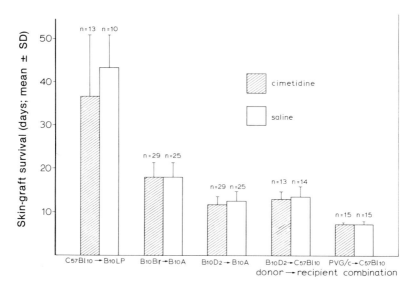

Fig. 5.   The effect of cimetidine and saline treatment on skin-graft survival in mice.

stimulation of lymphocyte cultures and responding capacity of patient lymphocytes in one-way mixed lymphocyte cultures) did not show any change. Changes in T-cell function induced by cimetidine are, therefore, unlikely.

B-cell function as tested by PWM stimulation and determination of immuno-globulin levels also showed no difference.

Several rather common drugs, such as acetylsalicylic acid and salazosulfapyridine, which are not known to produce immunological side-effects even after long-term clinical use, have been shown to induce obvious changes on the parameters evaluated in the present study [14, 15]. We therefore conclude it to be unlikely that an important clinical change in the immune response is associated with cimetidine treatment.

Skin-graft rejection in mice is primarily mediated by cytotoxic T cells [16, 17]. Furthermore, this model is very sensitive to small changes in the immune response [18, 19]. But even when histo-incompatibility was very weak, we found no effect of cimetidine on graft survival.

Based on our results, we conclude that neither an important clinical change in the immune response nor acceleration of graft rejection by cimetidine is likely.

Summary

The influence of treatment with cimetidine on the immune response was studied in 2 different models.

Nine patients with peptic ulcer disease were studied with 3 weeks' interval: before, during and 2 days after treatment with cimetidine 1.6 g/day. No change was observed in reaction to skin tests with *Candida albicans,* mumps, trichophyton, intermediate-strength purified protein derivative and streptokinase-streptodornase in patients, as compared to 11 controls. Nor did any change occur in total lymphocyte counts, nor in results of lymphocyte transformation tests stimulated by phyto-hemagglutinin, pokeweed mitogen and a cocktail of the antigens used for skin tests. Results of mixed lymphocyte cultures did not alter, and showed also un-changed stimulating and responding capacity of lymphocytes. No difference was observed in IgG, IgA or IgM levels, and all were in the normal range.

The influence of cimetidine on skin-graft survival in mice was studied in a well-defined transplantation model of inbred mice. Five different transplantation combinations with increasing antigenic disparity were studied. Cimetidine 25 mg/kg body weight was administered intraperitoneally with 8 hours' interval. No differences in graft survival were observed between cimetidine-treated groups and saline-treated controls in any of the combinations studied.

References

1. Plaut, M., Lichtenstein, L.M., Gillespie, E. and Henney, C.S. (1973): Studies on the mechanism of lymphocyte-mediated cytolysis. IV. Specificity of the histamine receptor on effector T-cells. *J. Immunol. 111*, 389.
2. Plaut, M., Lichtenstein, L.M. and Henney, C.S. (1975): Properties of a subpopulation of T-cells bearing histamine receptors. *J. Clin. Invest. 55*, 856.
3. Rocklin, R.E. (1976): Modulation of cellular immune response in vivo and in vitro by histamine receptor bearing lymphocytes. *J. Clin. Invest. 57*, 1051.
4. Avella, J., Madsen, J.E., Binder, H.J. and Askenase, P.W. (1978): Effect of histamine H_2-receptor antagonists on delayed hypersensitivity. *Lancet 1*, 624.
5. Wang, S.R. and Zweiman, B. (1978): Histamine suppression of human lymphocyte responses to mitogen. *Cell. Immunol. 36*, 28.
6. Zammit, M. and Toledo-Pereyra, L.H. (1979): Increased rejection after cimetidine treatment in kidney transplants. *Transplantation 27*, 358.
7. Primack, W.A. (1978): Cimetidine and renal allograft rejection. *Lancet 1*, 824.
8. McGregor, C.G.A., Cochran, A.J., Ogg, L.J., Gray, G.R., Smith, I.S., Gillespie, G. and Forrester, J. (1977): Immunological and other laboratory studies of patients receiving short-term cimetidine therapy. *Lancet 1*, 122.
9. De Pauw, B.E., Lamers, C.B.H.W., Wagener, D.J.Th. and Festen, H.P.M. (1977): Immunological studies after long-term H_2-receptor antagonist treatment. *Lancet 2*, 616.
10. Du Bois, M.J.G.J., Huismans, L., Schellekens, P.Th.A. and Eysvoogel, V.P. (1973): Investigations and standardisation of the conditions for microlymphocyte cultures. *Tissue Antigens 3*, 402.
11. Berden, J.H.M., Gerlag, P.G.G., Hageman, J.F.H.M. and Koene, R.A.P. (1977): Role of antiserum and complement in the acute antibody-mediated rejection of mouse skin allografts in strain combinations with increasing histoincompatibility. *Transplantation 24*, 175.
12. Bevan, M.J. (1976): H-2 restriction of cytolysis after immunization of minor H-congenic pairs of mice. *Immunogenetics 3*, 177.
13. Leguit, P. Jr., Meinesz, A., Huismans, L. and Eysvoogel, V.P. (1973): The use of an antigen cocktail in the lymphocyte transformation test. *Clin. Exp. Immunol. 14*, 149.
14. Opelz, G., Terasaki, P.I. and Hirata, A.A. (1973): Suppression of lymphocyte transformation by aspirin. *Lancet 2*, 478.
15. Holm, G. and Perlmann, P. (1968): The effect of antimetabolites on the cytotoxicity by human lymphocytes. In: *Advances in transplantation,* p. 155. Editors: J. Dausset and J. Hamburger. Munksgaard, Copenhagen.
16. Rygaard, J. (1974): Skin grafts in nude mice. *Acta Pathol. Microbiol. Scand. Sect. A Pathol. 82*, 80.
17. Pennycuik, P. (1971): Unresponsiveness of nude mice to skin allograft. *Transplantation 11*, 417.

18. Corry, R.J., Winn, H.J. and Russel, P.S. (1973): Primarily vascularized allografts of hearts in mice. *Transplantation 16,* 343.

19. Russel, P.S., Chase, C.M., Colvin, R.B. and Plate, J.M.D. (1978): Kidney transplants in mice. An analysis of the immune status of mice bearing long term H-2 incompatible transplants. *J. Exp. Med. 147,* 1449.

Discussion

Bertaccini: I would like to stress the importance of these studies of the immune response and histamine interactions with the various types of receptors, as they seem to be of great theoretical and practical importance. This is particularly true of the interaction of the 2 receptor types, which so far we have always regarded as independent and open to study under different experimental conditions, whereas here we clearly saw how often there are interactions between H_1- and H_2-receptors, and also saw the possibility of intervention of receptors which are different from the classical histamine receptors.

Surrenti (Florence): Does Dr. Festen have any immunological data after long-term treatment with cimetidine; for example, after one year's treatment?

Festen: Our data on this subject have been reviewed by Dr. Vickers. We have studied only 2 Zollinger-Ellison patients, treated for one year and 16 months respectively with an H_2-receptor antagonist. They were studied in the same way as the 9 patients I have just reported, and we could find no difference in those studies.

Smolen (Vienna): In view of some of the papers published by Plaut and by Matthysen's group on histamine Sepharose® beads, which showed that many of these results were not reproducible, could Dr. Vickers comment on some of the results she has shown from groups other than her own? Are they valid?

Vickers: All the experiments that have been done using separation of cells on histamine columns should be viewed with some caution. It has been shown that cells will bind to simple amines other than histamine, and these cells will respond in the same way as the cells which bind to histamine columns. I think that these results are interesting, but I would certainly not say that they are conclusive. They show that the cells which bind to these columns — whatever that means — have some important functions in immune responses. However, these studies are only a beginning.

Smolen: Would Dr. Vickers speculate on the possibility of an H_3-receptor in the immune system?

Vickers: No.

Smolen: Dr. Festen said that B-cell function was not altered during and after cimetidine treatment, based on pokeweed mitogen transformation and one-way mixed lymphocyte cultures, but I do not agree that these really reflect B-cell functions, and he did not look for B-cell differentiation or B-cell antibody production.

Festen: I apologise if I gave the impression that we studied all B-cell function. We studied some circumstantial evidence, and some aspects of the B-cell function — such as immunoglobulin, which was a very rough study. A French study has reported that these pokeweed stimulation and one-way mixed lymphocyte culture tests could decrease with cimetidine administration, which therefore indicates something about B-cell function but, I agree, not enough to tell us *all* about B-cell function.

Baron (London): If all advances in endocrine disease came from studying patients with excess production, would not the understanding of paracrine diseases come from studying patients with systemic mastocytosis and basophil leukaemia? What is the evidence for disturbances of immune behaviour in these patients?

Vickers: I know of no studies that have been done in these types of patients.

Festen: I know of none either.

Dr. Vickers' results in in vitro experiments and in lymphocyte transformation tests to phytohaemagglutinin, as well as the influence of histamine on those tests and the possible inhibition of this influence by cimetidine, are completely different from those reported in the literature. Our results, although obtained completely independently from Dr. Vickers' — in fact, we discussed them yesterday for the first time — are in total agreement with hers. We were unable to reproduce the results given in any of the literature reports. Does Dr. Vickers think that, at the least, a better definition of the receptor on lymphocytes is necessary after those reports by Plaut and Rocklin?

Vickers: Plaut and Rocklin have made a rather large jump in using one concentration of an antagonist, obtaining what in many cases is a small and not particularly reproducible displacement of a histamine response, and then claiming that this indicates an H_2-receptor involvement. There is not sufficient evidence to say either that an H_2-receptor is involved, or to say categorically that an H_2-receptor is not involved. We should be very cautious about attributing effects of histamine in these systems to action at an H_2-receptor.

Bertaccini: I saw with surprise that nordimaprit can be more active than dimaprit. We have tried many compounds similar to dimaprit without ever observing any activity, so we had the impression that the dimaprit molecule is fairly crucial for the maintenance of the biological activity, more so than the histamine molecule. Has Dr. Vickers any evidence of other activities of this nordimaprit molecule?

Vickers: As far as I know, nordimaprit is active only in immunological systems. In all the other systems it acts as the perfect control compound for dimaprit.

Bertaccini: It is very specific for this immunological test?

Vickers: Yes, it is.

Ciammaichella (Rome): After so many very interesting and modern concepts in an ultraspecialised field such as that of immunology, perhaps an internist might be allowed to voice his perplexity. Until yesterday I knew that histamine is the first protagonist in all allergic manifestations. Today, with great interest and with great amazement, we have seen and learned that histamine inhibits the formation of antibodies. I would like to ask Dr. Vickers whether, albeit very simplistically, she can clear up that apparent contradiction for us internists.

Vickers: I do not think it is a contradiction at all. It is clear that, when histamine acts as a mediator in various allergic reactions, the action is mediated via an H_1-receptor. The inhibitory actions of histamine which I have described are not mediated by stimulation of an H_1-receptor, but they may involve H_2-receptor stimulation. This is just another example of one compound producing 2 opposing effects, the net result being a balance between pro-inflammatory reactions and a limitation of those reactions. It is an acceptable concept that the agent which causes the inflammation will also act to limit that inflammation.

Bertaccini: I can add that histamine has been found in recent studies to act as an inhibitor of the release of slow reacting substances of the peptides which mediate inflammation. It seems that that is an action mediated through the H_2-receptors; thus, in this sense, histamine could function as an anti-inflammatory. We have always known it as an inflammatory agent, acting through stimulation of H_1-receptors, but this blocking of inflammation-enhancing peptides may be an anti-inflammatory action. Hence the theoretical possibility that the antagonists act as directly inflammatory agents. However, these are probably different receptors, and there may also have to be specific conditions for these effects to be modified.

Histamine receptors in the respiratory system: a review of current evidence

L.W. Chakrin and R.D. Krell

Section on Respiratory and Allergic Diseases, Department of Biological Research, Smith Kline & French Laboratories, Philadelphia, Pennsylvania, U.S.A.

Introduction

Some 14 years have passed since Ash and Schild first postulated the existence of at least 2 types of histamine receptor [1]. During this period, considerable interest has been shown in the second receptor type, termed the H_2-receptor, which presumably mediates histamine-induced secretion of gastric acid, increases in heart rate and inhibition of uterine contractions, among other physiologic functions. This interest resulted largely from the work of Black and associates, who provided pharmacological characterization to, and therefore substantiated the existence of, histamine H_2-receptors [2, 3].

When Lichtenstein and coworkers postulated a role for H_2-receptors on cells involved in hypersensitivity reactions [4, 5], research interest in H_2-receptors became focused on such target cells as basophils and mast cells, which are responsible, at least in part, for the release of the mediators of anaphylaxis. The receptors, it was thought, might mediate a histamine-induced elevation in cellular cyclic adenosine monophosphate (AMP) levels, which in turn would diminish endogenous histamine release and presumably, therefore, the pathophysiology of the anaphylactic reaction.

Equally interesting, the studies of Maengwyn-Davies in 1968 [6], Eyre in 1973 [7] and Fleisch and Calkins in 1976 [8] prompted a substantial research interest in histamine H_2-receptors in tracheobronchial smooth muscle.

This review will consider these 2 cellular locations for histamine H_2-receptors in the respiratory system, with particular focus on the evidence in support of their existence and their potential utility in respiratory diseases.

Pulmonary mast cell histamine receptors

If pulmonary mast cell histamine receptors function as modulators of mediator release, one of their potential therapeutic utilities would be in the management of asthma and related immediate-type allergic diseases.

Asthma is a disease marked by recurrent, quickly-developing bronchial obstruction leading to paroxysmal dyspnea. The condition results from a spasm of hypersensitive bronchial smooth muscle, generally in the segmental and smaller bronchi. The spasm is often accompanied by a mucosal edema and respiratory mucus hypersecretion. The symptomatology of immediate-type allergic diseases, including extrinsic asthma and allergic rhinitis, presumably results from the immunologically (antigen)-induced release of a variety of pharmacologically-active substances from mast cells, basophilic leukocytes and possibly other cells as well, previously sensitized with an antibody generally considered to be of the immunoglobulin E class.

In 1973, Lichtenstein and Gillespie suggested the existence of 2 receptors for histamine in the context of allergic or inflammatory responses [4]. Based on data accumulated with human basophilic leukocytes, they proposed that the H_1-receptor mediates vasodilation and the increased vascular permeability characteristics of the response to histamine, and that the H_2-receptor, located on the histamine releasing cell, mediates an inhibitory effect on the inflammatory response by increasing cellular cyclic AMP levels, which would diminish histamine release and, subsequently, the intensity of the response. The basis for this suggestion is as follows:

Histamine involved in immediate-type hypersensitivity reactions appears to be stored in discrete mast cell (or basophil) secretory granules as a complex with heparin and protein; this stored amine presumably undergoes slow turnover by comparison to the extra mast cell histamine of the gastrointestinal mucosa and the central nervous system.

It has been suggested that an early event in the release function from mast cells is an activation of a membrane-bound chymotrypsin-like proesterase (for review see [9]). The activation of the esterase presumably requires calcium ion and results in a dyflos-inhibitable enzyme. Later in the sequence there appears to be an energy-requiring step which is inhibitable by 2-deoxyglucose, an intracellular calcium ion-requiring step capable of being suppressed by edetic acid, and a step regulated by the relative levels of cyclic AMP and/or cyclic guanosine monophosphate (GMP). Presumably the mechanism of action of many of the compounds clinically effective in asthma is at the cyclic nucleotide step(s).

Further, several pharmacologically distinct receptors can, when activated, elevate mast cell cyclic AMP levels, and this effect has been associated with an inhibition of the release of the mediators of immediate type-I anaphylactic responses. The receptors involved include those sensitive to beta-adrenergic agonists [10] and some prostaglandins [11]. Similarly, it was suggested by Lichtenstein and Gillespie that receptors sensitive to histamine are also capable of regulating mediator release by elevating cyclic AMP levels [4]. These receptors were thought to be of the H_2 type, since burimamide but not mepyramine could prevent the alteration in cyclic AMP and the inhibition of mediator release produced by exogenous histamine.

Although species-specific, the data accumulated in our laboratory during the past few years is generally compatible with the hypothesis of Lichtenstein and coworkers [4, 5], since the data demonstrates a species-selective, mediator-selective enhancement of immunological histamine release from lung in the presence of the H_2-receptor antagonist metiamide. Alternatively, apparent enhancements of extracellular histamine may be realized by drug-induced inhibition of metabolism or tissue accumulation subsequent to release (for review see [12, 13]).

Nevertheless, we have demonstrated that high concentrations of metiamide enhance extracellular histamine from primate and canine, but not from rat lung in vitro. Moreover, the effect in primate and canine lung is mediator-selective, as metiamide has little effect on the release of slow-reacting substance of anaphylaxis (SRS-A), presumably Leukotriene C [12-14].

Over the course of the past 7 years, metiamide and other H_2-receptor antagonists and agonists have been evaluated in several in vitro models of immediate hypersensitivity, modified from the studies of Malley and Harris [15], Ishizaka et al. [16] and Kaliner et al. [17].

These systems involved passively sensitizing fragments of rhesus monkey lung and skin, rat lung, and canine lung in vitro for 90 minutes at 37°C in either dilutions of heat labile reaginic human serum in the case of the primate, dilutions of heat labile rat anti-ovalbumin serum for the rodent, or dilutions of canine anti-ascaris serum for the dog. Following sensitization, the tissues were rinsed and the fragments were randomly selected to form individual samples, each consisting of approximately 12 sections (275 mg) for lung and approximately 15 sections (350 mg) for skin. Where appropriate, drugs to be evaluated were introduced 5 minutes prior to challenge, and were present throughout the challenge period of 30 minutes at 37°C.

Immunological challenge of the sensitized tissues was achieved by incubation in a 'reversed type' anaphylactic reaction with anti-human IgE for the primate tissues, direct ovalbumin antigen solution for the rodent, and ascaris antigen for the dog. The amount of histamine released to the Tyrode's supernatant solution on challenge was evaluated either by the fluorometric method of Shore et al. [18] as modified with respect to citric acid by Anton and Sayre [19] or, in some instances, by bioassay utilizing the guinea-pig ileum preparation. The SRS-A released on challenge was estimated by bioassay utilizing guinea-pig ileum, following treatment of the preparation with mepyramine $(2.5 \times 10^{-6} M)$ and atropine $(3.7 \times 10^{-7} M)$ as described by Orange and Austen [20].

Metiamide enhanced the anti-human IgE-induced release of histamine from fragmented rhesus monkey lung as a function of its molar concentration, when that concentration was equal to or in excess of $1 \times 10^{-4} M$. When studied under these circumstances, metiamide produced 70-120% enhancement of amine release. Similar results were obtained with the primate skin preparation. It is presumptive that this enhancement of immunologic histamine release is due to a competitive antagonism of endogenous histamine at H_2-receptors on pulmonary (or cutaneous) cells responsible for such release. Metiamide was also evaluated for its effect on the release of SRS-A from rhesus monkey lung; while there was some significant enhancement at the highest concentration studied $(4 \times 10^{-4} M)$, the magnitude of the effect was considerably less than on histamine release.

Unlike the results with primate lung and skin, there was no significant effect of metiamide on the ovalbumin-induced release of histamine from passively-sensitized fragmented adult male rat lung, and isoprenaline also failed to consistently and significantly inhibit immunologic histamine release from rat lung. These 2 observations are consistent with the notion that beta-adrenergic agonists and histamine per se may not inhibit endogenous histamine release in the rat.

Finally, with respect to the canine, metiamide at concentrations in excess of $1 \times 10^{-4} M$ enhanced the ascaris antigen-induced release of histamine from fragmented, passively-sensitized canine lung and again disclosed mediator selectivity, as it had only modest effects on the release of SRS-A.

These observations with metiamide [12, 13] were later extended to cimetidine [14]. While this latter compound enhanced the anti-human IgE-induced release of histamine from fragmented passively-sensitized rhesus monkey lung, the extent of enhancement was not as great as seen previously with metiamide; at equimolar concentration, the enhancement with cimetidine was some 15% of that produced by metiamide. Somewhat greater enhancements were demonstrated for cimetidine as compared with metiamide in actively-sensitized guinea-pig lung challenged in

Table I.   The effect of H_2-receptor antagonists on immunologically-induced histamine release from pulmonary tissue in vitro.

Ref.	Species	Antagonist	Effect
[12]	Rat	Metiamide	No effect
[21]	Guinea-pig	Metiamide, cimetidine	'Enhanced' extracellular histamine
[13]	Dog	Metiamide	'Enhanced' extracellular histamine
[12]	Monkey	Metiamide	'Enhanced' extracellular histamine
[14]	Monkey	Cimetidine	Slightly 'enhanced' extracellular histamine
[22]	Man	Metiamide, cimetidine	No effect

vitro with ovalbumin by Dulabh and Vickers [21].

As in the case of metiamide, cimetidine failed to significantly enhance specific ovalbumin antigen-induced release of histamine from fragmented passively-sensitized rat lung. This observation is at least compatible with the hypothesis that agents which presumably alter the cyclic nucleotides, either directly or indirectly, may not regulate endogenous histamine release in the rat.

A summary of the in vitro studies with the H_2-receptor antagonists is given in Table I, documenting the species-specific 'enhancement' of histamine release from pulmonary tissue.

More recently, we have investigated a number of other H_2-receptor antagonists and agonists, utilizing the in vitro experimental models of immediate-type hypersensitivity reactions.

Beyond metiamide and cimetidine, our laboratory was especially interested in SK&F-91581 [23], a molecule in which the trione sulfur (= S) replaces the imino nitrogen (= NH) of guanidine and produces a compound which is devoid of agonist activity and, presumably, only very weakly active as an antagonist. The compound is an analog of the first-generation antagonist, burimamide. While it may possess some degree of H_2-antagonist activity on tracheobronchial smooth muscle [14], its activity in enhancing immunologically-induced histamine release from rhesus monkey fragmented passively-sensitized pulmonary tissues was quite unexpected and, in fact, greater than that seen with cimetidine.

If the H_2-receptor linked to the cyclic AMP system does modulate histamine release, then H_2-agonists would presumably be of therapeutic value, perhaps in such diseases as allergic rhinitis where histamine is thought to be a significant mediator of anaphylaxis. Accordingly, several H_2-receptor agonists were evaluated for their effect on immunologic histamine release from primate pulmonary tissue.

Dimaprit [24], a second-generation H_2-receptor agonist with even greater selectivity toward H_2-receptors than 4-methyl histamine, did not significantly alter the anti-human IgE-induced release of histamine from fragmented passively-sensitized primate lung. The data from primate lung is compatible with the observations of Kaliner [22], who demonstrated that dimaprit (and H_2-receptor antagonists) failed to significantly influence the immunologic release of mediators from human lung. Moreover, the recently disclosed third-generation agonist impromidine [25] was similarly evaluated in primate lung, and while some statistically-significant inhibition of histamine release was achieved at 4×10^{-5} M, this modest effect was surprisingly lost at higher concentrations.

Thus it would seem, on the basis of a variety of in vitro studies, that if H_2-receptors exist at all on pulmonary mast cells and are capable of mediating the autoregulation of histamine release, they have a unique structural specificity for the antagonists and, consequently, it will require more potent and selective H_2-agonists to demonstrate them convincingly.

Tracheobronchial smooth muscle histamine receptors

In 1968, Maengwyn-Davies reported a dual mode of action of histamine in the cat isolated tracheal chain [6]. This investigation suggested that histamine releases catecholamines which stimulate adrenergic beta-receptors to induce relaxation, an effect antagonized by pronetalol, and that histamine combines with its own specific receptors to induce relaxation, an effect blocked by mepyramine. This atypical or relaxant response to histamine was further described, and the bronchial response pharmacologically characterized, in cat tracheobronchial tissue by Chand and Eyre in 1977 [26]. It was in 1973, however, that Eyre reported the histamine-induced relaxation of terminal bronchi of sheep and cat trachea, an effect blocked by burimamide, thus suggesting a preponderance of H_2-histamine receptors in these tissues [7]. In 1976, Fleisch and Calkins studied the isolated rabbit trachea and bronchus and determined that, while bronchi contracted to histamine, the amine relaxed the carbachol-contracted rabbit trachea [8]. While the bronchial contractions caused by histamine were antagonized by mepyramine, the relaxation of the trachea caused by histamine was not affected by mepyramine, burimamide, metiamide or propranolol.

This work has prompted a significant research effort in recent years focused on an examination of tracheobronchial smooth muscle of several species (Table II). A substantial variability has been reported for both species and anatomic level of airway, which has made a review and analysis of the observations especially difficult. Nevertheless, the fundamental principles that would appear to apply across this variety of species are as follows: histamine, per se, will produce bronchospasm in man, guinea-pig and other species, and bronchodilation or no response in cat, rat, etc. [35]. Generally, however, in tracheobronchial smooth muscle, either spontaneously-contracted or contracted by a cholinergic agonist such as carbachol, histamine will produce a relaxation in the presence of mepyramine. In both human [30] and sub-human [14, 29] primates, guinea-pig trachea and horse bronchus, for example, the histamine relaxation appears to have been adequately antagonized by H_2-receptor antagonists, as for example metiamide, and mimicked by agonists such as dimaprit. These investigations would seem to have established the presence of bronchorelaxant H_2-receptors in these tissues. In lower species, as for example horse (trachea), rat, rabbit and ferret, the histamine relaxation generally was not blocked by the H_2-receptor antagonists nor, in fact, by a variety of other antagonists or metabolic inhibitors such as propranolol, indometacin, etc. (Table II). In these cases, the possibility of a third type of histamine receptor, which may be functionally similar to the classic H_2-receptor, has often been suggested (for review see [35]), since H_1- and H_2-receptor antagonists do not antagonize the relaxant effect of histamine. The possibility of this third histamine receptor type

Table II. The effect of antagonists on the tracheobronchial smooth muscle responses to histamine and related agonists in vitro.

Ref.	Species	Anatomic location	Agonist	Effect*	Antagonized by:
[27]	Horse	Trachea	Histamine	Relax	Not blocked by metiamide
		Bronchi	Histamine	Relax	Blocked by metiamide
[28]	Guinea-pig	Trachea + bronchi	Histamine	Contractions	Enhanced by metiamide
		Bronchi	2-methyl histamine	Contractions	No effect by metiamide
[7]	Sheep	Bronchi	Histamine	Relax	Blocked by burimamide
[14, 29]	Monkey	Bronchi	Histamine	Relax	Blocked by metiamide**
			Dimaprit		
			Impromidine		
[*]	Monkey	Trachea	Histamine	Relax	Blocked by metiamide
			Dimaprit		Not studied
[30]	Man	Bronchi	Histamine	Relax	Blocked by metiamide
[31]	Rat	Trachea	Histamine ⎫	'Relax'	Not blocked by cimetidine
			Dimaprit ⎭		
[6]	Cat	Trachea	Histamine	Relax	Partially by mepyramine and pronetalol
[26]	Cat	Trachea	Histamine		Not blocked by mepyra-
		Bronchi	2-methyl histamine ⎫ Relax		mine, burimamide, me-
			4-methyl histamine ⎭		tiamide, propranolol, indometacin
[8, 32]	Rabbit	Trachea	Histamine	Relax	Not blocked by mepyra- mine, burimamide, cime- tidine, metiamide, pro- pranolol, indometacin, phenoxybenzamine, etc.
[33]	Ferret	Trachea	4-methyl histamine ⎫ Relax		Not blocked by burima-
		Bronchi	Histamine ⎭		mide, cimetidine, metia- mide, propranolol, indo- metacin
[34]	Dog	Trachea	4-methyl histamine	No effect	None
		Bronchi			

* = often in presence of mepyramine; ** = K_B for metiamide varied with the agonist (see text); [*] = [Krell and Chakrin, unpublished observations].

should certainly be considered, but the relevancy of that possibility to other tissues or systems in the same species or to tracheobronchial smooth muscle in the higher species of primates remains to be determined.

While portions of the data supporting the species differences presently lack confirmation, it seems that, in several species at least, H_2-receptors clearly mediate a histamine-induced relaxation of tracheobronchial smooth muscle, as for example in rhesus monkey. Helical strips prepared from each primary bronchus were placed in an isolated tissue bath for measurement of isometric tension, with a resting tone of 2 g applied. The absence of a 'spontaneous' tone in these strips required the use of carbachol to induce a contraction in order to study the 'potential relaxant' activity of various agents. A concentration of 3×10^{-6} M carbachol was employed, and produced a contraction equivalent to an EC_{90} for this agonist.

Histamine produced a concentration-dependent relaxation of the smooth muscle equivalent to about 50% of that which could be obtained with 3×10^{-5} M dl-isoprenaline. As higher concentrations were used, contractions became superimposed on the relaxations. The H_1-receptor antagonist mepyramine, at a concentration of 1×10^{-5} M, prevented this reversal. The H_2-receptor antagonist metiamide shifted the histamine concentration-response curve determined in the presence of 1×10^{-5} M mepyramine to the right in a parallel manner. The K_B value for metiamide was 2.3×10^{-7} M, close to values reported in other tissues. SK&F-91581, at a concentration of 1×10^{-4} M, produced a modest shift to the right in the histamine curve and appeared to alter the maximum response.

Both dimaprit and impromidine can produce concentration-related relaxation of primate bronchial strips, effects that can be antagonized by metiamide. However, while metiamide 10^{-5} M can produce a parallel shift to the right in the dose-response curves of both agonists, the estimated K_B values (4.2×10^{-6} M for impromidine and 3.4×10^{-6} M for dimaprit) for metiamide versus these agonists were some 10 times higher than the reported K_B values for metiamide versus histamine in this and other tissues, at least suggesting that the agonists may produce relaxation of smooth muscle by other than merely H_2-receptor occupation. Similar results were reported by Drazen et al. in guinea-pig pulmonary tissue [36].

In vivo studies

In summary, from work reported during the past few years with H_2-receptors in both pulmonary mast cells and tracheobronchial smooth muscle in vitro, the potential exists for an enhanced, immunologically-induced bronchospasm as a consequence of H_2-receptor antagonist administration. This might be due to either enhancement of immunologically-induced histamine release from pulmonary 'mast cells' or potential blockade of H_2-relaxant receptors on tracheobronchial smooth muscle. A number of investigations have been undertaken to evaluate this possibility in vivo, in both small and large animal models of immediate hypersensitivity reactions.

In 1977, we reported that metiamide increased extracellular histamine in the medium surrounding passively-sensitized canine lung fragments which had been challenged with ascaris antigen [13]. In contrast, metiamide at doses up to 50 μmol/kg did not enhance ascaris antigen-induced pulmonary pathophysiology expressed as increases in pulmonary resistance or decreases in dynamic lung compliance in this species in vivo. Thus, insofar as a canine model of allergic asthma might be predictive of the human disease, it can be anticipated that the use of histamine H_2-receptor antagonists may not be deleterious to allergic asthmatics.

In 1978, Dulabh and Vickers demonstrated a metiamide or cimetidine enhancement of extracellular histamine induced with ovalbumin antigen from actively-sensitized guinea-pig lung in vitro [21]. While metiamide apparently did not potentiate the pulmonary anaphylaxis in vivo, and was thus consistent with the observations in the canine model, cimetidine *did* potentiate the anaphylactic reaction in vivo.

The effects of H_2-antagonists and the agonist 4-methyl histamine were also studied on the severity of guinea-pig anaphylactic reactions in vivo by Drazen et al. [37]. These investigators reported that both burimamide and metiamide increased the severity of the reaction, an effect apparently not shared by cimetidine. The agonist 4-methyl histamine significantly diminished the severity of the reaction in this species.

Thus, with some differences between studies, the guinea-pig appears to reflect the consequences of H_2-receptor antagonists in vivo.

Based on these studies, it is likely that the various animal models of allergic asthma may not provide consistent information on the in vivo activity of either the H_2-receptor antagonists or agonists, possibly due to the inconsistent role played by histamine, either directly or indirectly, in the allergic bronchospasm in vivo among the several species. Well-controlled clinical studies in man may, however, provide such information, and such studies are reported in other papers in this volume.

Acknowledgments

The authors express their appreciation to Drs. A. Misher, W. Duncan, P. Ridley, J. Weisbach and R. Brimblecombe for their interest and encouragement during the course of these studies. We also thank J. Mengel, R. Osborn, D. Young, L. Hostelley and S. Bostick for providing skillful technical assistance.

References

1. Ash, A.S.F. and Schild, H.O. (1966): Receptors mediating some actions of histamine. *Br. J. Pharmacol. 27,* 427.
2. Black, J.W., Duncan, W.A.M., Durant, C.J., Ganellin, C.R. and Parsons, M.E. (1972): Definition and antagonism of histamine H_2-receptors. *Nature (London) 236,* 385.
3. Black, J.W., Duncan, W.A.M., Emmett, J.C., Ganellin, C.R., Hesselbo, T., Parsons, M.E. and Wyllie, J.H. (1973): Metiamide, an orally active histamine H_2-receptor antagonist. *Agents Actions 3,* 133.
4. Lichtenstein, L.M. and Gillespie, E. (1973): Inhibition of histamine release by histamine controlled by H_2-receptor. *Nature (London) 244,* 287.
5. Lichtenstein, L.M., Plaut, M., Henney, C. and Gillespie, E. (1973): The role of H_2-receptors on the cells involved in hypersensitivity reactions. In: *International Symposium on histamine H_2-receptor antagonists,* p. 187. Editors: C.J. Wood and M.A. Simkins. Smith Kline & French Laboratories Ltd., Welwyn Garden City.
6. Maengwyn-Davies, G.D. (1968): The dual mode of action of histamine in the cat isolated tracheal chain. *J. Pharm. Pharmacol. 20,* 572.
7. Eyre, P. (1973): Histamine H_2-receptors in the sheep bronchus and cat trachea: the action of burimamide. *Br. J. Pharmacol. 48,* 321.
8. Fleisch, J.H. and Calkins, P.J. (1976): Comparison of drug-induced responses of rabbit trachea and bronchus. *J. Appl. Physiol. 41,* 62.
9. Kaliner, M. and Austen, K.F. (1975): Immunologic release of chemical mediators from human tissues. *Annu. Rev. Pharmacol. Toxicol. 15,* 177.
10. Orange, R.P. (1973): Immunopharmacological aspects of bronchial asthma. *Clin. Allergy 3,* 521.
11. Tauber, A.I., Kaliner, M., Stechschulte, D.J. and Austen, K.F. (1973): Immunologic release of histamine and slow reacting substance of anaphylaxis from human lung. V. Effects of prostaglandins on release of histamine. *J. Immunol. 111,* 27.
12. Chakrin, L.W., Krell, R.D., Mengel, J., Young, D., Zaher, C. and Wardell, J.R. Jr. (1974): Effect of a histamine H_2-receptor antagonist on immunologically-induced mediator release *in vitro. Agents Actions 4,* 297.
13. Krell, R.D. and Chakrin, L.W. (1977): The effect of metiamide in *in vitro* and *in vivo* canine models of type I hypersensitivity reactions. *Eur. J. Pharmacol. 44,* 35.
14. Chakrin, L.W., Bostick, S., Hostelley, L. and Krell, R.D. (1979): Effect of histamine H_2-receptor agonists and antagonists on pulmonary immunologically-induced histamine release and smooth muscle. *Pharmacologist 21,* 266.
15. Malley, A. and Harris, R.J. Jr. (1968): Passive sensitization of monkey lung fragments

with sera of timothy-sensitive patients. I. Spectrofluorometric analysis of histamine release. *J. Immunol. 100,* 915.

16. Ishizaka, T.K., Ishizaka, K., Orange, R.P. and Austen, K.F. (1970): The capacity of human immunoglobulin E to mediate the release of histamine and slow reacting substance of anaphylaxis (SRS-A) from monkey lung. *J. Immunol. 104,* 335.

17. Kaliner, M., Orange, R.P. and Austen, K.F. (1972): Immunological release of histamine and slow reacting substance of anaphylaxis from human lung. IV. Enhancement by cholinergic and alpha adrenergic stimulation. *J. Exp. Med. 136,* 556.

18. Shore, P.A., Burkhalter, A. and Cohn, V.J. Jr. (1959): A method for the fluorometric assay of histamine in tissues. *J. Pharmacol. Exp. Ther. 127,* 182.

19. Anton, A.H. and Sayre, D.F. (1969): A modified fluorometric procedure for tissue histamine and its distribution in various animals. *J. Pharmacol. Exp. Ther. 166,* 285.

20. Orange, R.P. and Austen, K.F. (1969): Slow reacting substance of anaphylaxis. *Adv. Immunol. 10,* 105.

21. Dulabh, R. and Vickers, M.R. (1978): The effects of H_2-receptor antagonists on anaphylaxis in the guinea pig. *Agents Actions 8,* 559.

22. Kaliner, M. (1978): Human lung tissue and anaphylaxis: the effects of histamine on the immunologic release of mediators. *Am. Rev. Respir. Dis. 118,* 1015.

23. Durant, G.J., Emmett, J.C. and Ganellin, C.R. (1977): The chemical origin and properties of histamine H_2-receptor antagonists. In: *Cimetidine: Proceedings of the second International Symposium on histamine H_2-receptor antagonists,* p. 1. Editors: W.L. Burland and M.A. Simkins. Excerpta Medica, Amsterdam-Oxford-Princeton.

24. Parsons, M.E., Owen, D.A.A., Ganellin, C.R. and Durant, G.J. (1977): Dimaprit [S-[3-(N,N dimethylamino)propyl]isothiourea] — A highly specific histamine H_2-receptor agonist. *Agents Actions 7,* 31.

25. Durant, G.J., Duncan, W.A.M., Ganellin, C.R., Parsons, M.E., Blakemore, R.C. and Rasmussen, A.C. (1978): Impromidine (SK&F-92676) is a very potent and specific agonist for histamine H_2-receptors. *Nature (London) 276,* 403.

26. Chand, N. and Eyre, P. (1977): Atypical (relaxant) response to histamine in cat bronchus. *Agents Actions 7,* 183.

27. Chand, N. and Eyre, P. (1977): Histamine reflexes constricted trachea and bronchi of horse. *Vet. Sci. Comm. 1,* 85.

28. Okpako, D.T., Chand, N. and Eyre, P. (1978): The presence of inhibitory histamine H_2-receptors in guinea-pig tracheobronchial muscle. *J. Pharm. Pharmacol. 30,* 181.

29. Krell, R.D. (1979): Pharmacologic characterization of isolated rhesus monkey bronchial smooth muscle. *J. Pharmacol. Exp. Ther. 211,* 436.

30. Dunlop, L.S. and Smith, A.P. (1977): The effect of histamine antagonists on antigen-induced contractions of sensitized human bronchus *in vitro. Br. J. Pharmacol. 59,* 475P.

31. Eyre, P. and Besner, R.N. (1979): Cimetidine fails to block functional antagonism of carbachol by histamine in rat trachea. *Res. Comm. Chem. Pathol. Pharmacol. 24,* 457.

32. Chand, N., Eyre, P. and DeRoth, L. (1979): Relaxant action of histamine in rabbit trachea: possible existence of third histamine receptor subtype. *Res. Comm. Chem. Pathol. Pharmacol. 23,* 211.

33. Chand, N. and Eyre, P. (1978): Histamine receptors of airway smooth muscle of ferret and rat. *Res. Comm. Chem. Pathol. Pharmacol. 21,* 55.

34. Bradley, S.L. and Russell, J.A. (1977): Distribution of histamine H_1- and H_2-receptors in dog airway smooth muscle. *Physiologist 20,* 11.

35. Eyre, P. and Chand, N. (1979): Preliminary evidence for two subclasses of histamine H_2-receptors. *Agents Actions 9,* 1.

36. Drazen, J.M., Schneider, M.W. and Venugopalan, C.S. (1979): Bronchodilator activity of dimaprit in the guinea-pig in vitro and in vivo. *Eur. J. Pharmacol. 55,* 233.

37. Drazen, J.M., Venugopalan, C.S. and Soter, N.A. (1978): H_2-receptor mediated inhibition of immediate-type hypersensitivity reactions *in vivo. Am. Rev. Respir. Dis. 117,* 479.

The effect of histamine antagonists on bronchoconstriction in man

Noemi M. Eiser, Jane G. Mills* and A. Guz
*Department of Medicine, Charing Cross Hospital Medical School, London; and
*The Research Institute, Smith Kline & French Laboratories Ltd., Welwyn Garden
City, United Kingdom*

H_1-receptor antagonists

Effect on bronchial provocation

More than 30 years ago, Curry [1] and Herxheimer [2] reported on the protective role of various antihistamines, now designated H_1-receptor antagonists, on both histamine- and antigen-induced asthma. Since then, a number of studies have confirmed these results.

Casterline and Evans exposed 11 asthmatics to inhalation challenges of increasing concentrations of histamine until the forced expiratory volume in 1 second (FEV_1) fell by 20% [3]. The challenges were repeated after pretreatment with diphenhydramine, and Figure 1 shows the results. The histamine response was reproducible, but in the presence of diphenhydramine a much larger dose of histamine was required to produce the same bronchoconstriction.

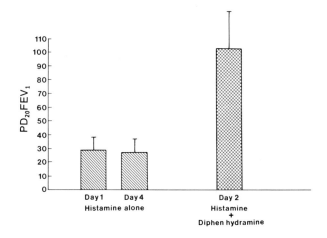

Fig. 1. *Histograms showing the mean (± SEM) dose of histamine which produced a 20% fall in FEV_1 ($PD_{20}FEV_1$) in 11 asthmatic subjects on 2 separate occasions, and the significant effect on $PD_{20}FEV_1$ produced by the inhalation of diphenhydramine 20 mg ($p < 0.005$). (Compiled from [3].)*

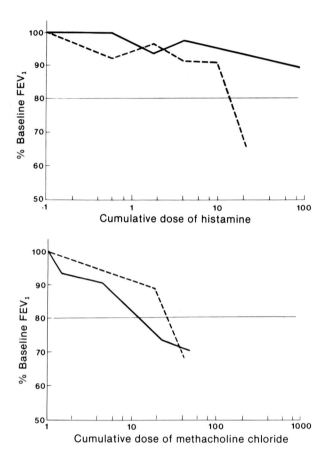

Fig. 2.   The effect of chlorpheniramine on the percentage fall in FEV₁ with cumulative doses of histamine (top) and methacholine (bottom), in a typical asthmatic subject. ——— = chlorpheniramine; --- = control. (Reproduced from [4] with the kind permission of The C.V. Mosby Co.)

Another study reported the effect of inhaled chlorpheniramine maleate 5 mg on histamine- and methacholine-induced bronchoconstriction in 9 asthmatics [4]. A typical result from one subject is illustrated in Figure 2. Chlorpheniramine prevented the response to histamine, but not to methacholine, suggesting that chlorpheniramine was acting as an H_1-receptor antagonist and not as an anticholinergic agent at this dose.

It is of interest that in the classical experiment by Schild et al. on excised bronchus and lung from an asthmatic [5], mepyramine was found to be 10^4 times more effective in protecting against histamine-induced bronchoconstriction than against antigen-induced bronchoconstriction.

Effect on bronchomotor tone

Evidence is conflicting on the effect of the H_1-receptor antagonists on bronchomotor tone. In vitro studies on guinea-pig tracheal chains by Hawkins suggested that,

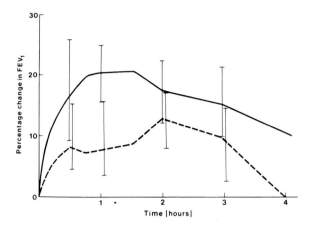

Fig. 3. Results of inhalation of clemastine (——) and placebo (---) in 12 asthmatic subjects (mean ± SEM). (Reproduced from [7] with the kind permission of the British Medical Journal.)

in this species at least, the effect was dose related, bronchoconstriction resulting from lower doses and bronchodilatation from higher doses of a number of H_1-receptor antagonists [6]. Nogrady et al. reported significant bronchodilatation in asthmatics following inhalation of clemastine as compared with placebo (Fig. 3); however, these subjects were not in a stable clinical state since they were recovering from acute exacerbations [7]. Both Popa [8] and Woenne et al. [4] reported bronchodilatation in asthmatics, following intravenous and inhaled chlorpheniramine respectively. In contrast, Maconochie et al. concluded that neither intravenous nor oral chlorpheniramine altered resting FEV_1 in normal subjects [9], and a recent study by Partridge and Saunders failed to confirm the results of Nogrady et al. with inhaled clemastine [10]. Several factors may explain these apparently conflicting results. Some H_1-receptor antagonists are local irritants in the bronchi and some, including chlorpheniramine and diphenhydramine, have been found to release histamine from passively-sensitised human lung in vitro [11]. The oral and intravenous antihistamines might not give adequate local concentrations to significantly affect bronchi.

H_1- and H_2-receptors in human lung

In vitro studies

With regard to the comparative roles of the H_1- and H_2-receptors in human airways, there is little published data at present. Dunlop and Smith reported on a series of experiments on isolated strips of human bronchi [12]. These strips were sensitised to *D. pteronyssius* and then challenged either with histamine or with antigen. The experiment was repeated in the presence of the H_1-receptor antagonist mepyramine and the H_2-receptor antagonist metiamide. The results suggested the presence of bronchoconstricting H_1-receptors and bronchodilating H_2-receptors.

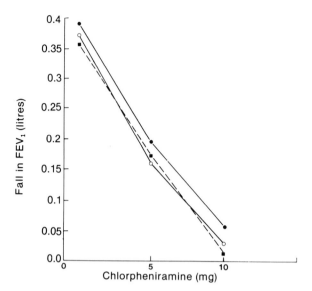

Fig. 4.   The dose-response relationship between intravenous chlorpheniramine and the fall in FEV₁ after histamine, after adding either placebo (•——•) or intravenous cimetidine 100 mg (○——○) or 200 mg (■--■). (Reproduced from [9] with the kind permission of MacMillan Journals.)

Studies in normal subjects

In vivo studies on normal subjects were undertaken by Maconochie et al., comparing the effects of oral and intravenous chlorpheniramine and cimetidine on the histamine response. Only chlorpheniramine prevented the histamine response. The addition of cimetidine to chlorpheniramine slightly increased the effect of chlorpheniramine, but this increase was not statistically significant (Fig. 4). These authors concluded that, in normal subjects, it is likely that only H_1-receptors are involved in histamine-induced bronchoconstriction.

Studies in asthmatic subjects

In a recent study on the effects of oral chlorpheniramine and cimetidine, Leopold et al. found that neither drug affected daily peak expiratory flow measurements nor exercise-induced asthma [13]. In antigen-induced asthma, Löwhagen and Lindholm found a slight protective effect with oral chlorpheniramine and no effect with oral cimetidine [14].

Studies on normal and asthmatic subjects

We have, also, studied the effect of intravenous injection of chlorpheniramine and cimetidine on histamine- and antigen-induced bronchoconstriction in man. Bronchial challenge with histamine was undertaken in 18 non-asthmatic and 18 asthmatic subjects. The bronchial response was monitored by serial measurements of specific airway conductance (sGaw), measured in a body plethysmograph. This measure of airways obstruction is highly sensitive and is effort-independent. Five breaths of histamine acid phosphate were inhaled from a Hudson nebuliser, attached to a breath-actuated dosimeter. The subject was instructed to inhale to a similar depth and at a similar flow rate, in order to ensure a standardised challenge. Every 3 minutes a further dose of histamine was delivered, at double the previous concentration, until a definite response occurred. A dose-response curve was then constructed for each challenge. On separate days the histamine challenge was repeated 10 minutes after intravenous injections of either a saline (placebo), cimetidine 200 mg or 400 mg, chlorpheniramine 20 mg, or cimetidine 200 mg with chlorpheniramine 20 mg. A similar protocol was used to challenge 9 atopic asthmatics with antigen, except that 10 minutes was allowed after each dose for a bronchial response to develop before sGaw was re-measured. Intra-subject and inter-subject comparisons of results were made simultaneously by analysis of variance.

The mean results for the histamine challenges are shown in Figure 5. The same pattern of response was seen in the normal subjects and in the asthmatics. Placebo did not significantly alter the histamine dose-response curve, but there was a small shift to the right with cimetidine, which only attained statistical significance at the highest dose of histamine with cimetidine 400 mg. There was a much larger shift to the right with chlorpheniramine and, similarly, with chlorpheniramine and cimetidine together. A similar pattern was seen with the antigen challenges. The antigen dose-response curve (Fig. 6) was not affected by placebo premedication, and was shifted markedly to the right by chlorpheniramine both alone and together with cimetidine. The antigen curve was shifted further to the right by cimetidine than the histamine curve had been, and the effect was greater with 200 mg compared with 400 mg cimetidine.

In conclusion, our results suggest the presence of both H_1- and H_2-receptors in the human bronchus, and suggest also that both types of receptor mediate bronchoconstriction. The pattern of these receptors appears to be the same in normal

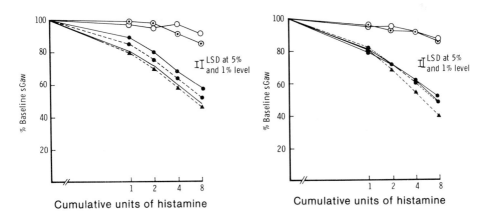

Fig. 5. Mean histamine dose-response curves for 18 normal subjects (left) and 18 asthmatic subjects (right). Challenges were made with histamine alone (——), histamine + placebo (▲--▲), histamine + cimetidine 200 mg (●--●), histamine + cimetidine 400 mg (●—●), histamine + chlorpheniramine 20 mg (○—○), and histamine + chlorpheniramine 20 mg and cimetidine 200 mg (⊙—⊙). The least significant differences (LSD) at the 5% and 1% levels, as calculated from an analysis of variance, are indicated.

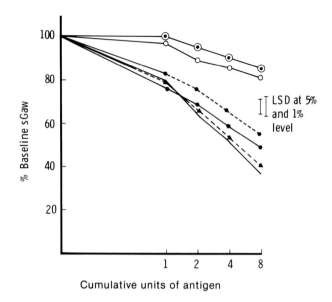

Fig. 6.   Mean antigen dose-response curve for 9 atopic asthmatics. For further information, see legend to Figure 5.

and asthmatic subjects. However, the effect of the H_1-receptors greatly predominates over that of the H_2-receptors. Since the antigen response was so effectively blocked by the H_1-receptor antagonist, it is likely that histamine is an important mediator in the Type I allergic response in human lungs. These results appear to be at variance with those of the authors previously mentioned. In the case of Dunlop and Smith this may be either a drug- or a dose-related phenomenon, since they used metiamide rather than cimetidine as their H_2-receptor antagonist and also used a very large dose. They did not demonstrate any dose-response relationships with their antagonists.

The blocking effect of cimetidine on the histamine response might have been significant in the study by Maconochie et al. if they had used a more sensitive measure of airways obstruction than FEV_1. This might also be true of the studies of Leopold et al. and Löwhagen and Lindholm. In these studies there was the added problem that oral doses of the antagonists might not have given sufficient local concentrations in the lungs to demonstrate what appears to be a small effect in our study.

Acknowledgement

We are much indebted to Smith Kline & French for their generous financial support.

References

1. Curry, J.J. (1946): The effect of antihistamine substances and other drugs on histamine bronchoconstriction in asthmatic subjects. *J. Clin. Invest. 25,* 792.
2. Herxheimer, H. (1949): Antihistamines in bronchial asthma. *Br. Med. J. 2,* 901.
3. Casterline, C.L. and Evans, R. (1977): Further studies on the mechanism of human histamine-induced asthma. *J. Allergy Clin. Immunol. 59,* 420.

4. Woenne, R., Kattan, M., Orange, R.P. and Levison, H. (1978): Bronchial hyperreactivity to histamine and methacholine in asthmatic children after inhalation of SCH 1000 and chlorpheniramine maleate. *J. Allergy Clin. Immunol. 62,* 119.

5. Schild, H.O., Hawkins, D.F., Mongar, J.L. and Herxheimer, H. (1951): Reactions of isolated human asthmatic lung and bronchial tissue to a specific antigen. *Lancet 2,* 376.

6. Hawkins, D.F. (1955): Bronchoconstrictor and bronchodilator actions of antihistamine drugs. *Br. J. Pharmacol. 10,* 230.

7. Nogrady, S.G., Hartley, J.P.R., Handslip, P.D.J. and Hurst, N.P. (1978): Bronchodilatation after inhalation of the antihistamine clemastine. *Thorax 33,* 479.

8. Popa, V.T. (1977): Bronchodilating activity of an H_1-blocker chlorpheniramine. *J. Allergy Clin. Immunol. 59,* 54.

9. Maconochie, J.G., Woodings, E.P. and Richards, D.A. (1979): Effects of H_1- and H_2-blocking agents on histamine-induced bronchoconstriction in nonasthmatic subjects. *Br. J. Clin. Pharmacol. 7,* 231.

10. Partridge, M.R. and Saunders, K.B. (1979): The effect of an inhaled antihistamine (clemastine) as a bronchodilator and as maintenance therapy in asthma. *Clin. Sci. Mol. Med. 56,* 10P.

11. Church, M.K. and Gradidge, C.F. (1979): Histamine H_1-antagonists and histamine release from human lung in vitro. *Br. J. Pharmacol. 66,* 68P.

12. Dunlop, L.S. and Smith, A.P. (1977): The effect of histamine antagonists on antigen-induced contractions of sensitised human bronchus in vitro. *Br. J. Pharmacol. 59,* 475P.

13. Leopold, J.D., Hartley, J.P.R. and Smith, A.P. (1979): Effects of oral H_1- and H_2-receptor antagonists in asthma. *Br. J. Clin. Pharmacol. 8,* 249.

14. Löwhagen, O. and Lindholm, B. (1979): Personal communication.

Discussion

Owen (Welwyn Garden City): In addition to histamine receptors on mast cells and on the respiratory smooth muscle, there are also histamine receptors on the pulmonary blood vessels. Is there any evidence that these receptors do or do not contribute to the overall response to histamine on respiratory function?

Eiser: There is not yet much data on the evidence for pulmonary vascular receptors in man. Such studies are very difficult to perform. It is theoretically possible that a vasodilatation in the pulmonary tree could change specific airways conductance, because it is such a sensitive measure of airways obstruction. This is why we have been so tentative in interpreting our results. It is possible that there is some contribution from the vasculature in changing airways obstruction, but it is not possible to differentiate using this measurement.

Boyce (Welwyn Garden City): During our studies with impromidine in normal subjects (some of whom were atopic — I would still call them normal), we have seen a nasal obstruction which appears to be dose-related and which is certainly either attenuated or abolished with cimetidine. It seems possible to get congestion or dilatation of the blood vessels in the nasal airway which can provoke symptoms rather like allergic rhinitis in some of these subjects. Dr. Chakrin speculated that an H_2-agonist may benefit allergic rhinitis, but our results provide evidence, although only anecdotal at present, that this is not so.

Does Dr. Eiser have any evidence of the effect of H_1- and H_2-antagonists on the late reaction?

Eiser: No. The late reaction is a very difficult one to investigate in man. As Dr. Boyce knows, it is quite variable in onset and quite difficult to reverse; I have gone out of my way to avoid using patients who have late reactions. I have no data on this at present, but it would probably be much more relevant to human asthma. The type I allergic response has relatively little importance in human asthma, except perhaps occasionally in industrial asthma. It would be much more important to look at the late reactions, although more dangerous and more difficult.

Baron (London): Dr. Eiser has shown remarkable prevention of both histamine- and antigen-induced bronchoconstriction by intravenous H_1-antagonists. What is the clinical evidence for their value? Have they been used extensively in the past 40 years?

Eiser: The popularity of the H_1-antagonists appears to have waxed and waned. Herxheimer and Curry advocated their use and claimed that they were very effective, but I think that, in practice, their use is limited, mainly by the central nervous system depression which occurs when they are given either orally or parenterally. Inhalation has been limited in some of the antihistamines by local irritation of the airways. In general, people have been quite disenchanted with the use of H_1-receptor antagonists. However, with the newer generation of compounds, there may again be a possibility for their use.

Histamine in the brain: its localization, functional role and receptors

Monique Garbarg, G. Barbin, A.M. Duchemin, C. Llorens, J.M. Palacios, H. Pollard, T.T. Quach, E. Rodergas, C. Rose and J.C. Schwartz
Neurobiology Unit, Centre Paul Broca I.N.S.E.R.M., Paris, France

Histamine is present in the mammalian brain, although it does not cross the blood brain barrier; it is held both in neuronal and non-neuronal cells, which exhibit different biochemical and pharmacological properties [1].

The non-neuronal cells constitute mainly a storage site for histamine, as indicated by a high level of the amine associated with a low activity of its synthesizing enzyme, L-histidine decarboxylase, as well as by its slow turnover; typical histamino-liberators such as compound 48/80 and polymyxin B release this pool of histamine, which sediments in heavy subcellular fractions similarly to mast-cell granules. These properties render it likely that this non-neuronal pool of histamine is localized in mast cells. In fact, mast cells or other closely-related cells have recently been identified in different brain regions, and Ibrahim et al. have shown that they are closely associated with blood vessels [2]. This localization suggests that brain mast cells, like peripheral mast cells, could participate in vascular control, immune responses or inflammatory processes.

Approximately half of the brain histamine is localized in neuronal cells, where it is generally accepted that it acts as a neurotransmitter [3, 4]. The visualization of such neurons could be of great help in understanding the functional role of histamine in the brain; however, fluorescence histochemical methods (which have been so useful in the study of catecholaminergic and serotoninergic neurons) are neither sensitive nor specific enough for histamine. Immunohistochemical methods are not available either.

Lesion studies, however, have proved to be a useful approach towards the uncovering of histaminergic pathways [5]. They have evidenced, in rat brain, the presence of an ascending histamine pathway, travelling along the medial forebrain bundle like the monoamines and widely innervating the whole telencephalon. Neuronal histamine is not held in monoaminergic neurons, as demonstrated by the fact that selective chemical lesions of either catecholamines or serotonin neurons do not result in significant changes in the histaminergic system [6]. The presence of histamine fibers in the medial forebrain bundle has been confirmed by the demonstration that electrophysiological effects recorded in the areas containing nerve terminals, such as the cortex or hippocampus, can be at least partially blocked by histamine antagonists after the stimulation of this bundle. Convergent results from various biochemical investigations have indicated that these neurons emanate from the upper part of the mesencephalon, either from the reticular mesencephalic formation or from the mammillary bodies [7]. Such an anatomical disposition (Fig. 1) recalls that of noradrenaline and serotonin and suggests that histamine, like the

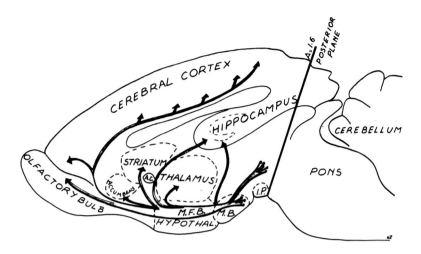

Fig. 1. Schematic drawing of the disposition of ascending histaminergic pathways in rat brain, as suggested by lesion studies. (Reproduced with permission from [26]).

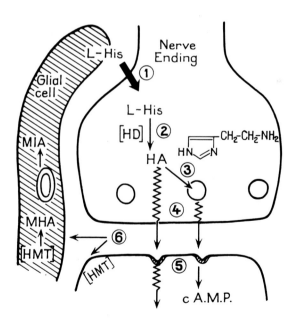

Fig. 2. A putative histaminergic synapse: the various steps in the metabolism of histamine (HA). 1: Uptake of L-histidine (L-His). 2: Synthesis of HA by the action of L-histidine decarboxylase (HD). 3: Storage of HA in vesicles. 4: Release of HA by nerve impulse. 5: Postsynaptic actions of HA. 6: Methylation of HA by histamine-N-methyltransferase (HMT) into 3-methyl histamine (MHA), which is then deaminated into methylimidazole acetic acid (MIA). (Reproduced with permission from [27]).

monoamines, might be involved in the general control of cortical activity.

Most of the criteria generally expected of a neurotransmitter are fulfilled by histamine [8]. A putative histaminergic synapse is shown in Figure 2. The amine is synthesized in a 1-step reaction which is catalyzed by a specific enzyme, L-histidine decarboxylase. This enzyme is distinct from the non-specific decarboxylase of aromatic acids, exhibits kinetic properties similar to those found for the L-histidine decarboxylase of rat gastric mucosa and is localized in the cytoplasm of nerve endings, whereas histamine is stored in synaptic vesicles by a reserpine-sensitive mechanism, a situation analogous to that found with other neurotransmitters. The half-life of histamine is less than 1 hour, indicating its dynamic state; moreover, its turnover can be rapidly altered in various physiological and pharmacological situations, thus reflecting the activity of histaminergic neurons. Indirect approaches provide evidence that histamine is released upon depolarization of nerve endings by a calcium-dependent process. Inactivation of the released amine is ensured only by an enzymatic process. Histamine is methylated by the action of histamine-N-methyltransferase, an enzyme localized both in neurons and in glial cells, and the 3-methyl histamine which is formed is a substance devoid of the biological activity of histamine.

The criteria of identity of action have not yet been demonstrated in mammalian brain. Nevertheless, Weinreich has shown that, in the mollusk Aplysia, exogenously-applied histamine mimics the activity of the natural transmitter released at defined synapses [9]. In mammalian brain, cerebral receptors responding specifically to histamine have been evidenced by electrophysiological and neurochemical approaches [10].

The microiontophoretic application of histamine in close vicinity of single neurons usually results in an inhibition of firing. Excitatory responses have also been reported, mainly in the hypothalamus [11]. These actions are mediated by specific receptors and imply the existence of 2 types of histamine receptor. More information as to the types of histamine receptor present on target cells has come from the biological responses induced by the amine and from the selective binding of radioactive ligands to the receptor recognition site.

The first biochemical evidence of the presence of histamine receptors in mammalian brain was provided by the histamine-stimulated increase of intracellular concentration of cyclic AMP: in a cell-free preparation of guinea-pig hippocampus, it is clear that the stimulation of adenylate cyclase, the enzyme responsible for cyclic AMP synthesis, is mediated by H_2-receptors [12, 13].

In intact cell preparations such as hippocampal slices, the cyclic AMP response is more complex. The involvement of H_2-receptors is indicated by the effect of different concentrations of the selective H_2-receptor antagonist metiamide on dose-response curves (Fig. 3). The parallel shift to the right, without modification of the maximal response, shows the competitive nature of this inhibition; when data are plotted according to Schild plot, a pA_2 value of 6.04 is obtained, which is in agreement with the value found for metiamide acting on a pure population of H_2-receptors on peripheral systems. On the other hand, several data strongly indicate that H_1-receptors are also involved in the cyclic AMP response to histamine [14]; when dose-response curves are constructed in the presence of the H_1-receptor antagonist mepyramine, a rather complex picture emerges (Fig. 4): for low concentrations of histamine, mepyramine is inactive, and for higher concentrations it induces an inhibition of competitive nature. When the data from the upper part of the curve

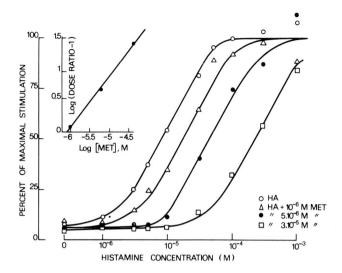

Fig. 3. *Inhibition by metiamide (MET) of the histamine (HA)-induced accumulation of cyclic AMP in slices from guinea-pig hippocampus. Inset: the Schild plot of the data. The* pA_2 *value, determined by linear regression, is 6.04. (Reproduced with permission from [14]).*

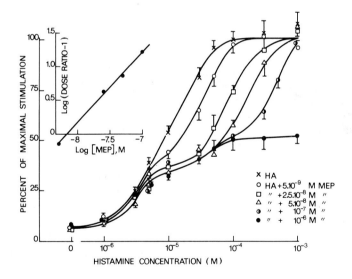

Fig. 4. *Inhibition by mepyramine (MEP) of the histamine (HA)-induced accumulation of cyclic AMP in slices from guinea-pig hippocampus. Dose-ratios were obtained graphically from the parallel displacement of upper parts of the curves (corresponding to 60-80% of the maximal stimulation). Inset: the Schild plot of the data. (Reproduced with permission from [14]).*

are plotted according to Schild plot, a pA_2 value of 8.2 is found. This value is far from that found for mepyramine acting on H_2-receptors ($pA_2 = 5.3$), but it agrees well with the values found in peripheral H_1 pure systems, such as guinea-pig ileum. Several other 'classical' antihistaminics also exhibit the same apparent affinities on this cyclic AMP generating system and on the guinea-pig ileum.

The complete blockade of the response to histamine by metiamide, whereas mepyramine blocks only a fraction of the response, suggests that the stimulation of cyclic AMP accumulation mediated by H_1-receptors is an indirect process which requires the stimulation of adenylate cyclase through H_2-receptors.

Such an indirect effect could be associated with a calcium translocation system, since the response mediated by H_1-receptors is dependent on the presence of external calcium [15]. Hence the stimulation of cyclic AMP induced by the H_1-receptor agonist 2-thiazolyl ethylamine in the presence of supra-maximal concentrations of dimaprit is largely prevented in the absence of extracellular calcium.

It is likely that a variety of biological systems linked to H_1-receptors might be coupled with a calcium channel. For example, histamine exerts a potent glycogeno-lytic effect on slices from mouse cortex [16] and stimulates cyclic GMP synthesis in neuroblastoma cells [17], both effects which have been shown to be mediated by H_1-receptors and which require the presence of external calcium.

The target cells bearing histamine receptors linked to adenylate cyclase are likely to be post-synaptic neurons, since the response to histamine is largely reduced after selective destruction of neuronal cell-bodies by kainic acid.

Nevertheless, histamine-sensitive adenylate cyclase has also been found to be present in a capillary-rich fraction [18]. In view of the post-synaptic localization of these histamine receptors, it was of interest to determine whether the interruption of histamine afferences to the guinea-pig hippocampus would be followed by changes in the responsiveness of target cells.

The lesions of the medial forebrain bundle which were performed to investigate this possibility were not followed by any detectable change of either H_1- or H_2-receptors linked to the cyclic AMP generating system [19]. This result contrasts with the clear-cut hypersensitivity evidenced in denervated hippocampus on micro-iontophoretic application of the amine. This lack of correlation between the biochemical and the electrophysiological effects of histamine raises the question whether the histamine receptors linked to adenylate cyclase are distinct from those mediating the electrophysiological effect of histamine.

A more direct approach to the characterization of receptors is provided by the technique of high-affinity labelling with radioligands. This procedure has been applied to histamine receptors by the use of the natural agonist ^{3}H-histamine and by the use of an H_1-antagonist, ^{3}H-mepyramine.

^{3}H-histamine binds to particulate brain fraction and labels a limited number of binding sites with a high affinity (K_D = 7 nM) and a maximal capacity around 0.1 pmole/mg protein [20]. This binding is reversible, and ^{3}H-histamine interacts with a single population of sites without cooperativity. That these binding sites are distinct from the recognition site of histamine-N-methyltransferase is evidenced by differences in their regional and subcellular distributions, in their ontogenetic development and in the potency of various inhibitors. Selective destruction of neuronal cell-bodies by kainic acid is accompanied by a large decrease in the ^{3}H-histamine binding sites, indicating that they might represent the recognition moiety of post-synaptic receptors. A pre-synaptic localization of the binding sites is ruled out by the lack of effect of the interruption of histaminergic afferences in rat striatum [21]. There is even a small but significant increase in the number of binding sites which could correspond to the denervation hypersensitivity already observed electrophysiologi-cally, but not on the cyclic AMP response to histamine. Although these data

Table I. Inhibition of ^{3}H-histamine binding by various agents, determined by incubation of ^{3}H-histamine 10 nM in the presence of the particulate fraction from cerebral cortex; the effects of at least 6 concentrations of each drug were determined (triplicate assays).

Agents	K_i (nM)
Histamine agonists	
Histamine	4
Nα-methyl histamine	5
Nα-Nα-dimethyl histamine	5
Impromidine	147
Dimaprit	200
4-methyl histamine	9,500
2-methyl histamine	19,000
2-thiazolyl ethylamine	25,000
2-pyridyl ethylamine	25,000
Histamine antagonists	
Triprolidine	12,600
Cimetidine	14,000
Promethazine	20,500
Mepyramine	36,200
Metiamide	40,000
Miscellaneous	
Amodiaquine	2,600
Putrescine	21,000
Clomipramine	23,500
Haloperidol	24,000
Inactive drugs	
3-methyl histamine (tele), imidazole, acetic acid, S-adenosylhomocyteine, histidine, clonidine, noradrenaline, dopamine, serotonin, 4-aminobutyric acid, carbachol, cadaverine, spermidine, mianserin, TRH, metoprine	> 50,000

$$K_i = IC_{50}/1 + \frac{[^3H\text{-histamine}]}{K_D}.$$ IC_{50} values were determined by log-probit analysis.

strongly suggest that those high-affinity binding sites represent true neuronal histamine receptors of some physiological relevance, they do not share the pharmacological properties of either H_1- or H_2-receptors (Table I).

The histaminergic specificity of these ^{3}H-histamine binding sites is strongly suggested by the lack of inhibitory potency of histamine metabolites and of other neurotransmitters, contrasting with the significant potency of agonists. However, they clearly differ from typical H_1- or H_2-receptors, as shown by the lack of correlation between the potency of agonists and their activity regarding biological systems, and by the very low inhibitory potency of H_1- and H_2-antagonists.

A possible explanation could be that these sites represent receptors conformationally-modified during the preparation of the particulate fraction, thus representing H_1- or H_2-receptors in a 'desensitized' state. However, one may as well speculate that ^{3}H-histamine labels a class of cerebral histamine receptors which are distinct from H_1- and H_2-receptors. More experimental work with other approaches is obviously needed to clarify this interesting possibility.

Table II. Inhibition of the in vivo binding of ^{3}H-mepyramine in mouse cortex by H_1-antihistamines in therapeutic dosages.

Drug	Dosage (mg/kg)	Inhibition (%)
Mepyramine	0.2	74 ± 7***
(+) Chlorpheniramine	0.1	69 ± 5***
(-) Chlorpheniramine	0.1	16 ± 3 (NS)
Cyproheptadine	0.5	73 ± 5***
Diphenhydramine	0.8	60 ± 6*
Promethazine	1.0	77 ± 6**
Triprolidine	0.4	70 ± 3**
Cinnarizine	1.2	40 ± 4**
Mequitazine	0.4	10 ± 17 (NS)

Groups of 5-10 mice received the various drugs intraperitoneally at the indicated dosage 1 hour before administration of ^{3}H-mepyramine 40 nCi/g, and were killed 3 minutes after. The homogenized cerebral cortex was filtered under vacuum and washed with 40 ml of NaK phosphate buffer 50 mM, pH 7.5. ^{3}H-mepyramine binding in the cerebral cortex of control mice was 4.2 ± 0.3 nCi/g. Inhibition was calculated from the values of controls in the same experiment.

*$p < 0.05$; **$p < 0.01$; ***$p < 0.001$; NS = not significant.

Finally, the specific labelling of H_1-receptors has been shown to be feasible by Hill and Young, using ^{3}H-mepyramine and a preparation of guinea-pig ileum [22]. This procedure was applied to label in vitro H_1-receptors from brain particulate fraction [23, 24]. ^{3}H-mepyramine labels a single population of sites, presenting a heterogeneous distribution and pharmacological properties of typical H_1-receptors.

Interestingly, ^{3}H-mepyramine can also be used to label H_1-receptors in vivo in the living mouse [25]. That H_1-receptors are labelled under such conditions is indicated by the saturable character of the process and by the similarities of the regional distribution and the pharmacological specificity with the in vitro binding of ^{3}H-mepyramine. The most interesting feature is that, at the therapeutic dosage, antihistaminics inhibit the binding of ^{3}H-mepyramine (Table II). Hence a significant proportion of H_1-receptors in the cerebral cortex of the mouse are occupied when they receive H_1-receptor antagonists systemically, at doses close to those used in therapy.

These observations suggest that the sedative properties of these compounds could result from blockade of H_1-receptors of histaminergic neurons in brain. The involvement of histamine in vigilance states would be consistent with the arousal reactions observed on EEG following intracerebral administration of histamine, and with the anatomical disposition of the ascending histaminergic pathway.

In conclusion, neurochemical studies have shown that histamine satisfies the criteria required for a neurotransmitter. Although little has been known about the role played by the histaminergic neurons in brain, current data indicate that histamine might be involved in the control of arousal mechanisms. The characterization and localization of histamine neurons and receptors might be helpful in elucidating the functional role of this amine.

References

1. Schwartz, J.C. (1975): Histamine as a transmitter in brain. *Life Sci. 17,* 503-518.
2. Ibrahim, M.Z.M., Al-Wirr, M.E. and Bahuth, N. (1979): The mast cells of the mammalian central nervous system. III. Ultra-structural characteristics in the adult rat brain. *Acta Anat. 104,* 134-154.
3. Schwartz, J.C., Barbin, G., Baudry, M., Garbarg, M., Pollard, H. and Verdière, M. (1979): Metabolism and functions of histamine in the brain. In: *Current developments in psychopharmacology,* pp. 173-261. Editors: B. Essman and L. Valzelli. Spectrum Publishers, New York.
4. Green, J.P., Johnson, C.L. and Weinstein, H. (1978): Histamine as a neurotransmitter. In: *Psychopharmacology: A generation of progress,* pp. 319-332. Editors: M.A. Lipton, A. Dimascio and K.F. Killam. Raven Press, New York.
5. Garbarg, M., Barbin, G., Feger, J. and Schwartz, J.C. (1974): Histaminergic pathway in rat brain evidenced by lesions of the MFB. *Science 186,* 833-835.
6. Garbarg, M., Barbin, G., Bischoff, S., Pollard, H. and Schwartz, J.C. (1976): Dual localization of histamine in an ascending neuronal pathway and in non-neuronal cells evidenced by lesions in the lateral hypothalamic area. *Brain Res. 106,* 333-348.
7. Pollard, H., Barbin, G., Llorens, C., Palacios, J.M., Schwartz, J.C. and Garbarg, M. (1980): Origin of histaminergic pathways projecting to the cerebral cortex and striatum investigated by lesions studies. (Submitted.)
8. Schwartz, J.C. (1977): Histaminergic mechanisms in brain. *Annu. Rev. Pharmacol. Toxicol. 17,* 325-339.
9. Gruol, D.L. and Weinreich, D. (1979): Two pharmacologically distinct histamine receptors mediating membrane hyperpolarization on identified neurons of Aplysia californica. *Brain Res. 162,* 281-301.
10. Schwartz, J.C. (1979): Histamine receptors in brain. *Life Sci. 25,* 895-912.
11. Haas, H.L. and Wolf, P. (1977): Central action of histamine: microelectrophoretic studies. *Brain Res. 122,* 269-279.
12. Green, J.P., Johnson, C.L., Weinstein, H. and Maayani, S. (1977): Antagonism of histamine-activated adenylate cyclase in brain by D-lysergic acid diethylamide. *Proc. Natl. Acad. Sci. U.S.A. 74,* 5697-5701.
13. Hegstrand, L.R., Kanof, P.D. and Greengard, P. (1976): Histamine-sensitive adenylate cyclase in mammalian brain. *Nature (London) 260,* 163-165.
14. Palacios, J.M., Garbarg, M., Barbin, G. and Schwartz, J.C. (1978): Pharmacological characterization of histamine receptors mediating the stimulation of cyclic AMP accumulation in slices from guinea-pig hippocampus. *Mol. Pharmacol. 14,* 971-982.
15. Schwartz, J.C., Barbin, G., Duchemin, A.M., Garbarg, M., Palacios, J.M., Quach, T.T. and Rose, C. (1980): Histamine receptors in brain: characterization by binding studies and biochemical effect. In: *Receptors for neurotransmitters and peptide hormones,* pp. 169-182. Editors: G. Pepeu, M.J. Kuhar and S.J. Enna. Raven Press, New York.
16. Quach, T.T., Duchemin, A.M., Rose, C. and Schwartz, J.C. (1980): ^{3}H-glycogen hydrolysis elicited by histamine in mouse brain slices: selective involvement of H_1-receptors. *Mol. Pharmacol.* (In press.)
17. Richelson, E. (1978): Histamine H_1-receptor-mediated guanosine $3'$-$5'$-monophosphate formation by cultured mouse neuroblastoma cells. *Science 201,* 69-71.
18. Karnyushina, I.L., Palacios, J.M., Barbin, G., Dux, E., Joo, F. and Schwartz, J.C. (1980): Studies on a capillary-rich fraction isolated from brain: histaminergic components and characterization of the histamine receptors linked to adenylate cyclase. *J. Neurochem.* (In press.)
19. Haas, H.L., Wolf, P., Palacios, J.M., Garbarg, M., Barbin, G. and Schwartz, J.C. (1978): Hypersensitivity to histamine in the guinea-pig brain: microiontophoretic and biochemical studies. *Brain Res. 156,* 275-291.

20. Palacios, J.M., Schwartz, J.C. and Garbarg, M. (1978): High affinity binding of ³H-histamine in rat brain. *Eur. J. Pharmacol. 50,* 443-444.
21. Barbin, G., Palacios, J.M., Rodergas, E., Schwartz, J.C. and Garbarg, M. (1980): Characterization of the high affinity binding sites of ³H-histamine in rat brain. *Mol. Pharmacol.* (In press.)
22. Hill, S.J., Young, J.M. and Marrian, D.H. (1977): Specific binding of (³H)-mepyramine to histamine H₁-receptors in intestinal smooth muscle. *Nature (London) 270,* 361-363.
23. Hill, S.J., Emson, P.C. and Young, J.M. (1978): The binding of (³H)-mepyramine to histamine H₁-receptors in guinea-pig brain. *J. Neurochem. 31,* 997-1004.
24. Tran, V.T., Chang, R.S.L. and Snyder, S.H. (1978): Histamine H₁-receptors identified in mammalian brain membranes with (³H)-mepyramine. *Proc. Natl. Acad. Sci. U.S.A. 75,* 6290-6294.
25. Quach, T.T., Duchemin, A.M., Rose, C. and Schwartz, J.C. (1979): In vivo occupation of cerebral histamine H₁-receptors evaluated with ³H-mepyramine: correlation with sedative properties of psychotropic drugs. *Eur. J. Pharmacol. 60,* 391-392.
26. Schwartz, J.C., Barbin, G., Garbarg, M., Llorens, C., Palacios, J.M. and Pollard, H. (1978): Histaminergic systems in brain. In: *Advances in pharmacology and therapeutics,* Volume 2, pp. 171-180. Editor: P. Simon. Pergamon Press, Oxford-New York.
27. Schwartz, J.C., Barbin, G., Garbarg, M., Pollard, H., Rose, C. and Verdiere, M. (1976): Neurochemical evidence for histamine acting as a transmitter in mammalian brain. In: *Advances in biochemical psychopharmacology,* Volume 15, pp. 111-126. Editors: E. Costa, E. Giacobini and R. Paoletti. Raven Press, New York.

Discussion

Brimblecombe: I thought that the evidence now is that the sedative effect of antihistamines is probably not correlated with their potency as antagonists at H_1-receptors. How does that fit in with your data, Dr. Garbarg?

Garbarg: Our data indicate that there is a correlation. Our experiments using the criterion of tritiated mepyramine binding in vivo indicate that antihistamines occupy H_1-receptors at these therapeutic doses.

Brimblecombe: But the link between that and sedation is not yet established, I suppose.

Sharpe (Welwyn Garden City): Kwiatkowski, when he first described the distribution of histamine in the brain in the 1940's, showed the highest concentrations in the cerebellum. Obviously, this is totally opposite to Dr. Garbarg's data, in that she has shown the lowest concentrations in the cerebellum. There were other differences also between his data and hers. Is there any explanation for these marked discrepancies?

Garbarg: It could be because of the technique used for the measurement of histamine. I do not remember how he measured histamine, but at that time I think that the only way to measure it was by the contraction of guinea-pig ileum, which is poorly sensitive. This could explain the discrepancies in the results.

Sharpe: I think it was a bioassay.

Garbarg: The mean concentration of histamine in the brain is about 50 ng/g, and I do not think that a bioassay was available at that time for such a determination. There are many other reports now which indicate that the cerebellum has a very low concentration of histamine.

Baron (London): Dr. Garbarg discussed the possible interaction of H_1- and H_2-receptors and calcium, but she did not discuss any possible interaction with other transmitters, such as acetylcholine and gastrin. Is it not possible to think of a brain cell as merely a relation of a gastric parietal cell?

Garbarg: In fact, there is a potentiation between noradrenaline and histamine on the cyclic AMP system. An indirect effect could, of course, be involved in the H_1-receptors' induced stimulation of cyclic AMP. This possibility is further strengthened by the fact that, in a cell-free preparation, only H_2-receptors can be demonstrated.

The effect of histamine H_2-receptor antagonists on plasma prolactin

P.C. Sharpe, M.A. Melvin, Jane G. Mills, W.L. Burland and G.V. Groom*

*The Research Institute, Smith Kline & French Laboratories Ltd., Welwyn Garden City; and *Tenovus Institute for Cancer Research, Welsh National School of Medicine, Cardiff, United Kingdom*

Introduction

The effect of the histamine H_2-receptor antagonist cimetidine on serum prolactin has been investigated, following occasional reports of breast pain, gynaecomastia and galactorrhoea occurring in patients undergoing treatment for peptic ulcer and related conditions, although raised plasma prolactin was found in only some of these subjects [1-4].

Previous studies in our unit have demonstrated rises in serum prolactin following the administration of cimetidine 400 mg as an intravenous bolus; oral cimetidine 800 mg did not affect serum prolactin, however, and the response to intravenous dosing was abolished by prior administration of bromocriptine [5].

We have now further investigated the effects of cimetidine by assessment of the effect of the simultaneous administration of impromidine, a specific histamine H_2-agonist which might be expected to inhibit effects of cimetidine at the H_2 receptor [6], and by comparison of prolactin responses to cimetidine and SK&F-92994, a compound shown in gastric secretory studies to be a specific competitive histamine H_2-antagonist with a potency on a molar basis, by the intravenous route, 8-10 times that of cimetidine on gastric acid output maximally-stimulated by impromidine. In the present paper, we will report on these 2 investigations.

Materials and methods

The effects of impromidine and cimetidine on prolactin secretion were studied in 5 healthy male subjects. On 3 separate occasions, at least 7 days apart, a cannula was inserted into a forearm vein in each arm at 8:30 AM, with the subject at rest. Venous blood samples for determination of serum prolactin were taken at 10-minute intervals for 1 hour prior to injection of cimetidine 200 mg or saline as an intravenous bolus, and then at 2.5, 5, 10, 15, 30, 45, 60, 75 and 90 minutes afterwards. Impromidine 10 μg/kg/hour or saline was infused intravenously for 120 minutes, starting 30 minutes prior to the injection of cimetidine or saline. This dose of impromidine has previously been shown to be equivalent to histamine acid phosphate 40 μg/kg/hour in its effect on gastric acid secretion [5]. Each subject received cimetidine alone once, impromidine alone once and both compounds together once; studies were carried out in single-blind randomised order.

The effects of cimetidine and SK&F-92994 were compared in 4 healthy male subjects. Studies were made as described above, but without concomitant infusions of impromidine or saline and with venous blood samples taken at 10-minute intervals for 30 minutes prior to intravenous injection of 200 mg of either cimetidine or SK&F-92994 and then at the times listed above. As before, treatment order was single-blind and randomised.

Prolactin was determined by radioimmunoassay [8] and blood cimetidine by H.P.L.C. [20]. Results were compared by an initial overall split-plot analysis of variance to test for differences between treatments, followed by separate analyses of variance at each time point.

Results

Cimetidine 200 mg administered intravenously increased serum prolactin in all 5 subjects by a mean of 113%, compared with the mean of the last 3 pretreatment samples. The peak mean concentration ($\pm$ SEM) of 209 $\pm$ 44 mU/l occurred at 10 minutes, and the mean value had returned to basal levels by 90 minutes (Fig. 1). Addition of impromidine infusion had no effect on the response to cimetidine, with an identical peak mean prolactin level of 209 $\pm$ 19 mU/l occurring at 5 minutes after injection of cimetidine. Impromidine infusion alone produced no significant alteration in serum prolactin.

In 4 subjects who received intravenous 200 mg doses of cimetidine and SK&F-92994, peak mean serum prolactin concentration of 360 $\pm$ 66 mU/l occurred 10 minutes after the injection of cimetidine (Fig. 2); SK&F-92994 did not affect serum prolactin concentration.

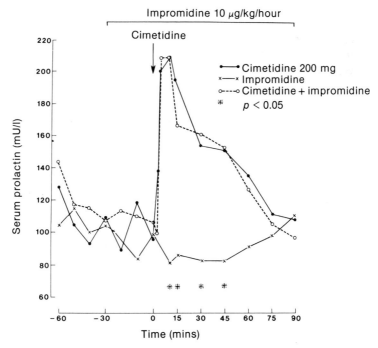

Fig. 1.   The effect of the intravenous administration of cimetidine and impromidine on resting serum prolactin. Mean of 5 subjects.

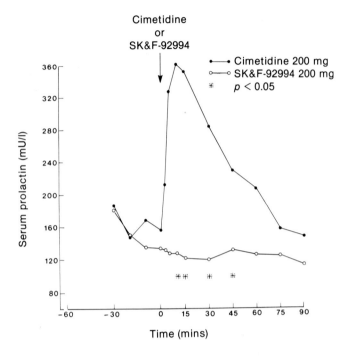

Fig. 2. *The effect of the intravenous administration of cimetidine and SK&F-92994 on resting serum prolactin. Mean of 4 subjects.*

Discussion

Prolactin is secreted from the anterior lobe of the pituitary following stimulation by a prolactin releasing factor which is secreted from the median eminence of the hypothalamus and is believed to be thyrotropin releasing hormone (TRH); secretion is inhibited by a postulated prolactin inhibitory factor (PIF), which may be dopamine secreted from dopaminergic neurones in the median eminence of the hypothalamus into the hypophyseal portal system. Since both the anterior pituitary and the median eminence of the hypothalamus lie outside the blood brain barrier, secretion of prolactin may be readily modified at these sites by pharmacological agents in the blood. However, the central pathways regulating PIF and TRH release may be assumed to lie *inside* the blood brain barrier, and, therefore, to be inaccessible to compounds which do not penetrate the barrier.

The failure of impromidine and SK&F-92994 to affect serum prolactin concentration, in contrast to cimetidine, may indicate either that the effect of cimetidine is peculiar to cimetidine and is unrelated to effects mediated via histamine H_2-receptors or, alternatively, that cimetidine acts at a site inaccessible to impromidine and SK&F-92994. Cimetidine is not thought to cross the intact blood brain barrier at normal therapeutic blood concentrations, but may well do so when very high blood concentrations are achieved immediately following intravenous injection of a bolus dose; it has been detected in the cerebro-spinal fluid in patients in hepatic or renal failure, in whom the barrier may be disrupted [9].

A central site of action of cimetidine would explain its failure to raise serum prolactin following oral administration. No information is available concerning penetration of the blood brain barrier by impromidine, although it seems unlikely that it crosses the barrier at the dose used in our study. Support for a central site of action is provided by the observation that the prolactin response to cimetidine is suppressed following elevation of brain dopamine by L-dopa, while the response to TRH remains intact [10]; it is possible that this might be a direct effect on dopamine receptors, as the response to cimetidine is also suppressed by bromocriptine. However, evidence against a direct effect on dopaminergic neurones was provided by Bohnet et al., who observed that cimetidine did not reverse the inhibitory effect of lisuride on prolactin secretion [11], and by Delitala et al., who demonstrated that the compound did not alter the inhibitory action of dopamine on isolated rat pituitary cells [12]. An effect mediated via hypothalamic TRH release can also be excluded, since intravenous bolus doses of cimetidine have been shown to have no effect on plasma TSH concentration [13, 14].

The possibility remains that cimetidine may affect prolactin secretion via a central histaminergic mechanism. Calcutt has reviewed the biochemical and physiological evidence and concluded that histamine may act as a central neurotransmitter [15], histamine has been demonstrated in the median eminence of the bovine hypothalamus [16], and histamine receptors have been shown to be involved in regulation of prolactin secretion in lactating rats [17]. Post-mortem studies on human brain have shown highest concentrations of both histamine [18] and histidine decarboxylase [19] in hypothalamus; in the latter study the enzyme was associated with sub-cellular fractions rich in nerve endings.

In the absence of experimental data on the ability of SK&F-92994 to cross the blood brain barrier, it is impossible to state whether the effect of cimetidine on prolactin is mediated via central histaminergic neurones, but this hypothesis is consistent with our findings and with those of other authors. However, similarities between the physicochemical properties of cimetidine and SK&F-92994 suggest that they are unlikely to differ significantly with respect to their ability to penetrate to the central nervous system and, therefore, if cimetidine can do so then SK&F-92994 may be expected to behave similarly when administered, as in our studies, under similar conditions and at similar doses. The possibility must, therefore, still be seriously considered that the effect on prolactin is a reflection of some specific feature of the cimetidine molecule; in that event, the site at which the compound is acting must remain the subject of speculation.

The clinical significance of these findings is unclear, but they may indicate that the rare occurrence of hyperprolactinaemia following oral cimetidine therapy results from individual variations in the permeability of the blood brain barrier, or from idiosyncratic reactions to the compound at another site.

Acknowledgements

Our thanks are due to Sister K. Wareham and to Miss C. Dutkowski for their assistance with these studies, and to Mr D. Daniel for the statistical analyses.

References

1. Delle Fave, G.F., Tamburrano, G., De Magistris, L. et al. (1977): Gynaecomastia with cimetidine. *Lancet 1,* 1319.

2. Hall, W.H. (1976): Breast changes in males on cimetidine. *N. Engl. J. Med. 295 (15),* 841.

3. Spence, R.W. and Celestin, L.R. (1979): Gynaecomastia associated with cimetidine. *Gut 20,* 154-157.

4. Bateson, M.C., Browning, M.C.K. and Maconnachie, A. (1977): Galactorrhoea with cimetidine. *Lancet 2,* 247-248.

5. Burland, W.L., Gleadle, R.I., Lee, R.M., Rowley-Jones, D. and Groom, G.V. (1979): Prolactin responses to cimetidine. *Br. J. Clin. Pharmacol. 7,* 19-21.

6. Hunt, R.H., Mills, J.G., Beresford, J., Billings, J.A., Burland, W.L. and Milton-Thompson, G.J. (1980): Gastric secretory studies in man with impromidine (SK&F-92676) — a specific histamine H_2-receptor agonist. *Gastroenterology.* (In press.)

7. Burland, W.L. and Mills, J.G. (Unpublished data.)

8. Groom, G.V. (1977): The measurement of human gonadotrophins by radioimmunoassay. *J. Reprod. Fertil. 51,* 273-286.

9. Schentag, J.J., Cerra, F.B., Calleri, G., De Glopper, E., Rose, J.Q. and Bernhard, J. (1979): Pharmacokinetic and clinical studies in patients with cimetidine-associated mental confusion. *Lancet 1,* 177-181.

10. Woolf, P.D., Leebaw, W.F. and Lee, L.A. (1977): Effects of CNS dopamine augmentation on stimulated prolactin secretion. *J. Clin. Endocrinol. Metab. 45,* 857-860.

11. Bohnet, H.G., Creiwe, M., Hanker, J.P., Aragona, C. and Schneider, H.P.C. (1978): Effects of cimetidine on prolactin, LH and sex steroid secretion in male and female volunteers. *Acta Endocrinol. (Copenhagen) 88,* 428-434.

12. Delitala, G., Stubbs, W.A., Wass, J.A.H. et al. (1978): Hypothalamic-pituitary effects of cimetidine. *Lancet 2,* 1054-1055.

13. Carlson, H.E. and Ippoliti, A.F. (1977): Cimetidine, an H_2-antihistamine, stimulates prolactin secretion in man. *J. Clin. Endocrinol. Metab. 45,* 367-370.

14. Morosini, P.P., Campanella, N., Chirelli, S., Pellegrini, F., Testa, I. and De Martinis, C. (1979): Cimetidine and hyperprolactinaemia. *Boll. Soc. Ital. Biol. Sper. 55 (1),* 14-17.

15. Calcutt, C.R. (1976): The role of histamine in the brain. *Gen. Pharmacol. 7,* 15-25.

16. Kizer, J.S., Palkovits, M., Tappaz, M., Kebabian, J. and Brownstein, M.J. (1976): Distribution of releasing factors, biogenic amines, and related enzymes in the bovine median eminence. *Endocrinology 98,* 685-695.

17. Arakalian, M.C. and Libertun, C. (1977): H_1 and H_2 histamine receptor participation in the brain control of prolactin secretion in lactating rats. *Endocrinology 100,* 890-895.

18. Lipinski, J.F., Schaumberg, H.H. and Baldesserini, R.J. (1973): Regional distribution of histamine in human brain. *Brain Res. 52,* 403-408.

19. Barbin, G., Palacios, J.M., Garbarg, M. and Schwartz, J.C. (1979): Characterisation of the histaminergic system in human brain. In: *Proceedings of the VII International Symposium of pharmacology.* Pergamon Press. (In press.)

20. Randolph, W.C., Osborne, V.L., Walkenstein, S.S. and Intoccia, A.P. (1977): High pressure liquid chromatographic analysis of cimetidine, a histamine H_2-receptor antagonist, in blood and urine. *J. Pharm. Sci. 66,* 1148-1150.

Discussion

Nelis (Zwolle): We studied 22 healthy volunteers (8 males, 8 pre-menopausal females and 6 post-menopausal females), who were given cimetidine and ranitidine on consecutive days in doses chosen for equivalency with regard to inhibition of gastric secretion. The order of giving the doses was randomly allocated. Cimetidine gave a very sharp peak of prolactin secretion at 15 minutes, in the same way as in Dr. Sharpe's study. Ranitidine did not influence prolactin secretion.

We wondered whether there was a difference between the subgroups, but all the subgroups were essentially the same.

Assuming that the new blocker described by Dr. Sharpe is structurally related to cimetidine, then a very daring hypothesis is possible: that there are 2 kinds of histamine H_2-receptors, both of which are blocked by cimetidine, whereas ranitidine and the new SK&F blocker selectively block one of them.

Festen (Nijmegen): Dr. Sharpe's data are very interesting, especially in combination with Dr. Nelis' data. Did Dr. Sharpe try using an intravenous bolus dose of nor-cimetidine which, as far as I am aware, is available to him? This would prove whether or not what is observed is a structurally-related effect.

Sharpe: I do not think we could administer that compound to man at the moment, although it would be interesting to try.

Bertaccini: We gave cimetidine to healthy volunteers, and there was no effect on basal prolactin with a dose of 100 mg given by continuous infusion. There was, however, an increase in the TRH response of prolactin during the administration of cimetidine. We had 3 cases of pituitary adenoma with hyperprolactinaemia. The injection of 4-methyl histamine in each of these 3 cases was followed by a certain amount of decrease in the hyperprolactinaemia. Three cases are insufficient to make any kind of statistical analysis, but the results suggest a probable role of H_2-receptors here.

Harvey (Bristol): Surely the most direct way of determining whether histamine pathways are involved in pituitary hormone release is to give some histamine and to measure the hormone response. That experiment must have been done — can Dr. Sharpe tell us about it?

Sharpe: There have been 2 reports on the effect of histamine, and they are contradictory. One said that it raised plasma prolactin, and the other that it did not. We have certainly got it in mind to investigate this ourselves. I suspect that the effect obtained may depend on the dose given.

Index of authors

(Numbers refer to pages)